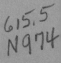

NURSE'S HANDBOOK OF

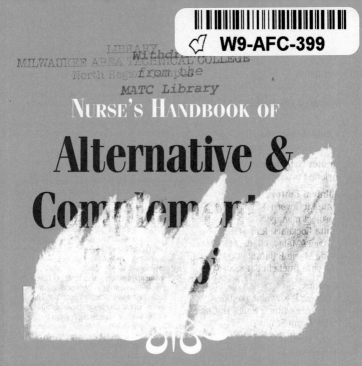

Alternative & Complementary Therapies

Second Edition

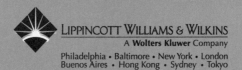

LIPPINCOTT WILLIAMS & WILKINS
A Wolters Kluwer Company

Philadelphia • Baltimore • New York • London
Buenos Aires • Hong Kong • Sydney • Tokyo

STAFF

Publisher
Judith A. Schilling McCann, RN, MSN

Editorial Director
H. Nancy Holmes

Clinical Director
Joan Robinson, RN, MSN

Senior Art Director
Arlene Putterman

Clinical Editors
Kate McGovern, RN, MSN, CCRN (project manager);
Anita Lockhart, RNC, MSN;
Patricia Malay, RN, BS, MSN, MA;
Anne Marie Palatnik, RN, MSN, CS;
Barbara Stiebeling, RN, MSN

Editors
Jennifer P. Kowalak (senior associate editor), Naina D. Chohan, Stacey Ann Follin

Copy Editors
Kimberly Bilotta, Scotti Cohn, Tom DeZego, Heather Ditch, Amy Furman, Shana Harrington, Judith Orioli, Carolyn Petersen, Marcia Ryan

Designers
Linda Franklin (book designer), Lippincott Williams & Wilkins (composition), Donna S. Morris

Cover Design
Larry Didona

Electronic Production Services
Diane Paluba (manager), Joyce Rossi Biletz (senior desktop assistant), Richard Eng

Manufacturing
Patrica K. Dorshaw (manager), Beth Janae Orr (book production coordinator)

Editorial Assistants
Danielle J. Barsky, Carol Caputo, Beverly Lane, Linda Ruhf

Librarian
Catherine M. Heslin

Indexer
Barbara E. Hodgson

NHACT2 – D N O S A
04 03 02   10 9 8 7 6 5 4 3 2 1

**Library of Congress
Cataloging-in-Publication Data**

Nurse's handbook of alternative & complementary therapies.— 2nd ed.
  p. ; cm.
Includes index.
1. Alternative medicine--Handbooks, manuals, etc. 2. Nursing—Handbooks, manuals, etc.
3. Holistic nursing—Handbooks, manuals, etc.
  [DNLM: 1. Complementary Therapies—Handbooks. 2. Nursing Care—methods—Handbooks. WB 39 N973 2003] I. Title:
Nurse's handbook of alternative and complementary therapies. II. Lippincott Williams & Wilkins.
R733 .N87 2003
615.5—dc21   2002007899
ISBN 1-58255-166-9 (pbk. : alk. paper)

Contents

Contributors and consultants

Angella Bascom, MSN, ARNP, Elliot Hospital/Regional Partners in Occupational Health; Manchester, N.H.

Mark A. Breiner, DDS, FAGD, FIAOMT, Dentist; Private Practice; Orange, Conn.

Michael Briggs, PharmD, Pharmacist/Co-Owner; Lionville Natural Pharmacy; Exton, Pa.

Donelle Bussom, RN, MSN, Senior Manager, Medical Affairs; ICON Clinical Research; North Wales, Pa.

Michael F. Cantwell, MD, MPH, Medical Director and Coordinator of Clinical Research; Health and Healing Clinic/California Pacific Medical Center; San Francisco

Elizabeth A. Chester, PharmD, BCPS, Clinical Pharmacy Specialist, Primary Care; Kaiser Permanente; Aurora, Colo.

Joanne D. Christophers, RN, BPS, CNAT, Coordinator of the Holistic Nursing Teaching Clinic; New York College of Health Professions; Education and Research; Syosset, N.Y.

Jeanneane L. Cline, RN, MS, CS, HTP, LCDC, LMFT, Instructor; School of Nursing; University of Texas at Arlington

Alan R. Cohen, MD, Medical Director; Harmony Health Care/Alan R. Cohen, MD PC; Milford, Conn.

Jason C. Cooper, PharmD, Pharmacist; Bon Secours/St. Francis Hospital; Charleston, S.C.

Ami Dansby, RPh, Pharmacist, Natural Medicine Consultant; Bruce's Pharmacy; Charlottesville, Va.

Lana Dvorkin, RPh, PharmD, Assistant Professor, Clinical Pharmacy; Massachusetts College of Pharmacy and Health Sciences; Boston

Jacob Farin, ND, Naturopathic Doctor; Center for Traditional Medicine; Lake Oswego, Ore.

Hope Farner, NMD, MS, Assistant Professor, Naturopathic Medicine; Southwest College of Naturopathic Medicine; Tempe, Ariz.

Marie Fasano-Ramos, RN, MA, MN, CMT, Holistic Nurse Practitioner; InterAge; Ventura, Calif.

June M. Ferrari, ND, CNC, Health Revolutions and Holy Redeemer Hospital Women's Center; Feasterville, Pa.

Tatyana Gurvich, PharmD, Clinical Pharmacologist; GAFPRP; Glendale, Calif.

Tiffani N. Hatcher, RN, MSN, CRNP-AC, Thoracic Surgery Nurse Practitioner; University of Maryland Medical Center; Baltimore

Anh Thu Hoang, PharmD, Scientific Associate; IntraMed Educational Group; New York

Susan Simmons Holcomb, RN-CS, MN, CCRN, FNP, Nurse Practitioner, Nutritional Counseling; Sastun Center of Integrative Healthcare; Mission, Kans.

Julia N. Kleckner, PharmD, Pharmacy Manager; Option Care; Upper Darby, Pa.

Robert J. Krueger, PhD, Professor, Pharmacognosy; College of Pharmacy; Ferris State University; Big Rapids, Mich.

Suzanne C. Lawton, ND, Naturopathic Doctor; Private Practice; Tigard, Ore.

Yun Lu, RPh, MS, PharmD; Cardiology/Anticoagulation Clinical Specialist; Hennepin County Medical Center; Minneapolis

Susan Luck, RN, BS, MA, CCN, HNC, Holistic Health Education, Clinical Nutritionist; Biodoron Immunology Center; Hollywood, Fla.

June H. McDermott, RPh, MBA, MS Pharm, FASHP, Clinical Assistant Professor; School of Pharmacy; University of North Carolina at Chapel Hill

Thomas M. Motyka, DO, Clinical Assistant Professor; School of Medicine; University of North Carolina at Chapel Hill

Jolynne Myers, RNCS, MSEd, MSN, ANP, Clinical Research Coordinator; Life Waves International; Kansas City, Mo.

Scott Olson, BA, ND, Naturopathic Doctor, Research Writer; Private Practice; Littleton, Colo.

Steven G. Ottariano, RPh, Clinical Staff Pharmacist; Veterans Affairs Medical Center; Manchester, N.H.

Robert Lee Page, II, PharmD, BCPS, Assistant Professor; School of Pharmacy; University of Colorado Health Sciences Center; Denver

June Riedlinger, RPh, PharmD, Assistant Professor, Clinical Pharmacy; Director, Center for Integrative Therapies in Pharmaceutical Care; Massachusetts College of Pharmacy and Health Sciences; Boston

Karin K. Roberts, RN, PhD, Associate Professor; Research College of Nursing; Kansas City, Mo.

Alean Royes, RNC, MSN, CNS, APN, Faculty; School of Nursing; University of Texas at Arlington

Anna Russo, NLP Practitioner, Master Practitioner, NLP International Trainer, Master Ericksonian Hypnotherapist, Master Trainer and President; Success Strategies NLP of (Troy) Michigan

Sharon Scandrett-Hibdon, RN, PhD, CHTI, CS, FNP, HNC, Family Nurse Practitioner; Groff Medical Clinic; Aubrey, Tex.

Jacob J. Schor, ND, Naturopathic Doctor; Denver Naturopathic Clinic

Elizabeth A. Seldomridge, RN, PhD, Chair and Associate Professor, Department of Nursing; Salisbury University; Salisbury, Md.

Marcia Silkroski, RD, CNSD, President; Nutrition Advantage; Chester Springs, Pa.

H. Robert Silverstein, MD, Medical Director, Preventive Medicine Center; Clinical Assistant Professor of Medicine; School of Medicine; University of Connecticut; Hartford

Ann McCloud Sneath, MSN, CRNP, Nurse Practitioner, Integrative Medicine; Private Practice; Paoli, Pa.

Katrina A. Steinberger, NMD, Medical Director; Scottsdale (Ariz.) Clinic for Alternative and Longevity Medicine

Ronald Steriti, NMD, PhD, Naturopathic Doctor; Naples, Fla.

Maria A. Summa, RPh, BCPS, PharmD, Assistant Professor of Clinical Pharmacy; Massachusetts College of Pharmacy and Health Sciences; Boston

Dorota K. Szarlej, BS, PharmD, Clinical Pharmacist, Drug Use Policy and Clinical Services; Thomas Jefferson University Hospital; Philadelphia

Timothy Taneda-Brown, ND, DC, Diplomate Acupuncture, Naturopathic Doctor; Ocean Pacific Natural Therapies; Surrey, British Columbia, Canada

Catherine Ultrino, RN, MSN, OCN, Nurse Manager; Hematology/Oncology; Boston Medical Center

Gail D. Vanark, RN, BSN, Staff RN; St. Joseph's Hospital/St. Joseph's Family Medical Center; Merrimack, N.H.

Diane Wind Wardell, PhD, RNC, HNC, Associate Professor; University of Texas;Houston

George L. White, Jr., PA-C, MSPH, PhD, Professor and Director, Public Health Programs; Department of Family and Preventive Medicine; School of Medicine; University of Utah; Salt Lake City

Laurie Willhite, PharmD, Clinical Pharmacy Specialist; Fairview University Medical Center; Minneapolis

Jared L. Zeff, ND, LAC, Naturopathic Doctor, Acupuncturist; Professor of Naturopathic Medicine; Bastyr University; Bothell, Wash.

We extend special thanks to the following people, who contributed to the previous edition:

IRENE BELCHER, RN, MS, CNS

JUDY A. CUSTER, RN, MS, CRNP, NP-C

CHARLOTTE ELIOPOULOS, RNC, MPH

JUNE M. FERRARI, ND

MILDRED I. FREEL, RN, MEd, CHTP, CHTT, HNC

LAURA K. HART, RN, PhD, CHTP

PAMELA POTTER HUGHES, RN, MSN, CNS

WILLIAM G. KRACHT, DO, FAAFP

ALICE L. KYLE, RN, MS, CS

GENEVIEVE G. MCCUNNEY, RN, BSN

KAREN E. MICHAEL, RN, MSN, PAHM

Sr. HELEN OWENS, OSF, RN, MSN

CATHLEEN M. RAPP, ND

KARIN K. ROBERTS, RN, PhD

MARY ANN T. ROMANO, PhD

MARCIA SILKROSKI, RD, CNSD

ARON SKRYPECK, RN, MSN, DOM

ROGER STEWART, DC

JEAN WATSON, RN, PhD, FAAN, HNC

JOHN T. ZIMMERMAN, PhD

Foreword

I n the short time since the first edition of *Nurse's Handbook of Alternative and Complementary Therapies* appeared, significant changes and growth have occurred in this field. More patients are trying therapies on their own, with or without the advice of their physicians and nurses and sometimes to the detriment of their conventional medical treatments. Clinicians are called on to answer patients' questions and give advice, and an increasing number are learning to administer clinically proven therapies and incorporating them into their conventional practices.

Nurses are facing new challenges as they journey down the path of incorporating alternative and complementary therapies into their practices, not the least of which is learning to use these therapies appropriately and effectively and to counsel their patients wisely.

Nurse's Handbook of Alternative and Complementary Therapies, Second Edition, eases the anxiety of this challenge by providing leading-edge information on a wide range of therapies in an interesting and concise manner. The contributors have done an outstanding job of sifting through reams of research and literature to provide readers with relevant summaries and practical guidelines for clinical practice.

Each entry in this comprehensive guide describes the subject therapy, its underlying principles, therapeutic goals, equipment used, the procedure itself, complications, supportive research, and the nurse's perspective on the therapy as well as important nursing considerations, including critical patient teaching.

The discussion of possible complications is especially helpful, as it equips nurses to promote safe use among patients, who often lack insight into the risks associated with what they perceive to be "natural" therapies. And the research summaries, highlighted in the entries for immediate reference, distill the available evidence — pro and con — on each therapy's efficacy.

An eye-catching graphic icon, *How it works,* calls attention to the function of certain therapies, such as acupuncture, biofeedback, and magnetic field therapy. Another icon, *Personal account,* identifies individuals' experiences with qigong exercises, Ayurvedic medicine for coronary artery blockage, and more.

The book's helpful appendices provide a list of many disorders and selected therapies used to treat them as well as an extensive compilation of support organizations and information resources for alternative and complementary therapies. Also included are patient teaching aids on specific therapies for patient handout.

Nurse's Handbook of Alternative and Complementary Therapies, Second Edition, covers its subject admirably. Be it identifying acupressure points that can relieve a headache or learning about the adverse effects of scores of herbal remedies, the ease with which nurses can retrieve a wide range of facts pertaining to alternative and complementary therapies supports this book's place as a valuable reference in every clinical setting.

When the now-famous 1993 research by Eisenberg and his colleagues was published, the term *unconventional* was used to describe therapies that fell outside the realm of Western medicine. Then came *alternative therapies,* which implied that these practices were used in place of mainstream approaches. Next, in recognition that these modalities could coexist with conventional health care practices, *complementary therapies* became the popular term. *Integrative care,* the term now in vogue, reflects the ideal orientation that all types of therapies can be used together to contribute to a unified approach to health care and the best outcome for the patient. Combining the best of both worlds creates a synergy with the potential to drastically change health care as we've known it.

Effective integration of alternative and complementary therapies into conventional medical and nursing care requires more than merely adding new therapies and products to the existing model of health care. Rather, new paradigms of practice are required to fully realize the potential of integrative care — paradigms that reflect the need for a holistic approach to health and healing.

This presents a wonderful opportunity for nurses because the nursing profession has a longer history than any other professional discipline of recognizing the need to address the individual's body, mind, and spirit through caregiving activities. Further, in their role as care planners and coordinators nurses have long been the hub of the wheel of health care services.

Nurses have a rightful place as leaders in the new paradigm of integrative care, and *Nurse's Handbook of Alternative and Complementary Therapies,* Second Edition, provides the knowledge that equips them to fill that place.

Charlotte Eliopoulos, RNC, MPH, PhD
President, American Holistic Nurses Association;
Specialist in Holistic Chronic Care Nursing
Glen Arm, Maryland

PART ONE

Understanding alternative and complementary therapies

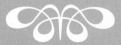

1

Fundamental facts

T his chapter covers the basics about alternative therapies — from their origins, availability, and research bases to the training practitioners receive and the coverage provided by medical insurance.

Alternative? Or complementary?

According to the *American Heritage Dictionary*, the term *alternative* means "offering a choice between two or more possibilities existing outside conventional institutions or systems." Alternative therapies are commonly thought to include all the treatments for disorders or health problems that haven't traditionally been recommended by medical doctors, taught in medical schools, or reported in the medical journals that most physicians read. They also include practices to maintain and promote health.

Alternative therapies are based on an approach to health that blends body and mind, science and experience, and traditional and cross-cultural avenues of diagnosis and treatment. Unlike Western medicine, alternative therapies don't rely solely on empirical science. (See *What to call it?*)

The term *complementary therapy* also refers to nontraditional therapies, and can be used in place of *alternative therapy*. The word *complementary*, which the *American Heritage Dictionary* defines as "completing or making up a whole," was adopted when research showed that most patients in the West

What to call it?

The terms *alternative, complementary, unconventional, nontraditional,* and *unorthodox* are used interchangeably in the media and in medical literature to denote healing practices that haven't traditionally been found in Western medical practice or taught in mainstream medical schools.

However, most practitioners of these therapies prefer the term *complementary* because they feel the other terms have negative connotations, implying the use of unproven practices.

Some practitioners make the following distinction. They define *alternative therapies* as those that are used *instead of* conventional or mainstream therapy — for example, the use of acupuncture rather than analgesics to relieve pain — and *complementary therapies* as those used *in conjunction with* conventional therapy — such as the use of guided imagery or meditation as an adjunct to drug therapy for pain control.

use nontraditional therapies in addition to, not instead of, traditional therapies. In fact, both of these combine in the term being used more and more today: *CAM,* an acronym that stands for complementary and alternative medicine.

Where CAM originated

Alternative therapies are used to treat a broad spectrum of signs, symptoms, and diseases. Many people also use them to promote relaxation, maintain health, and enhance overall well-being. Regardless of the problem for which they're used, these therapies address the whole person — body, mind, and spirit — not just the signs and symptoms.

Many alternative therapies practiced today have been used since ancient times and come from the traditional healing practices of many cultures, primarily those of China and India. In China, natural substances such as herbs have been used for thousands of years, and the Chinese government supports the use of herbal therapy. Acupuncture has also been used for centuries to relieve pain, and traditional Chinese medicine in general is thought to have evolved about 3,000 years ago. The

Indian principles of Ayurvedic medicine stem from the Vedas, the essential religious texts of Hinduism, which scholars believe are 5,000 years old.

Because of its blend of many cultures, the United States has a diverse store of healing modalities. Many immigrants who settled in the United States brought their native healing techniques with them. For example, Germans from the Rhineland and Switzerland brought a process called "sympathy healing" when they settled in what is now the eastern United States and Canada in the 17th and 18th centuries. And the practices of Native American medicine men influenced the early American colonists.

Who uses alternative therapies?

A landmark national survey published in 1991 by Harvard Medical School researcher David Eisenberg and colleagues found that about one-third of Americans who responded said they had used at least one unconventional therapy in the preceding year. The researchers estimated that Americans made 425 million visits to providers of unconventional therapy in 1990, a figure that exceeded the estimated number of visits to all primary care physicians (family practitioners, pediatricians, and internists) combined. These numbers were much higher than had previously been reported. Eisenberg and his colleagues performed a follow-up survey in 1997 to check the trends in alternative therapy use. They found that in 1997 Americans had visited alternative therapy providers 629 million times that year, an increase of more than 47%.

The 1990 survey showed that the use of alternative therapies was significantly higher among nonblack persons ages 25 to 49, those with some college education, and those with annual incomes more than $35,000. The follow-up survey showed that rates of use were up among all sociodemographic groups, and that more women (48.9%) than men (37.8%) used alternative therapy services in 1997. Nearly 90% of those who saw a provider of alternative therapy did so without the recommendation of their primary care physician, and a majority didn't inform their physician of their actions.

The original survey also showed that the most common conditions for which people turned to alternative therapies were back problems, anxiety, headaches, chronic pain, and cancer or tumors. By 1997, the reasons for seeing an alternative therapy provider had expanded somewhat, but back and neck problems were still the most common conditions for which people sought help.

A significant finding of the 1990 study was that alternative therapies usually were used as an adjunct to conventional therapy, not as a replacement for it. No respondents saw only an unconventional therapy practitioner for cancer, diabetes, lung problems, skin conditions, hypertension, or urinary tract problems. (See *Patient choices of alternative therapies,* page 6.) The researchers also inferred that many Americans are using alternative therapies for health promotion or disease prevention. The same was true of the follow-up study.

Reasons for increasing popularity

There are a number of reasons for the increased interest in alternative medicine. Most of the therapies are noninvasive. In addition, many people are encouraged by the research docu-

> **❝ Many people who seek unconventional treatments have chronic conditions for which conventional medicine has few, if any, effective treatments. ❞**

menting the effectiveness of specific therapies — such as acupuncture, meditation, guided imagery, and yoga — and by the fact that they have few or no adverse effects. Plus, many people who seek unconventional treatments have chronic conditions for which conventional medicine has few, if any, effective treatments, so they feel they have nothing to lose.

Another major reason for increased interest may be alternative medicine's holistic approach. More and more patients prefer alternative medicine's focus on treating the whole person to conventional medicine's tendency of treating only signs and symptoms. For example, in treating certain chronic disorders such as arthritis, Western medicine relies to a large degree on pharmaceutical treatments, many of which are associated with unpleasant adverse effects or fail to work after a certain period of time. Alternative therapy practitioners, in contrast, tend to tailor treatment plans to the individual and

Patient choices of alternative therapies

A 1991 study by Harvard Medical School researchers found that about one-third of all Americans had used alternative therapies in the preceding year. The chart below shows the 10 most common medical conditions reported by the study's respondents, the percentage who reported having those conditions, the percentage of those reporting who used alternative therapies, and the types of therapies they chose to use.

Condition	Percent reporting condition	Percent using alternative therapy	Most common therapies used
Back problems	20%	36%	Chiropractic, massage
Allergies	16%	9%	Spiritual healing, diet
Arthritis	16%	18%	Chiropractic, relaxation techniques
Insomnia	14%	20%	Relaxation techniques, imagery
Sprains or strains	13%	22%	Massage, relaxation techniques
Headaches	13%	27%	Relaxation techniques, chiropractic
Hypertension	11%	11%	Relaxation techniques, homeopathy
Digestive problems	10%	13%	Relaxation techniques, megavitamins
Anxiety	10%	28%	Relaxation techniques, imagery
Depression	8%	20%	Relaxation techniques, self-help groups

Adapted with permission from Eisenberg, D.M., et al. "Unconventional Medicine in the United States," *New England Journal of Medicine.* 328:246-52, January 28, 1993. ©1963 Massachusetts Medical Society. All rights reserved.

prefer to use natural substances such as herbs to minimize adverse effects. (See *Common underlying beliefs.*)

According to a 1993 British survey, the most valued aspect of alternative medicine is the time the practitioner spends with the patient and the attention paid to the patient's temperament, behavioral patterns, and perceived needs. In an increasingly stressful world, many people are searching for someone who'll take the time to listen to them and who'll treat them as people, not merely as bodies displaying signs and symptoms. Conventional physicians generally don't provide this kind of attention.

Some theorize that alternative therapies are enjoying a renaissance because modern society is spiritually malnourished and hungry for meaning and alternative therapy practitioners are more responsive to this need.

Another reason for the surge in use of alternative therapies stems from the movement to managed care and health maintenance organizations (HMOs) as the main providers of health insurance in the United States. This shift has placed a new emphasis on health maintenance and disease prevention. In part because of this emphasis, many Americans have decided

Common underlying beliefs

Despite their varying theories and practices, most practitioners of alternative therapies share the following fundamental beliefs:
  ▶ Each person is a unique individual consisting of body, mind, spirit, and emotions. These parts are integrated to make up the whole person and can't be separated.
  ▶ Good health is the state of balance between the physical, mental, spiritual, and emotional aspects of the person.
  ▶ The body has a natural ability to heal itself.
  ▶ Social and environmental conditions are as important as the physical and psychological makeup of the person. All these spheres of human existence need to be considered when diagnosing or recommending treatment.
  ▶ Treatment is a process that considers the root of the problem instead of merely treating the obvious signs and symptoms.
  ▶ The focus of treatment should be the patient's "perceived needs" rather than the medical diagnosis.

to take control of their health and are turning to alternative therapists in their search for good health and wellness.

Positive word of mouth is also leading patients to alternative therapies. Increasingly, thousands of health care professionals and millions of laymen are experiencing the effects of alternative remedies. They, in turn, are sharing this information with their relatives, friends, and patients. In addition, health care professionals are finding more professional journal reports on the benefits of alternative therapies, which has led many to incorporate individual therapies into their clinical practices.

What's considered alternative?

The National Center for Complementary and Alternative Medicine (NCCAM), a 1998 addition to the National Institutes of Health (NIH), has classified alternative medicine into five major categories, or *domains* of practice. These are: alternative medical systems, mind-body interventions, biological-based therapies, manipulative and body-based therapies, and energy therapies.

Alternative medical systems involve whole systems of theory and practice, many of which developed in other cultures around the world independently of Western medicine. Some examples of these are Asian systems, which include techniques such as acupuncture, and Ayurvedic medicine. Ayurvedic, which means "the science of life," is a system that evolved in India. Homeopathic and naturopathic medicine also fit into this domain.

Mind-body interventions are based on the belief in a profound interconnectedness of mind and body and the capacity of each to affect the other. Examples of mind-body interventions include biofeedback, meditation, hypnosis, dance therapy, music therapy, art therapy, yoga, t'ai chi chuan, guided imagery, and prayer and mental healing. Psychotherapy isn't considered alternative because it has a scientifically documented theoretical basis.

Biological-based therapies are therapies that are grounded in their direct biological effects on the human body. Interventions in this category include herbal remedies, special dietary regimens, orthomolecular therapy (megadose vitamins and minerals), and individual therapies (laetrile and shark cartilage, for example). Vitamin supplementation has been used in traditional Western medicine and isn't considered a CAM therapy.

Manipulative and body-based methods include manipulation or movement of the body. Examples of this are chiropractic therapy and massage therapy.

Energy therapies are those therapies that focus on energy fields believed to originate from either inside the body (biofields) or outside of it (electromagnetic fields). Examples of these kinds of therapies include qigong, reiki, and Therapeutic Touch.

Most widely used therapies

According to the 1990 Eisenberg study, the most popular forms of alternative therapy (excluding exercise and prayer) were relaxation techniques, chiropractic, and massage. Most respondents who saw alternative therapy providers sought treatment by acupuncture, chiropractic, hypnosis, and massage, in that order. The 1997 follow-up survey showed a greater variety of therapies in use, and there were large increases in the use of herbal medicine, massage, megavitamins, self-help groups, folk remedies, energy healing, and homeopathy.

Associated costs

The Eisenberg surveys estimated that Americans spent about $11.7 billion for alternative therapy services in 1990 (not including money spent for equipment, devices, books, or preparations such as herbs). In 1997, Americans spent $21.2 billion, an increase of more than 45%. These were out-of-pocket expenses. Third-party payment was most commonly granted for the services of herbal therapists, biofeedback providers, chiropractors, and megavitamin suppliers. However, both surveys showed that few health insurance plans reimbursed for alternative therapy services, and that about 60% of the costs were paid directly by patients.

The costs of alternative therapies vary according to the type of therapy. They also differ from region to region. As a general rule, most alternative therapy practitioners charge about the same as a physician for an office visit. Supplies, such as herbs or nutritional supplements, may make some therapies more costly.

Practitioner qualifications

Besides being provided by some physicians, alternative therapies may be provided by nurses, nurse practitioners, neighbors, friends, relatives, business people, and many others. The type of therapy practiced sometimes dictates the training and education of the therapist, but this isn't always true. Most alternative therapists aren't regulated by state licensure, so the level of expertise varies from one practitioner to another.

Few alternative therapies require the practitioner to have a college degree; those that do include osteopathy, chiropractic, naturopathy, and most types of psychotherapy. Many practitioners of alternative therapies have a college degree in their field of expertise and then have acquired alternative therapy training to enhance their professional skills. For example, many psychotherapists are known to practice hypnotherapy, biofeedback, or music therapy. Some nurses practice massage,

> 66 *Standardization of credentialing is likely to become an issue as alternative therapies gain greater acceptance.* 99

acupressure, acupuncture, or Therapeutic Touch. Some physicians practice acupressure or acupuncture. Physical therapists use acupressure, massage, and craniosacral and Feldenkrais techniques in their practices.

At present, any layperson can study and become licensed or certified to practice many alternative therapies. However, this is likely to change as more insurance companies and HMOs begin reimbursing for alternative therapies. These companies will probably require that practitioners have a certain level of formal education and some form of credentials before reimbursement is approved. Standardization of credentialing is likely to become an issue as alternative therapies gain greater acceptance.

Finding qualified practitioners

Patients should verify that the practitioner is licensed if the therapy they're seeking requires licensing. State licensing boards can provide this information. Some alternative therapies have national groups that certify those who have attended a recognized school and who have met the requirements established by that group. This type of information assures the patient that the practitioner has met the required schooling to practice in the field. (See *Educational and state requirements for practitioners.*)

Some practitioners will provide names of clients who may be contacted as references. Many health food store employees are familiar with alternative therapies and may be able to recommend qualified practitioners. Increasingly, physicians are becoming aware of alternative therapy practitioners in their respective areas and may be able to refer their patients to reputable ones.

Alternative therapies are offered in many settings that vary from one community to another. Wellness centers usually provide practitioners of several different therapies, including

Educational and state requirements for practitioners

The following chart provides a list of educational requirements and state licensure requirements for the practitioners of common alternative and complementary therapies.

Type of therapy	Education required	State license required
Acupuncture	Degree	28 states
Chiropractic	Degree	50 states
Herbology	Certificate	Varies
Homeopathy	Degree	Arizona, Connecticut, Nevada
Hypnotherapy	Certificate	Florida
Massage	Certificate	22 states
Naturopathy	Degree	9 states
Traditional Chinese medicine	Degree	Nevada, New Mexico
Osteopathy	Degree	50 states
Reflexology	Certificate	Arkansas, Florida, North Dakota, Texas, Washington

Therapeutic Touch, massage, diet and nutrition counseling, acupressure, acupuncture, and relaxation techniques. Many therapists offer their services from their homes or from free-standing offices. More and more physicians, particularly those in family practice, are acquiring alternative therapy skills and integrating them into their medical practice. This type of practitioner is more difficult to locate because medical practices don't commonly advertise the practice of alternative therapies. However, as alternative therapies become more accepted, this will probably change.

Many hospitals offer relaxation classes and self-help groups that are usually facilitated by hospital employees. Increasingly, hospitals are offering Therapeutic Touch classes to employees and to the community through their continuing education programs. In addition, some state and national therapy organizations maintain lists of facilities that provide their specialty. For example, the Nurse Healers–Professional Association has compiled a list of 72 health facilities in the United States that practice Therapeutic Touch.

> 66 *Many universities offer alternative therapy courses in their medical schools and master's level nursing curriculums.* 99

Disease-specific self-help groups and word of mouth are two common sources of information on alternative therapies. Internet discussion groups on alternative therapies may also be helpful.

Finding training

Some therapies, such as Therapeutic Touch, are fairly simple in theory and process but require many hours of practice to be effective; others, such as acupuncture, require extensive study. Many universities offer alternative therapy courses in their medical schools and master's level nursing curriculums, usually as elective courses. A study published in 1998 reported that 75 of 117 U.S. medical schools offered elective courses in alternative therapy or included such topics in required courses. Prominent examples include Boston University School of Medicine, Case Western Reserve University School of Medicine, Columbia University College of Physicians and Surgeons, Georgetown University School of Medicine, Johns Hopkins School of Medicine, Harvard University School of Medicine, and Stanford University School of Medicine. A 1995 survey found that about 40% of all family medicine departments offer some kind of instruction in alternative therapies.

Alternative therapy journals are helpful in listing courses offered in alternative therapies. Contacting organizations that represent specific therapies is another way to locate training courses.

Classes in alternative therapies that don't require a college degree or certificate are offered in the community at various locations. These are usually advertised by word of mouth, flyers, and newspaper ads.

Dangers associated with alternative therapies

Because alternative therapies are largely unregulated, they can pose legal and professional dangers to those who practice them as well as health-related dangers to patients who use them.

Professional hazards

Most alternative treatments are considered outside the accepted medical standards of practice. As a result, physicians who practice unrecognized therapies are subject to professional peer review, which can lead to disciplinary action.

Practicing outside the boundaries of accepted standards of care also leaves physicians, nurses, and other health care professionals vulnerable to civil liability in a malpractice case. Hence, referrals within or outside a medical practice should clarify that the therapy is alternative and not a part of the medical treatment regimen. All alternative therapy practitioners need to consult their state licensing boards to clarify that no laws restrict such practice.

Nurses who practice alternative therapies within a health care facility must make sure that the supervisory staff is aware of the practice and that the facility has a policy and procedure that addresses it, including any required legal safeguards.

When gathering a health history, all health care practitioners should ask patients if they're using any unconventional remedies or seeing any other health practitioners. If alternative therapists will be seeing the patient in the facility, the administration should be informed so that the medical and alternative therapies can be integrated.

Patient hazards

Patients seeking alternative therapies are vulnerable to "con artists" who prey on people who are ill. Health care professionals should encourage patients to research the literature, seek out qualified practitioners, and consult their medical providers before experimenting with health care alternatives. Besides avoiding questionable practitioners, they may also avoid the potential dangers of compound therapy. For example, many herbs and vitamins can adversely affect the medical outcome when used with prescription medications. People who take blood thinners can increase prothrombin time by taking vitamin E or garlic and decrease it by taking vitamin K. Also, misuse of certain herbs can produce toxic effects. Because few dietary supplements have been researched, their capacity to cause harm remains unknown.

Patients can also put themselves in danger when they reject medical treatments outright in favor of alternative therapies. For example, if a person newly diagnosed with cancer opts for unproven treatments instead of accepted treatments, this delay in treatment could affect his prognosis. Many believe the patient's needs are best met by integrating conventional and unconventional therapies.

One final concern, commonly expressed by traditional medical doctors, is that nontraditional practitioners won't recognize life-threatening illnesses when a person comes to an alternative therapy provider for services.

Response of the health care establishment

There's a growing open-mindedness among physicians about alternative medicine. The National Institutes of Health's (NIH's) creation of the Office of Alternative Medicine (OAM) in 1992, and the National Center for Complementary and Alternative Medicine (NCCAM) in 1998, has been instrumental in the growing professional acceptance of many alternative therapies and the integration of these therapies into conventional medicine.

In an unpublished survey of academic specialty-based physicians at Columbia University College of Physicians and Surgeons, more than 50% of the physicians stated that they personally used various alternative healing methods or referred patients for such therapies. A 1995 study found that 70% to 90% of family physicians in Maryland considered alternative therapies to be legitimate and made referrals for such treatments; 70% of those Maryland physicians expressed an interest in increasing their knowledge and training in these therapies.

Among physicians who actually administer alternative therapies themselves, the most common therapies are acupuncture, osteopathy, psychotherapy, homeopathy, and Therapeutic Touch. In addition, many health care providers practice alternative therapies, such as Therapeutic Touch and therapeutic massage, without recognizing them as such.

Many physicians are already well known for their contributions to the field of alternative therapy. Jon Kabat-Zinn organized successful meditation and stress-reduction classes for chronic pain control. Dean Ornish developed a diet and meditation program that has successfully reversed arteriosclerotic heart disease in many patients. Deepak Chopra's books explain the Ayurvedic lifestyle, and Andrew Weil's books espouse the benefits of integrative medicine — combining alternative and mainstream medical practices.

Holistic nursing and alternative therapies

Holistic care and holistic nursing fit well with alternative therapies. The words *holism* and *holistic* are derived from the Greek word *holos,* meaning health, entire, and whole. Holism is a philosophy of health care that views each person as an integrated whole consisting of body, mind, and spirit and that sees the whole as greater than the sum of its parts. Holistic practitioners look at the whole patient, not just the diseased part or system. They believe that good health isn't merely the absence of disease, but rather a dynamic process of well-being that requires the patient's active participation. They further believe that the body has an innate power to heal itself and that lifestyle factors play a major role in health and illness.

Although any health care provider can have a holistic outlook, this approach has primarily been associated with the nursing profession. Florence Nightingale expressed a holistic view of nursing when she said that nursing should "put us in the best possible conditions for nature to restore or to preserve health, to prevent or cure disease or injury." The holistic nursing movement is returning to these principles today.

> ❝Wisdom and healing come from the patient, not the practitioner. The practitioner helps the process of healing by creating an environment in which healing can happen.❞

The goal of holistic nursing is to promote health, facilitate healing, and alleviate suffering. To do so, the nurse focuses on treating the whole person — the body, mind, and spirit — when delivering care. According to holistic philosophy, wisdom and healing come from the patient, not the practitioner. The practitioner helps the process of healing by creating an environment in which healing can happen. (For more information, see chapter 3, Holistic nursing.)

Holistic nursing in conventional settings
Traditionally, nurses have found it hard to provide holistic care in institutions that are focused on the medical model. In this environment, care is typically symptom- and disease-oriented, focusing more on the diseased part than on the person with the disease.

However, some nurses today are changing this situation. One innovative program called the "Healing Web" was developed by a group of nurse-educators from South Dakota. This model teaches nursing students to listen reflectively, to trust their inner wisdom, and to foster interactions that recognize the value of all participants, whether they are patients, caregivers, or administrators. The core values of the model are collaboration, research, and integration of technology, mind, and spirit. Students are taught the Native American belief that each person has wisdom. They may call on experts to validate, clarify, or amplify, but they're encouraged to trust their intuition and know that wisdom comes from within each person, including the patient.

Becoming a holistic nurse

No formal education is required to implement many holistic nursing skills. The holistic approach requires only that the nurse learn to accept people as they are, without judgment and with compassion. This approach begins with self-acceptance, which can be achieved by focusing inward. Various methods, such as prayer, meditation, visualization, contemplation, and spiritual practices, can help a person develop this focus. According to the American Holistic Nurses' Association (AHNA), self-responsibility also leads the nurse to recognize the interconnectedness of all individuals and their relationship to the human and global community. This recognition and awareness facilitate healing.

In addition, the nurse can learn alternative therapy techniques to enhance patient care. The nurse can also become certified as a holistic nurse through testing endorsed by the AHNA.

One of the goals of holistic nursing care is to integrate holism into the nurse's life. Nursing then becomes an extension of the self rather than a job.

Research and NCCAM's role

Although many alternative therapies have been in use for thousands of years on various continents, there is little mainstream scientific research that documents how they work or whether they're effective. Alternative medicine's anecdotal evidence doesn't meet Western medicine's need for objective scientific proof. (See *The scientific method and holism,* page 18.)

Proponents of alternative therapies point out that only 15% of today's accepted medical treatments are supported by high-quality scientific evidence of efficacy. The U.S. Congress's Office of Technology Assessment reported that about 80% of medical practices used in the United States are unproved by rigorous randomized, double-blind controlled trials (the preferred method of conducting research in the West). Even so, these practices are commonly considered standard medical treatments.

The scientific method and holism

The scientific method of research as we know it today evolved over many centuries. The 17th-century philosopher René Descartes believed that every question could be broken down to its smallest part. This method, later referred to as *reductionism,* has inspired research to isolate factors that cause diseases.

The *scientific,* or *quantitative,* method was created so that results obtained in one study could be generalized to other patient populations and replicated in similar studies. Generalization and replication are usually done through randomized clinical trials in which people are assigned to treatment groups by chance.

The quantitative method's strength is its ability to predict and control outcomes. It formulates hypotheses by reducing the subject to its smallest part, testing the hypotheses, and rejecting or accepting (proving) the hypotheses. The success of this research method in the West has been instrumental in medicine's recognition as a scientific profession.

Quantitative vs. qualitative

Most alternative therapy practitioners believe that the quantitative method of research is incompatible with the *qualitative* holistic philosophy underlying most alternative therapies. They feel it seeks answers only to parts of the whole, whereas the holistic framework sees the whole as greater than the sum of its parts.

In addition, the different approaches to diagnosis and treatment of some of the alternative systems, such as traditional Chinese medicine and Ayurvedic medicine, make Western-style research difficult. One can't compare Western and traditional Chinese treatments for most conditions because health problems are diagnosed in completely different ways. For example, a patient diagnosed with pneumonia by a Western-trained doctor might be diagnosed by a doctor of Chinese medicine as having an excess of *qi* (a concept of vital energy that is foreign to the West).

The dearth of empirical data on alternative therapies has prevented them from being accepted by the mainstream medical profession. However, the nursing profession has joined other health care professionals in developing research to show the effectiveness of specific alternative therapies. For example, a cardiothoracic surgeon and a perfusionist who's an RN, cofounders of the Columbia-Presbyterian Complementary Care Center in New York City, are studying the use of relaxation during surgery to hasten recovery.

In 1992, Congress established the Office of Alternative Medicine (OAM) as part of the National Institutes of Health. OAM was charged with identifying and evaluating promising alternative treatments for serious health problems that affect the country, and for supporting and conducting research on unconventional health care practices to determine their effectiveness and providing information on them to the public and health care professionals. Further, OAM was established to help coordinate research and information on alternative therapies in the United States.

In 1998, Congress established NCCAM, which replaced OAM. NCCAM was given more authority to fund new research directly, design and support alternative therapies, and serve as a clearinghouse of information for the public.

To facilitate scientific evaluation, NCCAM funds a number of Specialty Research Centers at universities and health centers throughout the country. These centers are devoted to conducting ongoing research on the effectiveness of alternative therapies. Each center focuses on a specific health problem: human immunodeficiency virus infection and acquired immunodeficiency syndrome (AIDS), general medical conditions, women's health issues, stroke and neurologic conditions, cancer, aging, addictions, pain (two centers), and asthma, allergies, and immunology. These centers develop research agendas, provide technical assistance, and conduct research. NCCAM also awards grants for basic clinical research and supports doctoral and postdoctoral research in alternative therapies. In the year 2000, the agency funded more than 65 studies on various alternative therapies. (See *Alternative therapy research grants,* page 20.)

To disseminate research findings, NCCAM developed a national database of scientific literature on alternative and complementary practices. The NCCAM Clearinghouse provides information to the public, media, and health care providers. It also maintains a toll-free number (1-888-644-6226) and a Web site (*www.nccam.nih.gov*) to handle inquiries about alternative therapies. The Clearinghouse doesn't give advice or referrals.

Alternative therapy research grants

Between 1993 and 2001, the National Institutes of Health's National Center for Complementary and Alternative Medicine awarded grants for research on the following alternative therapies—although more and more individual studies are being approved:

▌ Acupuncture—for chronic sinusitis in human immunodeficiency virus (HIV) infection, postoperative oral surgery pain, premenstrual syndrome, osteoarthritis, depression, fibromyalgia, dental pain, hypertension

▌ Antioxidants—for cancer

▌ Ayurvedic herbal therapy—for Parkinson's disease

▌ Biofeedback—for pain, diabetes

▌ Chinese herbal therapy—for common warts, hot flashes

▌ Dance and movement therapy—for cystic fibrosis

▌ EEG normalization therapy—for mild head trauma

▌ Ginkgo biloba—for Alzheimer's disease, antidepressant-induced sexual dysfunction, insulin-resistance syndrome, vascular function, asthma

▌ Electrochemical treatment with direct current—for tumors

▌ Energetic therapy—for basal cell carcinoma

▌ Enzyme therapy—for metastatic breast cancer

▌ Guided imagery—for asthma

▌ Herbal medicines—to assess analgesic and antihyperalgesic effects

▌ Homeopathy—for mild traumatic brain injury

▌ Hypericum—for depression

▌ Hypnosis—for chronic pain, bone fractures

▌ Hypnotic imagery—for breast cancer

▌ Imagery—for breast cancer, acquired immunodeficiency syndrome

▌ Isoflavones—for alcohol abuse

▌ Laser acupuncture—for attention deficit disorder

▌ Macrobiotic diet—for cancer

▌ Massage therapy—for bone marrow transplant patients, HIV-1 patients, postsurgical outcomes; to assess effects on development of HIV-exposed babies

▌ Music therapy—for psychosocial adjustment to brain injury

▌ Nonpharmacologic analgesia—for invasive procedures

▌ Prayer (intercessory)—a pilot investigation

▌ Qigong—for late-stage reflex sympathetic dystrophy

▌ Spirituality—for living with HIV and AIDS

▌ Ta'i chi chuan—for balance disorders

▌ Therapeutic Touch—for stress

▌ Transcranial electrostimulation—for chronic pain

▌ Yoga—for obsessive compulsive disorder; to enhance methadone maintenance treatment.

Obstacles hindering research and acceptance

The 1994 report to NIH titled *Alternative Medicine: Expanding Medical Horizons* discusses a number of obstacles to research and acceptance. The report categorizes these obstacles as structural barriers (problems caused by definition, cultural, or language barriers), economic and regulatory barriers (financial and legal implications of state or federal regulations), and belief barriers (obstacles caused by misconceptions, stereotypes, or ideology). Although these barriers still exist, they're being steadily overcome.

Structural barriers

One of the fundamental problems in evaluating alternative medicine is the lack of clear definitions and classification methods. For example, health care professionals and laymen alike commonly use the terms *alternative, complementary, unconventional, unorthodox, nontraditional,* and *holistic* interchangeably, making classification difficult. Is a back massage considered an alternative therapy, a complementary therapy, or just a comfort measure? How should prayer and mental healing be classified? These problems as well as the general inability of Western scientists to understand foreign diagnostic concepts, such as the traditional Chinese concept of *qi* (discussed in chapter 4, Alternative systems of medical practice), make it difficult to devise fair scientific methods of evaluating these therapies.

Economic barriers

Another research barrier is the limited amount of money to perform such studies. Currently, drug companies and private contributors provide most of the money spent on medical research in the United States. Major drug companies spend billions of dollars on research in the hope of discovering new marketable medications. They have no incentive to fund studies of nonpharmaceutical therapies.

Compared to this funding, resources for alternative therapy studies are limited. This situation has begun to change, however, since the creation of NCCAM. In fact, NCCAM is the best current source of research funding for the study of alternative therapies. Its annual research budget has grown from predecessor OAM's $2 million in 1992 to NCCAM's $12 million in

1997 and more than $32 million for 2001. Another, unexpected contributor has been the Department of Defense, which funded a University of Alabama study on the effect of Therapeutic Touch on burns. In addition, national groups representing specific alternative therapies commonly receive small grants to conduct approved research studies.

Financial constraints also affect consumers, who now must pay out of pocket for most unconventional treatments. However, increasing numbers of HMOs see health promotion and preventive care as a method of reducing health care costs and are beginning to cover such treatments as chiropractic care, acupuncture, osteopathy, therapeutic massage, Therapeutic Touch, and biofeedback. As these therapies become more popular and research substantiates their effectiveness, more insurance companies are likely to cover them.

Regulatory barriers

The regulatory requirements of the Food and Drug Administration (FDA) hamper the development and evaluation of alternative therapies. According to the 1994 report to NIH, "because the costs of developing, evaluating, and marketing new drugs are so prohibitive, pharmaceutical companies are not likely to invest time and effort in therapies, such as nutritional or behavioral approaches, that cannot be patented" and thus allow the companies to recoup their investment.

On the other hand, the general absence of regulations in the field of alternative medicine may limit its acceptance by consumers and health care professionals. Although the FDA regulates the development and sale of drugs, it has little control over the production or sale of nonpharmaceutical remedies, including vitamin and mineral supplements and herbal products. In 1994, Congress passed the Dietary Supplement Health and Education Act, which allows companies to sell whatever supplements they please as long as the label makes no claim to treat disease. There are no regulations requiring that the ingredients listed on the label actually be in the product or even that each pill in the bottle contains the same amount of the active ingredient.

The lack of regulations may also pose legal problems for practitioners in certain states. Practitioners who claim to treat human diseases or disorders and use alternative therapies in states that don't license those therapies may be subject to legal action for practicing medicine without a license. However, as more and more HMOs and other insurance providers begin reimbursing for alternative therapies, the public and Congress are likely to demand increased regulations to ensure that patients are protected from harm by unqualified practitioners.

Belief barriers

According to the 1994 report to NIH, conventional physicians have a number of misconceptions and biases that prevent them from accepting alternative therapies. These include:

▶ comfort in the status quo (Physicians prefer established therapies to unconventional ones that haven't been validated by the scientific method.)

▶ reliance on high technology (Physicians regard high-tech procedures such as medical imaging as state-of-the-art and tend to view the "low-tech" alternative therapies as ineffective.)

▶ belief in mainstream medicine as the only true healing profession. (MDs [and their professional organization, the American Medical Association (AMA)] believe that only holders of medical degrees from approved institutions should be allowed to practice medicine. For years, the AMA's Committee on Quackery attempted to eliminate competition from such alternative practitioners as chiropractors and doctors of osteopathy, homeopathy, and naturopathy and forbade AMA members from dealing with them. This practice has decreased since the Supreme Court's 1991 ruling in the case of *Wilk et al. v. the AMA*, which found the AMA's practices a violation of federal antitrust measures.)

Some of these same beliefs apply to the general public. Many laymen are more comfortable with traditional medical practice than with alternative and complementary therapies. They tend to think that current medicine is "tried and true" and, therefore, safe and effective, whereas alternative therapies are supported only by anecdotal evidence and may be more dangerous. However, NCCAM has begun subjecting more and more of these therapies to rigorous scientific testing; this ongoing research should go a long way toward correcting misconceptions and myths and reassure those who are waiting for proof before using alternative therapies.

Finally, the media in the United States have brought a lot of alternative therapies to the public's attention. However, faced with sometimes conflicting, inaccurate, or unreliable information, consumers may be left more confused than enlightened.

Preferred research methods

A 1995 report of NCCAM's Practice and Policy Guidelines Panel describes the traditional hierarchy for rating the evidence of research studies. Randomized, controlled trials carry the greatest weight, followed by controlled observational studies (such as controlled cohort studies and case-control studies), uncontrolled studies (such as case series), single-case reports, and expert opinion.

Studies that examine health concerns and outcomes that are important to patients and provide accurate measures (such as the incidence of heart attacks, strokes, and death) are considered more reliable than studies with physiologic endpoints (such as renal function) or studies that use poorly validated measures that are variable (such as some scales for emotional well-being and functional status).

Support for qualitative rather than quantitative methods

The main barrier to research in alternative therapies is the belief that studies of these therapies must fit into a quantitative model. NIH's support for finding a better way of measuring the

> ❝ Expecting alternative therapies to provide evidence of their effectiveness in a way that conventional Western medicine approves is a false premise. ❞

effectiveness of alternative therapies will go a long way toward acceptance of qualitative methods, which often use outcome studies, as a legitimate research tool.

Indeed, some health care professionals are proposing less reliance on randomized clinical trials and more reliance on outcomes research. They argue that expecting alternative therapies to provide evidence of their effectiveness in a way that conventional Western medicine approves is a false premise. NCCAM's Practice and Policy Guidelines Panel hasn't found universal acceptance of the assumption that alternative and complementary medicine must wait for clinical trial evidence of their effectiveness.

According to R. Edwards, outcomes research provides a multifaceted method for understanding how medical intervention affects patients' lives from the patient's perspective. Outcome studies can be used to demonstrate effectiveness, tolerability, and cost-effectiveness of alternative therapies — the criteria for which the government and insurance companies are looking. Edwards believes that use of the randomized clinical trial as the gold standard in medical research needs to be reexamined in light of a broader concept of health and being. He suggests that the real challenge is to know which research framework will best fit the treatment being studied.

The role of nursing research

Nursing research into such therapies as Therapeutic Touch has proliferated in the past 8 years, primarily in the form of master's theses and doctoral dissertations. Most of these studies have been outcome studies that address the patient's response. The holistic measures used in alternative medicine, which emphasize overall well-being, the patient's personal experience, and the quality and character of the relationships that contribute to the healing process, may best be studied using qualitative measures. Increasingly, nurse educators are approving qualitative methods of research for theses and dissertations.

Organizations that support CAM

Over the years, many groups have emerged that started as a few people gathering to learn about specific alternative therapies. As interest in these therapies has increased, many of these groups have grown into national and international organizations. An example of this growth is the Nurse Healers–Professional Association, which was started by the nurses who learned Therapeutic Touch from its founders, Dolores Krieger and Dora Kunz. Today, this group has members from many countries and maintains files on all members and the alternative therapies that they practice and teach.

Another organization, already mentioned, is the American Holistic Nurses' Association, which promotes holistic nursing and offers certification in Healing Touch.

Services usually offered

Many organizations establish practice guidelines and recommendations for training. Some also have an official certifying process for members who have achieved a certain level of expertise.

In addition, these organizations offer information in the form of newsletters and articles regarding alternative therapies and other holistic concepts. These newsletters list classes on alternative therapies, tell consumers where they can find alternative therapy practitioners, and provide information on different therapies. They also advertise national and regional conferences.

Many organizations offer addresses of their members so that members can network with each other, and many now have Web sites where consumers and health care providers can browse for information.

Locating professional groups

Libraries have resource guides for locating professional groups associated with alternative therapies. Searching the Internet is another way to find information on alternative therapies. (See the appendix, Alternative therapy organizations, for a detailed list of therapy-specific organizations.)

Selected references

Astin, J.A. "Why Patients Use Alternative Medicine: Results of a National Study," *JAMA* 279(19):1548-553, May 1998.

"Complementary and Alternative Therapies," *Holistic Nursing Practice* 13(3):vii-viii, April 2000.

Dossey, B.M. "Holistic Nursing: Taking Your Practice to the Next Level," *Nursing Clinics of North America* 36(1):1-22, March 2001.

Edwards, R. "Our Research Approaches Must Meet the Goal of Improving Patient Care," *Alternative Therapies in Health and Medicine* 3(1):100, January 1997.

Eisenberg, D.M., et al. "Trends in Alternative Medicine Use in the United States, 1990-1997: Results of a follow-up National Survey," *JAMA* 280(18):1569-575, November 1998.

Eisenberg, D.M., et al. "Unconventional Medicine in the United States: Prevalence, Costs, and Patterns of Use," *New England Journal of Medicine* 328(4):246-52, January 1993.

Eliopoulos, C. "Using Complementary and Alternative Therapies Wisely," *Geriatric Nursing* 20(3):139-42, May-June 1999.

Eskinazi, D., and Hoffman, F.A. "Progress in Complementary and Alternative Medicine: Contribution of the National Institutes of Health and the Food and Drug Administration," *Journal of Alternative and Complementary Medicine* 4(4):459-67, Winter 1998.

Herdtner, S. "Using Therapeutic Touch in Nursing Practice," *Orthopedic Nursing* 19(5):77-82, September-October 2000.

National Institutes of Health. *Alternative Medicine: Expanding Medical Horizons. A Report to the National Institutes of Health on Alternative Medical Systems and Practices in the United States prepared under the auspices of the Workshop on Alternative Medicine, Chantilly, Virginia, September 14-16, 1992.* NIH pub. 94-066. Washington, D.C.: U.S. Government Printing Office, 1994.

Tyler, V.E. "Herbal Medicine: From the Past to the Future," *Public Health Nutrition* 3(4A):447-52, December 2000.

Umbreit, A.W. "Healing Touch: Applications in the Acute Care Setting," *AACN Clinical Issues* 11(1):105-19, February 2000.

Weil, A. *Spontaneous Healing: How to Discover and Enhance Your Body's Natural Ability to Maintain and Heal Itself.* New York: Knopf, 1995.

PART TWO

Alternative therapies and nursing practice

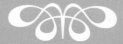

2

Impact on nursing practice

The implementation of alternative therapies has given nurses a greater degree of autonomy and independence from physicians and institutionalized facilities and a way of enriching their own fields of practice. Among the many alternative therapies that nurses now practice are Therapeutic Touch, music and sound therapies, art therapy, aromatherapy, and relaxation techniques, to name just a few. Some of these alternative therapies have their roots in Florence Nightingale's book *Notes on Nursing*. Many of them can be viewed as nursing interventions rather than areas of practice requiring a physician's order to implement.

Some nursing care activities now labeled as alternative are the very aspects of care that patients are requesting and seeking on their own. Thus, the public's increasing use of alternative therapies requires nursing to become prepared to practice in this arena, or at least be knowledgeable, so that collaboration and referrals can be professionally conducted to serve the interests, expectations, and requests of patients, families, and the community.

Alternative therapy or nursing intervention?

Redefining some common alternative therapies as focused clinical nursing interventions may remove the need to label them alternative. Such focused clinical interventions are rooted in nursing's history and derived from nursing arts and conventional nursing care approaches. These therapies seek to offer pain control, symptom management, and comfort measures. Such therapies help to create a sense of health and well-being in the patient, leading to self-control, self-knowledge, self-care, self-recovery, self-healing, and wholeness outcomes.

Two commonly used therapies in nursing practice and research are Therapeutic Touch and guided imagery. Therapeutic Touch has been used by nurses for the past 25 years. It's now being introduced to other practitioners, including conventional medical practitioners, as the basis of energy medicine. These and other caring-healing therapies have long been within the purview of nursing practice.

When certain alternative practices are recognized as part of nursing's framework rather than solely alternative therapies, they can be seen as fundamental to nursing practice and essential aspects of human caring.

Because nurses deal with intimate issues of patients, families, and communities, they may be able to discuss alternative therapies for given conditions. In many instances, nurses are now able to formally carry out selected complementary or alternative interventions with their patients.

Although the American Nurses Association (ANA) doesn't have a formal position on alternative nursing practice, there are growing developments within the profession. Moreover, the ANA's latest social policy statement puts forth some common values and assumptions that mesh well with both holistic nursing and alternative medicine frameworks. (See *The ANA and alternative practices*, page 32.)

This changing perspective on alternative therapies, within the field of nursing and among the public, can now be reframed as conventional nursing care and healing modalities, nursing arts, and nursing therapeutics. This change expands and enriches nursing's current practice models, rather than detracting from them.

New options for nurses

Because the fields of alternative medicine, mind-body medicine, and holistic nursing are expanding into scientific, professional, and public circles, new options now exist for collaborative interdisciplinary education, practice, and research. This

The ANA and alternative practices

In its 1995 social policy statement, the American Nurses Association addresses holistic philosophy and the incorporation of complementary and alternative practices for the patient. The statement includes values, assumptions, and philosophical perspectives that are congruent with holistic approaches, holding that:

▶ humans manifest an essential unity of mind, body, and spirit
▶ human experience is contextually and culturally defined.

The policy statement and definition of nursing goes on to acknowledge four essential features of contemporary nursing practice:

1. attention to the full range of human experiences and responses to health and illness without restriction to a problem-focused orientation
2. integration of objective data with knowledge gained from an understanding of the patient's or the group's subjective experience
3. application of scientific knowledge to the processes of diagnosis and treatment
4. provision of a caring relationship that facilitates health and healing.

growing field opens up opportunities for individual nurses, as well as nursing collectively, to advance along clinical career lines, in contrast to being confined to a specific level of practice or a traditional medical or nursing specialty area. No longer is the nurse limited to hospital or home care. In the past, nurses had to abandon clinical practice and move into administration or education in order to advance. Now, career-long, clinical progression has become a new opportunity for nurses. The field of alternative therapies permits nurses — and nursing — to sustain and excel in advanced clinical nursing activities. Yet, exploring alternative medicine allows a nurse to continue to follow her individual interests and talents, while practicing in various settings and populations.

These new options have helped reestablish the nurse's role as a holistic care provider. Further, health care practices are becoming increasingly interdisciplinary, as a new cadre of alternative practitioners has arrived on the health care scene. The intersection between some of nursing's traditional caring and healing arts and the evolution and emergence of the new field of alternative medicine allows practitioners from different backgrounds to come together in a common, shared perspective: that of treating the whole patient.

Some controversy remains about whether complementary and alternative care should be supervised by an attending primary care physician. Because this issue is still a matter for public debate, nurses can take the lead in creating a role for themselves in making this decision. What's more, the use of alternative medicine can help nursing mature in its mission and expand its scope of practice, all of which enhances, rather than conflicts with, professional nursing practice.

Incorporating alternative therapies into your practice

The task of incorporating alternative therapies into nursing practice can be complex. In addition to learning specific techniques, you must be able to establish congruence between your own cultural beliefs and biases and the culture, values, and belief systems of your patient.

Understanding the alternative approach

For many people, conventional medicine is the only approach to illness they have ever known. But because of this country's cultural diversity, many others bring traditional healing practices, folk medicine, and beliefs from their cultural backgrounds. To them, conventional medicine is the "alternative." Their culture may have a broad acceptance of certain practices that are still regarded with suspicion by the medical mainstream in the United States. These disparate feelings regarding alternative therapies challenge nurses to find a middle ground that takes into account their own biases as well as their patient's while also evaluating the overlapping value of various therapies.

Each complementary or alternative practice has its own vision, theory, therapeutics, style, structure, and body of evidence for healing. These diverse systems commonly compete not only with conventional medicine but also with each other. However, there are also commonalities among different therapies. These commonalities include nature, vitalism, science, and spirituality.

Nature

Nature is a central focus for many complementary and alternative therapies. Many practitioners view nature as the original perfect state of being, ultimately benign and pure. Therefore, natural therapies are felt to be superior to technologically generated interventions, such as chemicals, drugs, and mechanical or surgical procedures. As these "generated" interventions are seen as artificial, *externally* generated, and po-

> 66 *Self-generated, natural healing therapies are usually preferred across most systems of alternative therapy. This preference is manifested in the use of natural foods and herbs, and energy. However, "natural" doesn't mean nontoxic; death can be as natural as a poisonous mushroom.* 99

tentially toxic, the *self*-generated, natural healing therapies are usually preferred across most systems of alternative therapy. This preference is manifested in the use of natural foods and herbs. However, "natural" doesn't mean nontoxic; death can be as natural as a poisonous mushroom.

Vitalism

The notion that nature and life processes aren't controlled by mechanical forces alone but instead may be self-determining is called *vitalism*. This belief system ascribes animate rather than inanimate properties to biological or scientific models. For example, people who adhere to vitalistic reasoning believe that manipulation or enhancement of the body's vital energy is one explanation for the success of alternative therapies. Vitalism is considered part of a vital force of nature, subtle but real. Vitalism also refers to a psychic or mental force, a spiritual presence, and an organizational principle or informational network. Homeopathic practitioners believe in a vital spiritual force; chiropractic practitioners refer to "innate intelligence" and "psychic force." Other therapies, such as hypnosis, biofeedback, and Therapeutic Touch, have hints of this perspective of vitalism.

Science

In many areas of alternative medicine, a wide chasm separates practitioners and scientists. For example, pharmacognosists (scientific herb researchers) have advanced degrees and understand the scientific method, yet they have no direct experience with patients. Conversely, practicing herbalists have this experience but, lacking a rigorous scientific foundation, they thus may rely on folklore to explain the genuine benefit that patients derive from their herbal remedies. Much of the conflict within the area of science arises from these differences between practitioners and researchers.

Although most practitioners of both conventional and alternative therapies consider themselves to be scientific, their definitions of what constitutes science may not concur. Alternative medical science tends to be more observational, qualitative in nature, and less controlled and experimental than conventional biomedical science. Furthermore, many alternative practitioners lack experience with controlled, experimental designs and common deductive methods.

> ❝ *Alternative medical science tends to be more observational, qualitative in nature, and less controlled and experimental than conventional biomedical science.* ❞

Because alternative medicine may lack empirical evidence, Western scientists generally scoff at apparently effective treatments or methods. What's more, when both groups agree that a treatment is valid, they may disagree on the reason. Their differing explanations arise naturally from the biases of the practitioners.

Spirituality

Most practitioners of alternative medicine operate from a view of science, nature, and spirituality that isn't based in the realm of practical experience alone. Beyond material medicine, the role of human freedom, belief systems, choice, and spirit comes into greater play. For example, prayer, religion, and Eastern beliefs, such as psychic healing, ritual, and the spiritual world, play a part in alternative medicine. In general, practitioners of alternative medicine seem to place more importance on spirituality in their practice of healing than do traditional medical practitioners.

Integrating alternative and conventional

More and more common medical conditions (mainly chronic conditions) are being treated by both conventional medical science approaches *and* alternative therapies. Currently, many patients are seeking alternative therapy on their own initiative in addition to seeing their medical doctors. However, as alternative therapies gain acceptance and supportive evidence, some physicians are beginning to integrate alternative therapies into their practices and in some cases referring patients to alternative therapists.

Responding to the increased patient demand, hospitals are increasingly incorporating new practice models such as integrated practice. These practice models respond to patient choices and requests for alternative options as part of a holistic approach to healing.

Educating yourself

Conventional practitioners of medicine and nursing shouldn't enter into alternative practices lightly. Although some of the basic complementary approaches, (various forms of touch, imagery, sound, diet, environment, and relaxation approaches) are traditional nursing skills, they haven't always been incorporated at an advanced level in conventional nursing educational programs. In addition, some approaches, such as acupuncture, homeopathy, energy work, and manual healing therapies, require advanced training, supervised practice, and hours of clinical experience as well as formal education and, in some cases, certification.

With a framework of traditional nursing skills and experience, you can add alternative therapy skills directly to your practice or use them to expand or transform the nature of your work. By becoming more familiar with a range of alternative therapies, you'll be in a better position to respond to increasing demands from the public.

You can do the following to incorporate new therapies into your practice:

▶ Become more familiar with the overall field, specific therapies that interest you, and reputable practitioners.

⚫ Acquire advanced practice skills or certification in selected alternative practices.

You can become more educated and experienced in various therapies by doing additional reading, consulting with colleagues already practicing in the field, or pursuing various professional development programs.

Nursing programs

The number of nursing schools in the United States offering course work in alternative therapies is difficult to determine because some, if not most, of the less invasive alternative therapies are described as holistic, caring-based nursing arts or nursing therapeutics. Thus, these therapies aren't referred to as alternative course work. However, a growing number of undergraduate and graduate nursing programs include alternative therapies in their curriculum.

An informal international survey revealed that more than 80 schools of nursing already teach some level of Therapeutic Touch to their students. A more formal report found 76 schools of nursing in the United States and 12 in Canada that have curriculum content in this specialty. Additionally, 71 health care facilities in the United States and 28 in Canada provide Therapeutic Touch as a treatment option, according to the *Journal of Holistic Nursing*.

Moreover, a 1996 survey conducted by the National League for Nursing (NLN) indicated that 57 baccalaureate nursing programs offered some courses in acupressure, aromatherapy, imagery, sound therapy, massage, Therapeutic Touch, relaxation, visualization, and various other therapies. Forty-one master's-level nursing programs reported some form of course work in these same therapies. Furthermore, 75% of the nurse administrators responding to the survey agreed that in the next decade there would be a marked increase in alternative or nontraditional medicine.

Advanced degree programs

Several schools have designed advanced degree programs in holistic nursing or alternative therapies. Schools that offer formal academic master's degrees or graduate level studies in holistic nursing and alternative therapies include:

⚫ Beth El College of Nursing (Colorado Springs)
⚫ University of Colorado (Denver)

▶ College of New Rochelle (New York)
▶ University of Louisville School of Nursing (Kentucky)
▶ Florida Atlantic University (Boca Raton)
▶ University of Tennessee (Memphis).

Also, the University of Colorado Center for Human Caring offers a professional development certificate in advanced practices, such as the caring-healing relationship, caring-healing arts, and Therapeutic Touch. Additional programs are being developed as the demand for alternative therapies continues to expand.

Assessing the patient's knowledge

Before introducing alternative therapies to your patients or their families, you'll need to assess the person's knowledge, values, beliefs, and cultural interests in such therapies. In many instances, patients seeking an alternative therapy are well informed and knowledgeable. Patients commonly request such options as music, massage, acupuncture, or chiropractic interventions as part of their health care.

66 *Informed choice for nurse and patient is fundamental to introducing or intervening with alternative therapies. Educating the patient may further help him come to a comfortable decision based on his interests and desires.* 99

A midwestern hospital's recent community study found familiarity with and use of complementary and alternative therapies. Of the survey respondents, more than 60% indicated general familiarity. (See *Gauging patient knowledge.*)

Sometimes, the nurse may be aware of various options that can facilitate a patient's treatment and recovery, but the patient may be uninformed or suspicious of the treatment. This is why informed choice for nurse and patient is fundamental to introducing or intervening with alternative therapies. Educating the patient may further help him come to a comfortable decision based on his interests and desires.

Staying within the patient's frame of reference is important when working within this growing field. What is considered alternative to one person may be considered a natural choice by another. Let the patient and your knowledge of the field guide

Gauging patient knowledge

A 1997 study, conducted in the Rocky Mountain region, reported that local communities already used and had extensive familiarity with alternative and complementary therapies. Of the respondents, 60% or more indicated general familiarity with complementary therapies; 89% with chiropractic; 84% with massage therapy; 83% with acupuncture; 79% with prayer; 79% with relaxation techniques; 78% with herbal medicine; and 78% with vitamin therapy. Also, 61% of the respondents indicated they had used at least one complementary therapy.

you. Also, remember to consider the nature of your relationship with the patient and family when making a treatment decision.

Answering questions about research

Your patient may inquire about scientific evidence to support a particular alternative therapy. Part of your response should be an explanation of how standards differ between the alternative medicine, conventional medicine, and nursing research approaches. (See *Comparing research approaches,* page 40.) These different approaches can be summed up as experimental (randomized, controlled trials) in conventional medicine and as observational (outcome, or evidence-based, studies) in alternative medicine. Although these two opposing approaches raise different questions about the subjects in the minds of researchers and highlight their differing approaches to investigation, you can add to your explanation the fact that both sides are moving toward a more common research approach.

With the recent rise of outcome studies and evidence-based practices by governments, health care systems, research institutes, and insurance agencies, the two differing perspectives toward research are beginning to merge by necessity. The same evidence-based practice momentum is now gaining momentum within nursing practice, especially for those interventions that are considered alternative.

The current shift in research is toward evidence-based practice, which relies on outcome studies. This approach seeks to carry out, analyze, and summarize the best available

Comparing research approaches

Alternative medicine practitioners accuse conventional scientists of being too mechanical and reductionist, while conventional physicians and scientists charge alternative practitioners with being too anecdotal and relying on folklore rather than hard science. This chart outlines differences in these practices.

Alternative medicine	Conventional medicine
Observational	Experimental (empirical)
Vitalistic and naturalistic	Mechanical-technical
Case histories	Laboratory science
Holistic	Reductionist

evidence so that it can be identified as the basis for clinical guidelines for practitioners and the public.

Even though nurses are considered essential to health care delivery and are primary caregivers when patients are hospitalized, the results of evidence-based practice or patient-outcome indicators have yet to become the norm in nursing. Research that has been completed in the area of evidence-based practice has largely been confined to patient outcomes related to satisfaction with care, infection control, successful early discharge, and numerous other desirable health outcomes. The reason for this narrow focus in research may be the pivotal role nurses play in quality improvement and outcome management.

The traditional research emphasis on randomized, controlled trials has been criticized by many nurses. This criticism is generally unsympathetic toward scientific experimentation and includes arguments for the need for evidence-based practice. A great deal of contemporary and progressive nursing research is grounded in approaches that value qualitative data and the use of interpretation. As nursing practice has diverse origins, diversity of research is necessary. Ideally, a combination of traditional research, evidence-based practice, and qualitative research could be used to provide the most comprehensive results.

The establishment in 1992 of the National Institutes of Health's (NIH) Office of Alternative Medicine (OAM) has fostered collaboration within NIH that has benefited nursing research. From 1993 to 1994, OAM gave nine research awards, totaling more than $2 million, to the National Institutes for

> *Research that explores complementary and alternative nursing practices helps provide a rich, broad specific database of selected clinical interventions that translate scientific advances into up-to-date, patient-focused, cost-effective, multidisciplinary health care practices.*

Nursing Research (NINR). In addition to other research projects, NINR is gathering information on intervention studies that overlap with alternative therapies. Nursing interventions being researched through NINR funding include guided imagery, pain management, and caregiver touch. (See *Common themes of nursing research,* page 42.)

Nursing interventions that fit conceptually with alternative and complementary interventions consist largely of noninvasive, natural, self-generating, and human-environmental interventions. These interventions promote pain control, symptom management, wound healing, comfort, and a state of well-being. In practice and research, such nursing interventions focus on self-centered care, recovery, knowledge, and healing. Additional interventions surround healing, health promotion, and quality-of-life approaches. Research that explores complementary and alternative nursing practices helps provide a rich, broad scientific database of selected clinical interventions that translate scientific advances into up-to-date, patient-focused, cost-effective, multidisciplinary health care practices.

Future investigations should increase the depth of nursing science in this area. Continuous research, both qualitative and quantitative, is needed to sustain public trust, which allows the nursing profession to continue to excel in providing patient-focused health care.

Common themes of nursing research

With money increasingly available for research, alternative approaches in nursing care have been under investigation. Recent nursing intervention studies have examined some of the following themes:
▶ comfort
▶ evaluation of educational programs
▶ guided imagery
▶ pain management
▶ patient management
▶ self-care
▶ self-management
▶ touch.

Answering insurance questions

Whether your patient's health insurance provider will reimburse him for an alternative or a complementary therapy depends on the provider and the type of policy. Until recently, alternative practices — labeled as nonessential and unscientific — were unlikely to be covered by medical insurance. This is rapidly changing today, as approaches once considered unconventional are gaining mainstream acceptance. Studies now show that Americans pay more visits to alternative health care providers than to traditional providers. The World Congress on Complementary Therapies in Medicine, held in Washington, D.C., in 1996, was chaired by former U.S. Surgeon General C. Everett Koop, which shows additional mainstream acceptance.

In an even more dramatic turn, a 1995 survey of the United States' largest health maintenance organizations (HMOs), which are traditionally conservative in their reimbursement practices, found that 86% cover chiropractic, 69% cover lifestyle modification weight-loss programs, 31% cover acupuncture, 28% cover relaxation therapies, 17% cover mental imagery therapy, and 14% cover massage therapy and hypnosis.

A recent community survey found that one-fourth of the respondents had some form of insurance coverage for complementary therapies. Of those individuals whose insurance didn't cover complementary therapies or those who were uncertain, 45% indicated they would switch to an insurance plan that covered both traditional and complementary medical treatments. This survey indicates that as the usage of complementary therapies becomes more widespread, patients will begin to seek insurance programs that cover these therapies.

Clearly these shifts indicate that covering some of these less invasive, self-care therapies is gaining momentum both with the public and with insurance companies. Some practices are covered because of public demand and because they cost less than more invasive, conventional medical-surgical interventions. This trend is expected to continue. When the public requests alternative care, nurses will be available to provide it. What's more, the availability of health care coverage for complementary and alternative treatments will make it practical for nurses already practicing in multiple settings to provide these treatments.

Answering questions about availability

You can tell your patients that the availability of complementary and alternative therapies in traditional health care venues is increasing. Some systems have been slow to change for fear of medical staff resistance and, in some instances, patients' reservations. For example, the nursing practice of Therapeutic Touch in conventional hospitals in the late 1980s and early 1990s resulted in some patient complaints and a reexamination of how Therapeutic Touch was being used. More recently, this therapy has been offered along with a range of other therapies by mainstream academic health science centers, including Columbia University Hospital; New York University Hospital; Stanford Children's Hospital (California); Queen's Medical Center, Honolulu; and The Children's Hospital, Denver.

Just as HMOs are modifying their policies to include such therapies in their coverage, hospitals and health care facilities are also offering specific therapies or entire clinics devoted to complementary and alternative care. Even the most conservative conventional systems are now yielding to public demand and to consumers' willingness to spend their own money to seek care elsewhere.

Although many institutions are offering alternative therapies under the umbrella of research centers, others are responding to cost incentives and reaching out directly to the public. To bring mainstream clinicians into the process, some facilities are using terminology such as "patient choice," "options," and "integrative practice" as a way to bring two disparate systems into one coherent practice mission.

Some hospitals have conducted community surveys as a means of educating their professional staff about what patients are seeking and expecting from their health care system. The results have been surprising. In one such survey, respondents were asked whether the local community hospital should permit complementary therapists to administer to patients in the hospital. The majority of respondents indicated that they would support complementary therapies, with the most enthusiastic support coming from those who had received such therapy in the past. Even among those who had never used complementary therapy, there was a reasonable level of support for such a policy.

The therapies rated as most appropriate for the hospital in this survey were acupuncture, massage therapy, chiropractic, nutritional therapy, and relaxation techniques. Other therapies that received support included vitamin or nutritional supplement therapy, herbal medicine, homeopathic or naturopathic medicine, and spirituality or prayer. Approaches such as aromatherapy and yoga were seen as less important than the other therapies for use in a hospital setting. (However, use of aromatherapy in hospitals, including the use of essential oils, is becoming more widespread, especially in the United Kingdom, Australia, and New Zealand.)

As a result of the survey, that local community hospital is now offering practice privileges to an acupuncturist, who is also a medical doctor. The physician is board-certified in family medicine and is also prepared in acupuncture, stress-reduction, meditation, and yoga. He has incorporated all of these natural healing therapies into his practice, thus allowing the hospital to make these therapies available for hospitalized patients. This extension of staff privileges for acupuncture, specifically, is consistent with new policy recommendations from the NIH. The NIH recently backed acupuncture use when clear evidence of its effectiveness exists — for example, in nausea and vomiting, dental surgery pain, lower back pain, headaches, asthma, and menstrual cramps.

Informed consent

Most alternative therapies are offered in the context of a caring-healing relationship. Consent is necessary for either direct practice of alternative therapies or referral and recommendations for them. Depending on the nature of the therapy, formally obtaining informed consent may not be necessary. For example, if you were seeking a patient to participate in a formal research program investigating a specific therapy, you would need to obtain informed consent. If you were introducing a specific noninvasive therapy such as Therapeutic Touch, use of calming words and caring expressions of support, or relaxation imagery, no formal informed consent would be expected.

However, if you were planning to introduce a more intrusive therapy, such as aromatherapy, you'd have to obtain a clinical informed consent as it's considered a patient choice option. Also, because aromatherapy may affect other patients in addition to the one you are treating, you must be sensitive to the wishes of your patient's roommate if you're practicing in a hospital or other large facility.

In summary, you should be able to distinguish when a cooperative, mutual agreement of clinical consent is sufficient (for supportive, calming, comforting therapies offered within the context of a caring relationship) and when you need more formal consent (for more intrusive therapies or for research or advanced clinical intervention purposes). In all instances, you're expected to make an ethical commitment to your relationship with your patient, so that any intervention fits with the patient focus and the patient's general consent. (See "Professional liability," page 51, for further discussion of this topic.)

> ❝ You may find using alternative therapies valuable because it changes your perspective as a caregiver from the conventional, fragmented, physical, medical care emphasis to one of a more integrated, holistic, and spiritual dimension. ❞

Advantages of alternative therapies

As a nurse, you should be aware that scientific evidence increasingly suggests that some alternative therapies (such as acupuncture) should be medically recommended and used as a low-cost option in pain and symptom management in designat-

ed cases. A consensus panel at the NIH made such recommendations to the public and the health care community in 1997.

You may find using alternative therapies valuable because it
changes your perspective as a caregiver from the conventional, fragmented, physical, medical care emphasis to one of a
more integrated, holistic, and spiritual dimension. Clearly, this
is the kind of care that consumers are seeking and for which
they're willing to pay.

Avoiding risks of some alternative therapies

Whatever you believe about the scientific validity of some complementary therapies, you'll probably agree that some therapies (such as Therapeutic Touch) can be beneficial even
though they may not have been fully endorsed scientifically.
The primary risks arise when the patient uses such therapies
as a *substitute* for accepted medical treatments — thus risking
disease progression — or seeks care from several practitioners without informing his primary and secondary health care
providers.

Preventing delays in treatment

As a practitioner, you're aware that perhaps the biggest risk in
using alternative therapies is that patients may delay obtaining more conventional and effective therapies when they're indicated. In nursing practice, commonly used therapies, such
as Therapeutic Touch and relaxation techniques, are never
considered substitutes for conventional medicine. You can't go
wrong when you use these therapies as complements to established approaches or preventive interventions. In addition, as
a first-line practitioner, with the trust of your patient, you can
encourage those who are reluctant to seek conventional treatment to do so when necessary.

As the public becomes more selective and educated in its
own care system and self-care programs, patients will become
discriminating enough to combine the best of both therapies.
Most people who use alternative therapies do so in conjunction with conventional medicine. Nevertheless, you should be
vigilant about preventing delay or prolonged use of alternative
therapies when conventional treatment is necessary.

Preventing fragmentation of care

When patients seek care from several unrelated providers, they risk fragmenting their care. Providing comprehensive, integrated care is one reason for medical and nursing practitioners and hospitals to integrate alternative practices into mainstream care. This integration avoids a fragmented, uncoordinated approach in which conventional and alternative therapies may counteract or interfere with each other.

The public may still reject the idea of having medical or nursing staff control their freedom of choice. As a nurse, you can persuade your patients that communicating with their health care provider about their use of alternative therapies is important for both their safety and their comfort.

Because consumers are increasingly using alternative therapies on their own, outside of conventional systems of care, you have a responsibility as a nursing practitioner to seek information from your patients about their use of other therapies. Gathering such information is critical in order to minimize medical risks and improve the overall quality of patient care and confidence in the profession.

Incorporating alternative therapies into the care plan

Before you begin incorporating alternative therapies into a patient's care plan, you'll need to examine your readiness. The following questions can serve as guidelines to assist you with your self-assessment.

◗ Are you familiar with and prepared to use the therapy under consideration?

◗ Do you have evidence that this therapy may assist your patient? For example, research suggests that women in labor can benefit from guided imagery or massage to help relax them.

◗ Is the patient or family requesting or expressing interest in a given therapy? For example, is your patient with chronic pain inquiring about acupuncture?

◗ Have you had any personal or clinical experience in using this therapy or observing its use by other practitioners?

◗ Do you need any additional training, professional development course work, clinical experience, and supervision before incorporating the therapy into your care plan? Are you willing to seek out such training?

▶ Are you familiar with local practitioners who are qualified and hold appropriate credentials?

Other issues to consider before incorporating therapies into the care plan include factors mentioned earlier, such as patients' beliefs and value systems, cultural customs and habits, interests, and knowledge of general or specific practices. Certainly, if a patient requests such therapies, you have an obligation to obtain as much information as possible before giving advice. (See *Before discussing alternative care.*)

You'll also need to consider the nature of the caring relationship and context for the care plan: the patient's history, the patient's health concerns, previous care, prevention, and treatment plans.

Establishing a journal

You should obtain information about the patient's own self-care practices that incorporate alternative therapies to assess them for safety and efficacy, evaluate the patient's preferences, and find out which experiences have worked.

For a patient who is already using an alternative therapy on his own, you may wish to suggest keeping a journal as a personal record of how the therapy is working. During follow-up visits, review the patient's journal, if possible, and discuss both subjective and objective outcomes with the patient.

Documenting the patient's self-care

Always document the patient's use of an alternative or complementary therapy, including whether any nursing interventions involved such care. Documentation is critical because without knowledge of a patient's use of alternative therapy, the conventional practitioner — the patient's physician or you — may unknowingly prescribe or administer a potentially dangerous drug. The prescribed drug could have adverse or toxic effects when combined with an alternative therapy. For example, if the patient is regularly taking a strong herbal tea, carrying out a regimen of megadose vitamins, or using a special diet from an alternative practitioner, the risk of overdose or drug interaction increases.

Before discussing alternative care

When your patient asks about alternative care, you must first understand his background, including cultural viewpoints and expectations about conventional and nontraditional medicine. Other considerations are the patient's symptoms, medical and nursing diagnoses, and the nature of the patient's experiences associated with the health problem.

Answer your own questions before the patient's
Before deciding on your nursing care plan, ask yourself these questions:

▶ Is the patient's condition chronic or acute?
▶ Is the condition related to a diagnosed medical condition?
▶ Is the alternative treatment for an adverse effect of a medical treatment?
▶ Is the presenting concern associated with pain, comfort, back problems, stress, alleviation of suffering (for example, nausea and vomiting, migraine headaches, and other general and specific conditions that aren't effectively treated by conventional methods)?
▶ Have conventional medical options been used or ruled out as appropriate therapies?
▶ Could alternative approaches be used in conjunction with conventional therapies?

Ultimately, you'll have to rely on your own professional judgment and competency in an area before introducing or referring a patient for a specific alternative therapy.

Answering patients' questions

When responding to patient questions and concerns about complementary and alternative therapies, remember that you must first establish the caring nature of the relationship before effective communication and information can be processed. In this way, you'll maintain communication and trust and foster participation in a genuine ongoing dialogue with the patient. True healing occurs in the human-to-human caring relationship. No alternative, conventional, or complementary therapies can be effective without it.

With the relationship firm, follow these guidelines:

Understanding transcultural issues

The type of questions your patients ask may depend on their cultural background. Some patients may question you about treatment effectiveness and practitioner credentials because they may be suspicious of alternative medicine. Some ethnic populations, on the other hand, may be widespread users of alternative medicine but reluctant to disclose their practices. Their distrust may arise from previous experience with skeptical medical practitioners.

Native Americans and Mexican-Americans, for instance, are statistically more likely to use alternative medicine. For example, a 1996 study found that 44% of Mexican-American participants used an alternative therapy one or more times during the previous year, and 66% of them never reported these visits to their established primary care provider.

Leininger's transcultural nursing theory
Madeleine Leininger's transcultural nursing theory serves as an effective guide to explaining care uses and meanings. Her theory makes the patient's cultural perspective a formal aspect of any plan of care. This model ensures that the patient's values, beliefs, and lifestyle provide the base for planning, implementing, and evaluating culture-specific care. Without formally incorporating the subjective cultural meaning of care for a given patient in a specific care situation, you can inadvertently affect the patient's care needs adversely or even violate the patient's basic beliefs.

Becoming familiar with the views of the patient population you serve can help you individualize your care. *Note:* Be careful not to make generalizations about what a patient may prefer based on stereotypes of gender, ethnicity, or culture. Just because a patient has an Irish-sounding name, don't assume she's a practicing Catholic who would want a priest to attend her. Similarly, just because a patient appears to be Asian or Asian-American doesn't mean he's comfortable with acupuncture.

▶ Pay attention to which person initiates the dialogue. Did the question come from the patient or did a family member raise the issue? Sometimes you might face inquiries from another practitioner or a neighbor, friend, or coworker.

▶ Find out how informed the patient is. How much information does the patient already have about the issues?

▶ Ask if the patient already engages in self-care practices that are considered alternative. How effective are they?
▶ Learn whether the patient is interested in or receptive to alternative care. How does he feel about adding to the care he's already receiving?

Be prepared to answer specific questions about your own philosophy, experience, and knowledge. You may be asked whether you're qualified to administer or refer for alternative therapies.

Knowledge of different therapies and trust in the practitioner often affects the nature of patient questions and how much a patient will disclose about his use of alternative therapies. Your goal is to provide culturally congruent as well as clinically safe care, regardless of your own cultural background and that of the patient. (See *Understanding transcultural issues.*)

Professional liability

Claims against alternative providers have been influenced by the nature of patient-practitioner relationships. A caring relationship, which fosters communication and patient involvement and choice in decision making, contributes to high-quality standards of care and is associated with a decrease in claims.

Alternative practitioners have a history of engaging in just such relationships — personalized and caring; this is one of the reasons that patients seek them out. Patients need to be listened to, to feel they're being heard, to be treated as individuals, and to be understood. All of these factors contribute to patient satisfaction and make a difference with respect to legal claims against any practitioner.

When claims are made specifically against physicians who provide alternative treatments, they usually arise because of departures from generally accepted standards of care, unprofessional conduct, violation of a specific law or regulation, or evidence of a pattern of practice that constitutes fraud or negligence.

Other factors that affect professional legal issues include lack of consensus within the medical community on use of alternative therapies or circumstances surrounding the decision to use these therapies. Interestingly, some state laws (in North Carolina, New York, Oklahoma, and Washington, for instance) actually prohibit bringing charges of unprofessional conduct based solely on the use of alternative therapies. Other states will likely follow this trend.

Reducing your liability

To reduce professional liability, remember to use informed consent when it's indicated. Even though you may have difficulty obtaining truly informed consent—for example, because of the absence of consistent and accurate data regarding the risks and benefits of alternative treatments, it's always wise to provide the best information available. Also, by maintaining open and honest patient communication and building trust within a caring relationship, you should be able to obtain an authentic informed consent.

Preventing liability issues from arising depends on good communication skills and thorough documentation. (See *Minimizing your professional liability*.) This process is carried out most effectively in genuine dialogue and in partnership with the patient.

Licensure and regulation

Requests for qualifications and credentials are growing, which places demands on the community of alternative practitioners. You may need to obtain additional credentials, education, clini-

---

Minimizing your professional liability

The foundation of a healthy professional relationship is trust between the caregiver and the patient. You can also minimize professional liability in these ways:
- Consult with other colleagues when in doubt about performing a particular therapy or when you have any questions about care.
- Document nurse-patient communication.
- Build a record of clinical dialogues, encounters, advice, and recommendations.
- Encourage patients to keep their own records of specific therapies used and their effects.
- Seek to sustain a current relationship through open communication and genuine dialogue.

cal supervision, and even licensing. These requirements are increasingly necessary for all alternative practitioners, including nurses.

At the most basic level, the aim of regulating nursing practice is to protect the public. Licensure, registration, and credentials, including new forms of certification and professional development certificate programs, are all part of a growing movement to help make sure that health care providers meet the required levels of competency to practice. These requirements are also a form of liability protection for you.

Although the scope of practice and the specific regulations for different practices vary from state to state, a common foundation exists across the United States. For example, the basic nursing functions of teaching, counseling, and prevention serve as a core upon which nursing practice can be built.

Toward increased flexibility

The rapid changes occurring in the health care delivery system are, in some instances, creating more flexible models for all health professionals. Some of these changes are related to recommendations from national study groups and foundations dedicated to improving policies and reforming health care. For example, the 1994 Pew Health Professions Commission recommended fundamental shifts in educational requirements for all health professions, emphasizing relationship-centered care as the basis for all reform. In 1995, the Commission further proposed regulatory reform for all health professions. While still allowing flexible scopes of practice, the Commission stressed the need for rigorous competency requirements.

One of the factors motivating reform at all levels is the public's demand for quality health care choices, along with reduced costs and improved access. However, certain existing regulations can create barriers to access, especially for a number of therapies now considered complementary or alternative that have long been part of nursing's practice skills. These barriers are constructed in two ways. The listing of an act in the regulation of one health profession can be interpreted as making it the exclusive purview of that profession. Conversely, the absence of an act can be interpreted as making that act outside the scope of a profession.

Indeed, legal challenges have been brought against health care providers who engage in nontraditional health care practices. The argument in these legal actions is that the alternative therapy is outside the scope of their practice.

More recently, however, individual states have begun to permit physicians to incorporate alternative healing approaches into their conventional practices, provided the physicians are qualified. These state regulations have begun to include acupuncture, acupressure, massage, homeopathy, and other alternative therapies.

No single profession has exclusive domain over the diverse range of alternative therapies, and the boundaries between the roles and practices of health professionals and qualified laypersons are increasingly being blurred. The danger to nursing in this area of new regulations is that, as new regulations are developed for other professions, a specific therapy may become the domain of one or two given professions. Nurses must be aware of the possibility that the profession could be excluded from a particular mode of caregiving, even though that therapy may already be incorporated into nursing's caring and healing practices.

Nurse practice acts

Nurse practice acts across most of the United States address professional nursing. Although the nurse practice acts differ from state to state, the overall legal base for practice is noticeably uniform.

Nurse practice acts don't include language specific to alternative therapies, although some do explicitly forbid prohibiting such activities under certain circumstances. For example, under the Arizona Nurse Practice Act, "caring for the sick in accordance with the practice of religious principles or tenets of any well-recognized church or denomination which relies upon prayer, or spiritual means of healing" must not be prohibited. Thus, selected nurse practice acts provide legal protection for nurses practicing in these areas of alternative and complementary therapies. The Colorado Nurse Practice Act (1995) offers an example of language that's open to a range of therapies that fall within the scope of practice. (See *Nurse practice acts and alternative medicine*.)

Any professional definition of nursing describes the nature and components of the field and its attempts to meet and address the needs of the public. Many state nurse practice acts and definitions of nursing remain intentionally vague, allowing state-to-state variability in interpretation and application.

The 1995 American Nurses Association (ANA) definition of nursing reflects the general nature of nursing by highlighting four features of contemporary practice:

▶ attending to the full range of human experience
▶ integrating objective and subjective information
▶ applying scientific knowledge to diagnosis and treatment

Nurse practice acts and alternative medicine

Most state nurse practice acts don't mention alternative medicine. Colorado's act doesn't specifically mention it either, but it does provide a broad range of practice options. Compare the language in your own nurse practice act to that in the Colorado act:

"The practice of professional nursing means the performance of both independent nursing functions and delegated medical functions in accordance with accepted practice standards. Such functions include the initiation and performance of nursing care through health promotion; supportive or restorative care; disease prevention; and diagnosis and treatment of human disease, ailment, pain, injury, deformity, and physical or mental condition using specialized knowledge, judgment, and skill involving the application of biological, physical, social, and behavioral science principles required for licensure as a professional nurse.

"The practice of professional nursing shall include the performance of such services as:

▶ evaluating health status through the collection and assessment of health data
▶ health teaching and health counseling
▶ providing therapy and treatment that is supportive and restorative to life and well-being either directly to the patient or indirectly through consultation with, delegation to, supervision of, or teaching of others
▶ executing delegated medical functions
▶ referring to medical or community agencies those patients who need further evaluation or treatment
▶ reviewing and monitoring therapy and treatment plans."

▶ providing a caring relationship.

Although the ANA doesn't have a position statement or refer specifically to complementary and alternative practices, the revised 1995 policy statement provides a useful framework

> 66 *In general, current state regulation of nursing doesn't preclude nurses from practicing many alternative therapies, even though state practice acts don't specifically address these options.* 99

that's philosophically consistent with this emerging field of practice.

In general, current state regulation of nursing doesn't preclude nurses from practicing many alternative therapies, even though state practice acts don't specifically address these options. Alternative and complementary therapies provide opportunities for professional nurses to expand their practice, particularly with those therapies that reside within nursing's framework and research tradition, such as Therapeutic Touch, relaxation techniques, imagery, and the creation of healing environments.

Advanced nurse practice acts

The implementation of advanced practice nursing and advanced nurse practice acts is a relatively new phenomenon in the field of professional nursing. Some of this terminology emerged during the debate surrounding the Clinton health care reform proposals. Part of the rationale for this new terminology was to provide a means to recognize and reimburse professional nurses and specialized nurse practitioners, especially those with graduate degrees and advanced education.

Now, however, advanced practice registries are appearing within state nurse practice acts, along with definitions and scopes of practice for professional nursing in general. The Colorado Nurse Practice Act is representative of the activities in the field with respect to nurse practice acts, advanced practice movements, and the emerging developments in complementary and alternative therapies. (See *A sample of advanced practice nursing law.*) At one level, some of the therapies already fall within the scope of general professional nursing; at another level, some of these therapies may require evidence of either national accreditation or certification and graduate degrees in the field.

The emergence of certification in holistic nursing is indicative of the momentum gathering in this field. A core curriculum in holistic nursing already exists. Trends such as those seen in the holistic nursing field are expected to expand and encompass other alternative fields as well. The opportunities for professional clinical expansion into alternative and complementary arenas become greater every day.

The current and emerging nurse practice acts and advanced nurse practice initiatives are flexible enough to permit nurses to practice alternative therapies. Nevertheless, nurses need to remain attentive to the changing practice acts of both nursing and other health professional groups to assure that nursing's

---

A sample of advanced practice nursing law

The Colorado Nurse Practice Act of 1995 contains an example of advanced practice nursing regulation. It defines advanced practice and recognizes the need for registry. The act says:

"The general assembly hereby recognizes that some individuals practicing pursuant to this article have acquired additional preparation for advanced practice and hereby determines that it is appropriate for the state to maintain a registry of such individuals."

It goes on to define the advanced practice nurse as "a professional nurse who is licensed to practice...who obtains specialized education or training...and who applies to and is accepted by the board for inclusion in the advanced practice registry."

Because the category of advanced practice is new, the Colorado practice act points out that "on and after July 1, 1995, until July 1, 2008, the requirements for inclusion in the advanced practice registry shall include the successful completion of a nationally accredited education program for preparation as an advanced practice nurse or a passing score on a certification examination of a nationally recognized accrediting agency, or both." After July 1, 2008, however, the requirements for advanced practice nurse registry include the "successful completion of a graduate degree in the appropriate specialty."

right to practice is protected and appropriately expanded within nursing regulation.

According to Harvard professor Jessie Gruman, licensure, certification, clinical practice guidelines, and reimbursement are the formal gateways through which innovation in health care becomes standard. Each requires a level of evidence and organization that hasn't characterized alternative practices to date. At a time when all of medicine is being called to account for its effectiveness through rigorous scientific evaluation, advocates for alternative practices must expect that no less will be required of them.

Ethical considerations

The ethics of alternative practice reside within the individual practitioners and the systems in which they're practicing. Anyone who is truly committed to reforming health care and creating models of caring, healing, and health in contrast to expensive cure models has an ethical responsibility to consider both the advantages and disadvantages of alternative practices.

If nurses approach practice from an authentic commitment to attend to patients and accommodate their cultural practices and beliefs, then not taking alternative practices into account might be considered unethical.

In alternative therapy practices, as with conventional practices, the responsibility to be truthful, seek informed consent, and maintain open communication and partnership for the care plan is crucial. Many questions about health care choice, access, and quality are confronting policymakers and health care providers. With public demand for alternative therapies increasing at its current rate and scientific evidence about their effectiveness growing, ignoring complementary and alternative practices clearly becomes unwise if not unethical. If you can't make any of these therapies a part of your own practice,

66With public demand for alternative therapies increasing at its current rate and scientific evidence about their effectiveness growing, ignoring complementary and alternative practices clearly becomes unwise if not unethical. 99

you should at least consider becoming part of a referral network.

Reinventing the profession

The latest outcome of these changes in health care practice is the shift toward multiprofessional, interdisciplinary collaboration. All health care professionals should recognize the need for intentional, purposeful collaboration to create a seamless, integrated system for the public. Ideally, a new system will emerge that combines the best of conventional medicine with the best of alternative practices.

> 66 *The goal for the medical community is to identify and apply practices that promote healing and health, not just treatment and elimination of disease. That kind of philosophical shift requires intense interprofessional dialogue.* 99

The goal for the medical community is to identify and apply practices that promote healing and health, not just treatment and elimination of disease. That kind of philosophical shift requires intense interprofessional dialogue as well as dialogue between health care professionals and the public. Moving in this direction requires new working relationships beyond existing hospital models and the established systems of the moment.

Engaging the community

Some institutions engage the community at large in shaping the policy of the institution with respect to offering alternative therapies. Public demand for these services can therefore influence such future planning. Other policy shifts that allow alternative practices and practitioners within conventional systems emerge as a result of such community requests.

Finally, policy shifts are coming from practitioners themselves. Conventional physicians and nurses increasingly choose to obtain additional skills in selected alternative therapies that can easily be integrated into traditional practices.

Still other systems provide access through research initiatives. They approach access to complementary and alternative therapies in their facilities by setting up demonstration units that incorporate clinical interventions and research and evaluation of different therapies.

Shaping public opinion

Changing policies, politics, and practices are all under way in the United States and abroad. These changes will eventually result in mainstreaming of complementary and alternative therapies in all treatment programs and systems.

With the health care environment evolving and public and governmental changes under way, the climate is ideal for new treatment initiatives and policy directions for alternative medicine. Hospitals, insurance companies, HMOs, and other related systems should make these therapies more commonly available. The cost implications of ignoring them are too high. If self-care, health promotion, and preventive health care are part of a wider public agenda, then health care professionals must respond and adapt. With an opportunity and a professional responsibility to help shape public opinion and policy, nurses can and should continue to lead this movement.

Selected references

Berger-deRada S. "The Next Step for Nurses Performing Complementary Therapies," *Pelican News* 56(1):4, March 2000.

Braun, J.A., and Rabar, M.E. "Courtroom Tactics: Malpractice Issues in Complementary and Alternative Medicine: Going to Trial," *Medical Malpractice Law & Strategy* 17(12):6-9, October 2000.

Buckle, J. "Ask the Physician. Aromatherapy in Nursing." *Alternative Medicine* (27):36-40, January 1999.

Cohen, M.H. "Complementary Medicine: Legal Status of the Non-Licensed Provider in the USA," *Complementary Therapies in Nursing & Midwifery* 6(2):98-101, May 2000.

Filshie, J. "A Time for Change," *Acupuncture in Medicine* 18(2):87, December 2000.

Gilliland, I. "Case Report. Using Aromatherapy as a Therapeutic Nursing Intervention," *Journal of Hospice & Palliative Nursing* 1(4):157-8, October-December 1999.

Green, J.A. "Collaborative Physician-Patient Planning and Professional Liability: Opening the Legal Door to Unconventional Medicine." *Advances in Mind-Body Medicine* 15(2):83-110, Spring 1999.

Kaltsas, H. "Politics of Medicine: The Struggle for Freedom of Medical Choice. Help Get Acupuncture Covered under Medicare," *Alternative Medicine* (36):20-22, July 2000.

Kendall, M.L. "Integrative Medicine: Taking the Lead in Holistic Palliation," *Journal of Hospice & Palliative Nursing* 1(2):56-61, April-June 1999.

Kenny, C. "Quest for Healthy Alternatives...Complementary and Alternative Medicines," *Nursing Times* 96(49):10-11, December 2000.

Salladay, S.A. "Healing is Believing: Postmodernism Impacts Nursing," *Scientific Review of Alternative Medicine* 4(1):39-47, Spring-Summer 2000.

Simon, J.M. "The Explosion of Complementary and Alternative Therapies," *Nursing Diagnosis* 10(3):91, July-September 1999.

Thompson, E., "Washington Insurers Must Cover Alternative Care," *Modern Healthcare* 30(6):36, February 2000.

3

Holistic
nursing

More than 100 years ago, Florence Nightingale, the founder of modern nursing, recognized the healing power of nature. In her book, *Notes on Nursing*, she propounded the healing benefits of sound, color, light, fresh air, warmth, and cleanliness and wrote, "Nursing is putting the patient in the best condition for nature to act upon him."

Today, the holistic nursing movement is returning to Nightingale's point of view. After decades of seeing medicine and nursing

> 66 *Nursing is putting the patient in the best condition for nature to act upon him.* 99 — *Florence Nightingale, Notes on Nursing*

reduced to a series of technological procedures focused on treating malfunctioning body parts, more and more nurses are returning to their roots as nurturers, working in tandem with natural processes and the patients themselves to promote healing.

Concept of holism

The word *holism* derives from the Greek word *holos*, meaning "health," "entire," and "whole." Holism views health as a dynamic state that's much more than simply the absence of disease signs and symptoms. In holism, health is a constantly evolving process of well-being in which an individual's mind, body, emotions, and spirit are balanced in relation to each other and are in harmony with, and guided by, an awareness of self, society, nature, and the universe. No single aspect of an individual's interactions with others is seen as all-important or as more important than another. The World Health Organization (WHO) defines *health* holistically as "a state of complete physical, mental, and social well-being, not merely the absence of disease or infirmity."

Viewed holistically, feelings, attitudes, and emotions aren't isolated events but are translated into changes that simultaneously affect all parts of the body. Pain and illness aren't inherently negative but are a natural part of life and are valuable signals of an internal conflict that needs to be addressed. To be healthy is to be whole, and healing is the process of achieving health or wholeness.

Based upon this fundamental view of holism, all interventions delivered by all health care systems and their practitioners, regardless of their individual worldviews, are holistic in impact. All interventions affect some part of the human system and, therefore, affect the whole system.

The Newtonian/Cartesian worldview, which has informed allopathic medicine, perceives the mind and body as separate entities and perceives the individual to be distinct and separate from nature and the universe. In contrast, the holistic perspective views the world as a harmonious and indivisible whole. The individual isn't separate from nature or the cosmos, but rather is a microcosm. There's a belonging and wholeness to the universe, separation without separateness. This holistic model, which is gaining prominence in scientific thought as well as in the health field, implies that we're all interconnected with one another and with all things in the universe. What's more, humans are constantly changing and inherently moving toward wholeness. (See *Comparing allopathic and holistic outlooks*, page 64.)

> ❝ Holism requires an individual to accept responsibility for his own well-being — his own physical, mental, emotional, and spiritual health; his personal choices; and the health of his relationships. ❞

Comparing holistic and allopathic outlooks

Holistic health care providers see their approach to health and illness as radically different from that of conventional (allopathic) practitioners, as shown in the chart below.

Holistic model

▶ Emphasis is on achieving optimal body-mind health and finding the root causes of the disease.

▶ Disease or disability is seen as a process.

▶ Pain and disease may be valuable signals of internal conflict.

▶ Body and mind are viewed as interconnected; psychosomatic illness is the province of all health care providers.

▶ Mind is a primary or equal factor in all illness.

▶ Placebo effect is evidence of mind's role in disease and healing.

▶ When assessing a patient, health care provider relies primarily on qualitative information (such as his own intuition and patient's reports); quantitative data are an adjunct.

▶ Treatment considers the whole patient.

▶ Minimal interventions with appropriate technology are complemented by noninvasive techniques (such as diet and exercise).

▶ Patient is viewed as autonomous.

▶ Health care provider is viewed as a therapeutic partner.

▶ Health care provider's care is viewed as a component of healing.

Allopathic model

▶ Emphasis is on eliminating symptoms and disease.

▶ Disease or disability is seen as an entity.

▶ Pain and disease are viewed as wholly negative.

▶ Body and mind are seen as separate; psychosomatic illness, as a mental problem for referral to a psychiatrist.

▶ Mind is a secondary factor in organic illness.

▶ Placebo effect is evidence of power of suggestion.

▶ When assessing a patient, health care provider relies primarily on quantitative information (charts, tests, etc).

▶ Treatment is aimed at eliminating symptoms or disease.

▶ Primary interventions are drugs or surgery.

▶ Patient is viewed as dependent on health care providers.

▶ Health care provider is considered the authority.

▶ Health care provider should be emotionally neutral.

Adapted from Ferguson, M. *The Aquarian Conspiracy.* ©1982 by Marilyn Ferguson. Used by permission of Jeremy P. Tarcher, a division of Penguin Putnam Inc., New York.

Holism requires an individual to accept responsibility for his own well-being — his own physical, mental, emotional, and spiritual health; his personal choices; and the health of his relationships. Choice refers to maintaining a controlling influence over the flow of one's life while participating in the natural give and take of life. Maintaining this control involves responding to the needs of others while reaching for what's needed for oneself, all from a position of strength, confidence, and empowerment. Relationships that are in balance involve the giving and receiving of respect, care, and love.

Choosing to maintain control over one's life requires self-responsibility for the direction of that life, and self-responsibility is basic to achieving wellness. It's the cornerstone of the healing process and assumes self-awareness and awareness of others. Holism is a process that aims to achieve higher levels of awareness and self-realization.

Roots of holistic medicine

Although the holistic concept of health care has recently reemerged in the West, it has been present in other cultures for thousands of years. Early healers in both Eastern and primitive cultures treated their patients holistically — they viewed the body as interconnected with the spiritual and natural worlds. Shamans believed physical illness resulted from a spiritual or mental imbalance. Healers in Eastern cultures have for thousands of years focused on the concept of a vital energy, or life force, within each human being that must be kept in balance to maintain health and well-being.

These healers developed natural forms of healing based on this life force, many of which (acupuncture, meditation, herbal therapy, and others) are used today. The ancient Chinese and Indian civilizations developed sophisticated holistic health care practices based on healthy lifestyles to promote optimum health and prevent disease. Traditional Chinese medicine employs combinations of acupuncture, meditation, herbal therapy, massage, diet, and gentle exercise (tai chi chuan) to adjust or maintain the body's energy balance. In India, Ayurvedic medicine advocates a combination of natural living, herbal therapy, meditation, and yoga to achieve a balanced state of inner harmony, health, and natural well-being.

In the West, early allopathic physicians — such as Hippocrates (4th century B.C.), Galen (2nd century A.D.), and

Paracelsus (16th century A.D.) — treated their patients holistically. Hippocrates was the first to use the word *holos* to refer to the treatment of the total person. He advanced a theory about the close relationship of disease and the physical environment that was commonly accepted until the advent of the germ theory of disease in the late 19th century. The concept that diseases are caused by specific agents led to spectacular advances but at the cost of fragmenting human illness into a plethora of treatment specialties. Medicine became focused on the problem rather than the whole person.

The term *holism* was coined in 1926 by Jan Christian Smuts, a South African statesman, biologist, and philosopher. He proposed an alternative to the reductionist science of the time. Smuts believed there was a process, which he called *holism*, that enabled the human organism to maintain its balance in a fluctuating environment. He theorized that nature tends to bring things together to form whole organisms and that the determining factors in nature and evolution are whole organisms rather than their constituent parts.

Rise of health and wellness

The holistic philosophy of health and illness reemerged in Western medicine in the 1940s with Flanders Dunbar's work on psychosomatic medicine. Dunbar identified personality traits typical of patients suffering from a particular disease. This approach to medicine, which linked disease to the patient's state of mind and emotions, was further developed by Hans Selye in the 1950s.

Selye's theory of stress was based on what he termed the *general adaptation syndrome.* This syndrome involves activation of the hypothalamic-pituitary-adrenal axis in response to varying degrees of stress that simultaneously affect all body systems, evoking an alarm reaction (the fight-or-flight response). If stress comes to an end, the body should be able to use its coping mechanisms to return to a normal state, leading to recovery. However, if the stress doesn't stop, the body can no longer respond appropriately, and exhaustion sets in, followed by organ damage and disease.

In the 1960s, researchers Thomas Holmes and Richard Rahe established the relationship between lifestyle and the onset of illness by showing that the more changes — positive and negative — that a person experienced during a particular time, the more likely he was to become sick. This assessment tool is called the Social Readjustment Rating Scale. In 1961, Halbert Dunn published his watershed book, *High-Level Wellness.* Dunn defined *high-level wellness* as "an integrated method of functioning which is oriented toward maximizing the potential of which the individual is capable within the environment in which he is functioning." He stated that, although it was easier to fight *against* something like a disease, it was healthier and more positive to fight *for* something like optimal wellness. The wellness movement changed the focus of health care from recovery from disease to the support of wellness and the prevention of illness.

In 1974, the Canadian Ministry of Health and Welfare presented evidence that linked lifestyle and environment to health and illness. The report introduced a broader vision of health care that included the environment, lifestyle habits, and health care organizations. It also recommended moving the power for health care away from the medical profession to a broader variety of health care providers.

In 1976, the United States Select Senate Committee issued a report that confirmed the relationship between diet and disease. This report led to changes in Americans' food consumption patterns, such as reduced intake of red meat and fats and increased intake of whole grain products and fruits and vegetables. Changing public demand also led to increased production of lean meats.

During the 1970s, holistic health practitioners, whose numbers were increasing, began to emphasize that health was linked to a lifestyle that included proper nutrition, physical awareness, stress reduction, and self-responsibility. In the late 1970s and 1980s, holistic health associations were formed in an attempt to centralize advocates of holistic health. These associations provided useful educational and networking functions for health care advocates and consumers.

Building on the work of Smuts, D.C. Phillips, a sociobiologist and philosopher, identified the following principles of holism in 1976:

▶ The analytic approach, as typified by the physiochemical sciences, proves inadequate when applied to a biological organism, to society, or to reality as a whole.

▶ The whole is more than the sum of its parts.

▶ The whole determines the nature of its parts.

▶ The parts can't be understood in isolation from the whole.

▶ The parts are dynamically interrelated or interdependent.

At the Alma-Ata Conference in 1977, the WHO declared its international health care goals in its report, *Health For All By The Year 2000.* In addition to spelling out the WHO's landmark definition of *health,* the report called for equitable distribution of primary health care to provide for promotive, preventive, curative, and rehabilitative services.

The United States followed suit in 1979, when the Surgeon General released a report called *Healthy People* that focused on health promotion and disease prevention. In 1980, the Department of Health and Human Services outlined 226 measurable health objectives in another report, *Promoting Health/ Preventing Disease: Objectives for the Nation.* Both documents urged improving health and reducing mortality rates in the areas of maternal-neonatal health, nutrition, physical fitness, family planning, sexually transmitted diseases, and occupational safety and health.

> *Healers need to heal themselves in order to change an ailing and failing health care system.* — Charlotte McGuire, American Holistic Nurses' Association

Holism in nursing

In 1980, the American Holistic Nurses' Association (AHNA) was founded by Charlotte McGuire, a Texas nurse who was disillusioned with the state of the health care system, including the lack of respect nursing received and hospital administrators' focus on making profits rather than on providing quality patient care. McGuire observed that many nurses were feeling "burned out" on the job, and she realized that "healers need to heal themselves in order to change an ailing and failing health care system."

America began responding more ardently to health promotion in the early 1990s, primarily in response to the ever-increasing costs of a health care system based on treating disease. A decade after *Healthy People* was released, the Public Health Service joined with numerous health care organizations and professionals to issue *Healthy People 2000.* This document set three major health care goals to guide system reform in the 1990s: increasing the span of healthy life for all Americans, reducing disparate health levels among socioeconomic groups, and providing access to preventive services for all Americans.

During this same time, the Pew Health Professions Commission issued an analysis of future health care needs and of how America's health care system should prepare to serve those needs in its report, *Healthy America: Practitioners for 2005.*

In another report, *Agenda For Action,* issued in 1991, the Commission identified 9 characteristics needed to build a new health care system, together with 17 competencies that would be required of new practitioners entering the system.

In 1991, the American Nurses Association responded to the Pew report with its *Agenda for Health Care Reform.* The cornerstone of this proposal was enhancing delivery of health care services by giving nurses expanded roles as primary care nurses in the community. Although care for special populations and preventive services composed a significant part of this proposal, promotion of healthy lifestyles, self-responsibility for health, and responsible decision-making were strongly advocated.

In 1992, Congress established the Office of Alternative Medicine (OAM) within the National Institutes of Health to facilitate the fair, scientific evaluation of complementary and alternative therapies, including the holistic approach.

A logical fit

Holistic nursing has as its fundamental responsibilities promoting health, facilitating healing, and alleviating suffering. In working toward these goals, holistic nurses look at the whole person — body, mind, and spirit — rather than merely a specific symptom or illness. They view each person as a whole greater than the sum of his parts — a whole that's constantly interacting with and being acted upon by external and internal factors. They don't see disease as bad and health as good but rather both as natural, necessary components of lifelong growth and learning and movement toward self-awareness and wellness. The nurse is a therapeutic partner who works with the patient to facilitate the healing process.

Nursing is the logical discipline to promote holistic practices. The essence of nursing has always been nurturing, caring, and healing rather than curing. Curing is the process of eliminating the signs and symptoms of disease, whereas healing is the process of restoring balance to body, mind, and spirit.

Whether nursing is being delivered holistically isn't a function of the type of activity occurring or the outcome of the intervention. It's the process itself, the interaction and the principles that underlie that interaction. The nurse who functions holistically includes in care delivery the principles of therapeutic presence, centering, the movement of energy, and respect for and use of all resources. These are explained below.

Therapeutic presence
Acknowledgment of and respect for others is the foundation of holistic practice. Therapeutic presence means that the holistic nurse acts as a facilitator-participant in the healing process, respects the patient's identity and autonomy, supports his choices, and encourages him to express his fears, needs, and expectations. The characteristics of therapeutic presence are touching, silence, intimacy, caring, listening, and recognition.

A holistic nursing assessment tool can help in collecting data about a patient's nine human response patterns (communicating, valuing, relating, perceiving, knowing, feeling, moving, exchanging, and choosing). For an example of such a form, see *Using a holistic nursing assessment tool.*

Centering
The process of centering directs awareness inward, relaxing and balancing responses of the sympathetic nervous system. Attention shifts toward self-observation and away from involvement with the external environment. A nurse who's centered feels totally integrated and focused and operates more easily from heart-centered decisions, functioning lovingly, intuitively, creatively, and spontaneously. The process of operating from the heart is evidenced by the presence of caring and compassion.

Movement of energy
Holistic nursing regards the universe and everything in it as energy vibrating at different frequencies. Different frequencies create different patterns. Sensitivity to energy movement allows the nurse to be aware of the patient's body, mind, and spiritual patterns and to promote balance and harmony in the patient. This process can be measured by the patient's movement into a relaxed, peaceful state conducive to healing.

Using a holistic nursing assessment tool

Below you'll find the first page of a typical holistic nursing assessment tool. It's based on the nine human response patterns to ensure that all parts of the whole person are assessed. Note the addition of the term *transcending* to the *valuing* human response pattern. This was done to ensure that the spiritual dimension of life is adequately assessed.

Name: _Barbara Rogers_   Age: _40_   Sex: _F_
Address: _31 Montecristo Dr._   Telephone: _609-555-0056_
          Erial, N.J. 08064
Significant other: _Gary (husband)_   Telephone: _same as above_
Date of admission: _1/4/02_   Medical diagnosis: _Cholecystitis_
Allergies: _Iodine, silk tape, shellfish_   Dyes: _yes_

Communicating — A pattern involving sending messages

Possible nursing diagnoses:

Read, write, understand English (circle):
Circle all to indicate that the patient can
read, write, and speak English.
Other language: _Spanish_
Intubated: _No_
Speech impaired: _yes - lisp_
Alternate form of communication: _None_

Impaired verbal communication

"Valuing-Transcending" — A pattern involving spiritual growth

Religious preference: _Baptist_
Important religious practices: _Goes to church on Sunday_
Cultural orientation: _None_
Cultural practices: _None_
Meaning and purpose in life: _To be the best person she can be, to do no harm, to raise her children to be happy and healthy adults_
Inner strengths: _Faith in God, responsibility to those who depend on her_
Interconnections (self, others, universe, higher power): _God, family, a few good friends_

Spiritual distress (Distress of the human spirit)

Readiness for enhanced spiritual well-being

Use of all resources

Holistic nursing respects and uses all possible resources to aid the patient. The OAM has classified alternative therapies into seven major categories of interventions: mind-body interventions, bioelectromagnetic applications in medicine, alternative systems of medical practice, manual healing methods, pharmacologic and biological treatments, herbal medicine, and diet and nutrition in the prevention and treatment of chronic disease. Holistic nurses can use any of these interventions in their practice except for those health care systems or therapies (such as psychotherapy and hypnotherapy) that require a license to perform. However, a holistic nurse can legally use the techniques of these licensed systems or therapies (specific psychotherapeutic communication techniques or body manipulation techniques from massage therapy) as long as they aren't delivered as a complete course of psychotherapy or massage therapy. The alternative modalities commonly used by holistic nurses include mind-body interventions, manual healing methods, and diet and nutrition. Herbal therapy is also used, but only after changes in diet have been ineffective. Herbs are considered medicinal.

> *The holistic nurse has the advantage of being active and accepted in the allopathic and alternative therapy health care arenas and is uniquely prepared to counsel patients about a wide range of complementary and alternative therapies.*

The holistic nurse has the advantage of being active and accepted in the allopathic and alternative therapy health care arenas and is uniquely prepared to counsel patients about a wide range of complementary and alternative therapies, such as Therapeutic Touch and acupressure.

American Holistic Nurses' Association

The AHNA's mission is to educate nurses and the public in the concepts and practice of holistic health care. Its major objectives are:

▶ to encourage nurses to be models of wellness
▶ to improve the quality of health care by promoting education, participation, and self-responsibility for wellness; inter-

acting with other health-related organizations; and encouraging and reporting the research of holistic concepts and practice in nursing

▶ to function as an empowering network for those persons interested in holistic nursing

▶ to explore, anticipate, and influence new directions and dimensions of health care, especially within the practice of nursing.

Membership in the AHNA is open to all persons who support the mission of the organization.

The AHNA's underlying philosophy is that nursing is an art *and* a science. In 1994, the organization adopted a formal description of holistic nursing, which is as follows:

▶ Holistic nursing embraces all nursing practice that has healing the whole person as its goal. Holistic nursing recognizes that there are two views regarding holism: Holism involves studying and understanding the interrelationships of the bio-psycho-social-spiritual dimensions of the person, recognizing that the whole is greater than the sum of its parts, and holism involves understanding the individual as an integrated whole interacting with and being acted upon by internal and external environments. Holistic nursing accepts both views, believing that the goals of nursing can be achieved within either framework.

▶ Holistic practice draws on nursing knowledge, theories, expertise, and intuition to guide nurses in becoming therapeutic partners with patients in strengthening the patients' responses to facilitate the healing process and achieve wholeness.

▶ Practicing holistic nursing requires nurses to integrate self-assessment and self-care into their own lives. Self-responsibility leads the nurse to a greater awareness of the interconnectedness of all individuals and their relationships to the human and global community and permits nurses to use this awareness to facilitate healing.

In 1993, the leaders of the AHNA and the certificate programs of Holistic Nursing and Healing Touch participated in a Delphi study of basic principles and corresponding care goals of holistic nursing practice. A high level of consensus was reached regarding 17 basic holistic principles and 92 related care goals. These principles addressed the concepts of health, healing, unity, energy, and the holistic patient-practitioner relationship. (See *Basic principles of holistic nursing practice,* page 74.)

Basic principles of holistic nursing practice

The following basic principles of holistic nursing practice were discussed in a research forum by members of the American Holistic Nurses' Association in 1993:

▶ Human beings are energy fields.

▶ Unity and interdependence exist within the mind, body, and spirit.

▶ Health involves a sense of unity (connectedness or oneness) with the self and cosmos.

▶ Health is a process that may include disease.

▶ Health is the dynamic evolution (continuous process of emergence) toward balanced integration.

▶ Healing, when viewed holistically, is unpredictable in terms of time frame, cause, or outcome.

▶ Energy fields are constantly interacting.

▶ The Source is experienced or known through joy, beauty, love, light, peace, power, and life.

▶ Change in health can occur through *experiential learning*, which is defined as a change in behavior that occurs as a result of living through an activity, event, or situation.

▶ Spiritual health is necessary for physical, mental, and emotional well-being.

▶ The human spirit is the core of the person.

▶ Energy fields can become unbalanced as a response to stress in any one of the three domains of body, mind, and spirit.

▶ Healing involves a transformational change that encompasses the whole person; it requires the involvement of the spiritual, emotional, and intellectual domains as well as the physical body.

▶ Wellness encompasses increasing openness (acceptance of diversity) and increasing harmony (coherent, high-frequency energy fields).

▶ The patient-practitioner relationship is one of equal partnership with differing responsibilities.

▶ One's health and disease are manifested in one's lifestyle, habits, and conscious awareness as well as the body's physical being and energy.

▶ Each health system should be respected for the resources and tools it offers, while being challenged to prove its credibility.

Adapted with permission from Estby, S.N., et al. "A Delphi Study of the Basic Principles and Corresponding Care Goals of Holistic Nursing Practice," *Journal of Holistic Nursing* 12(1):402-13, March 1994.

Standards of holistic nursing practice

In 1994, the AHNA adopted the *Standards of Holistic Nursing Practice,* which established the scope of holistic practice. The standards are based on the philosophy that nursing is both "...an art and a science that has as its primary purpose the provision of services to help individuals achieve the wholeness within them." Any nurse can practice holistic nursing. These standards provide a means of measuring the quality of holistic care provided to patients. The standards were revised in 1997 and form the framework of the *Core Curriculum for Holistic Nursing.*

The standards of care and practice are organized around nine concepts: holistic philosophy, holistic foundation, holistic ethics, holistic nursing theories, holistic nursing and related research, holistic nursing process, meaning and wholeness, patient self-care, and health promotion. (See *AHNA Standards of Holistic Nursing Practice,* pages 76 to 79.)

Certification programs in holistic nursing

It's possible to become board certified in holistic nursing. The American Holistic Nurses' Certification Corporation is the arm of the AHNA responsible for administering the certification program. Certification promotes the professional advancement of holistic nursing, validates a nurse's knowledge of holistic nursing, and documents competence in the practice of holistic nursing.

To be eligible to take the examination involves three prerequisites: a baccalaureate degree, 1 year of practice implementing the principles of holistic nursing, and 48 hours of continuing education within the 2 previous years. A nurse who has met these conditions may take the examination, which is given once a year at sites across the country.

Certificate programs in holistic nursing are open to all nurses, including administrators, educators, students, and practicing nurses. The program prepares nurses for holistic nursing practice and helps unify holistic nursing care. The four programs that the AHNA endorses are: aromatherapy, Healing Touch, Amma therapy, and imagery. After successful completion of one of these programs, the nurse is awarded continuing education credit units, which may be used toward fulfilling the continuing education requirement for the certification exami-

(Text continues on page 79.)

AHNA Standards of Holistic Nursing Practice

The Standards of Holistic Nursing Practice, as adopted by the American Holistic Nurses' Association (AHNA), consist of two parts divided into nine concepts, with general standards of care proposed for each of the nine concepts. Specific standards of practice ensure that each standard of care can be accomplished. In this partial sampling, the parts, concepts, and standards of care are given.

Part I: Discipline of holistic nursing practice

Concept I: Holistic philosophy
▶ Holistic nurses shall be committed to the development of the art and science of holistic nursing practice.
▶ Holistic nurses shall actively participate in professional activities to promote competency in practice and to assure quality of care to patients.

Concept II: Holistic foundation
▶ Holistic nurses shall be committed to personal development of holism.

Concept III: Holistic ethics
▶ Holistic nurses shall adhere to a professional ethic of caring and healing that seeks to preserve the dignity and wholeness of the patient receiving care.
▶ Holistic nurses shall participate in establishing and promoting conditions in society in which holistic health can be achieved.
▶ Holistic nurses shall actively participate in professional activities to assist in responding to changes occurring in the practice environment.
▶ Holistic nurses shall participate in the ethics of caring and identify a linkage of caring to public policy.
▶ Holistic nurses shall participate in holistic ethics by a commitment to practices that respect, nurture, and enhance an integral relationship with the earth's functioning.
▶ Holistic nurses shall act politically to protect, foster, and advocate for the interspecies of life on the planet.
▶ Holistic nurses shall teach, share, and serve as resources in considering the holistic nature of the universe.

AHNA Standards of Holistic Nursing Practice *(continued)*

Concept IV: Holistic nursing theories
▶ Nursing theory shall provide the framework for documenting professional nursing practice.

Concept V: Holistic nursing and related research
▶ Patients and significant others shall receive advice on nursing interventions and holistic therapies based on research findings.
▶ Patients and significant others shall receive care by nurses who deliver nursing care grounded in a nursing theory/conceptual model.

Concept VI: Holistic nursing process
▶ Patients shall be assessed holistically and continually.
▶ The patient's actual and high-risk problems/patterns/needs or opportunities to enhance health and well-being, and their priorities, shall be identified based upon collected data.
▶ The patient's actual or high-risk problems/patterns/needs or opportunities to enhance health and well-being shall have appropriate outcomes specified and revised as appropriate.
▶ The patient's outcomes will reflect a concern of persons as a total system and a view of health that identifies both internal and external environments that maximize his potential for functioning within the environment.
▶ The patient shall have an appropriate plan of holistic nursing care formulated, focusing on health promotion or health maintenance activities.
▶ The patient and significant others shall be told the degree to which information is or isn't known regarding all nursing recommendations for care.
▶ The patient's holistic nursing care plan shall be implemented according to the priority of identified problems/patterns/needs or opportunities to enhance health and well-being.
▶ The patient's holistic nursing care plan shall be implemented within the context of assisting him to progress forward and upward toward a higher potential of functioning.
▶ The patient's response to holistic nursing care shall be continuously evaluated.

(continued)

AHNA Standards of Holistic Nursing Practice *(continued)*

Part II: Caring and healing of patients and significant others

Concept VII: Meaning and wholeness

▶ Patients and significant others experience the presence of the nurse as a shared humanness that includes a sense of connectedness and attention to them as unique persons.

▶ Patients and nurses experience a sense of valued interchange (authenticity).

▶ Patients and significant others shall receive care consistent with their cultural backgrounds, health beliefs, and values.

▶ Patients' and significant others' cultural diversity and its importance to the global community will be respected, protected, and enhanced.

▶ Patients and significant others shall receive care consistent with their values and beliefs.

▶ Patients shall be cared for as whole, spiritual beings.

▶ Patients and significant others shall receive support for their spiritual growth.

Concept VIII: Patient self-care

▶ Patients and significant others shall be facilitated and supported in managing self-care to maximize quality of life (such as treatments and adverse effects, activities of daily living, and changes in relationships and lifestyle).

▶ Patients and significant others shall have the information and resources needed for ongoing holistic health care.

▶ Patients shall receive care aimed at empowering them to accept responsibility for their own health and well-being.

▶ Patients and significant others shall receive care in a safe environment.

▶ Patients and significant others shall receive care in a respectful and healing environment.

▶ Patients and significant others shall be cared for in as healthy an environment as possible, with clean air and water, nutritious food, and with environmentally "friendly" life-sustaining practices.

AHNA Standards of Holistic Nursing Practice *(continued)*

Concept IX: Health promotion
▶ Patients and significant others possess the knowledge they want and need to be involved in decisions about health care, work, home life, and recreation.
▶ Patients and significant others receive health care based on priorities of care that contribute to desired outcomes.
▶ Patients and significant others are active partners in health care planning and decision making based on individual desires.
▶ Patients and significant others shall recognize patterns that place them at risk for health problems (such as personal habits, personal and family health history, or age-related risk factors).
▶ Patients and significant others shall practice preventive measures (such as immunizations, breast self-examination, fitness/exercise programs, or belief practices [prayer]).

nation. The skills learned through the program may be legally integrated in nursing practice in accordance with the nurse practice acts in the United States.

The Certificate Program in Holistic Nursing is open to all nurses, including administrators, educators, students, and practicing nurses. The program prepares nurses for holistic nursing practice and helps unify holistic nursing care. It consists of four phases, with three phases each lasting 3½ to 4½ days and the practicum phase lasting 8 to 12 months. This core curriculum covers a wide range of alternative and traditional therapies, including relaxation, imagery, music therapy, touch, nutrition, spirituality, and energetic healing. After successful completion of the program, the nurse is awarded a certificate and is qualified to take the certification examination.

Other AHNA services and activities
The AHNA also offers a Healing Touch certification. It publishes a monthly newsletter, *Beginnings,* as well as the quarterly *Journal of Holistic Nursing,* which contains peer-reviewed

scholarly articles. The organization also sponsors seminars and conferences on holistic healing as well as local and regional networking support groups and maintains an Internet Web site.

Selected references

"Complementary and Alternative Therapies," *Holistic Nursing Practice* 13(3):vii-viii, 1-78, April 2000.

Dossey, B.M., et al. *AHNA Standards of Holisic Nursing Practice: Guidelines for Caring and Healing.* Gaithersburg, Md.: Aspen Pubs., Inc., 2000.

Dossey, B.M. "Holistic Nursing: Taking your Practice to the Next Level," *Nursing Clinics of North America* 36(1):1-22, March 2001.

Dunbar, F. *Psychosomatic Diagnosis.* New York: Paul B. Hoeber, Inc., 1943.

Dunn, H. *High-Level Wellness: A Collection of Twenty-nine Short Talks on Different Aspects of the Theme "High-level wellness for man and society,"* Arlington, Va.: R.W. Beatty Co., 1961.

Freeman, L. *Best Practices in Complementary and Alternative Medicine: An Evidenced-based Approach with Nursing CE/CME.* Gaithersburg, Md.:Aspen Pubs., Inc., 2001.

Frisch, N., et al. *AHNA Standards of Holistic Nursing Practice: Guidelines for Caring and Healing.* Gaithersburg, Md.: Aspen Pubs., Inc., 2000.

Herdtner, S. "Using Therapeutic Touch in Nursing Practice" *Orthopedic Nursing* 19(5):77-82, September-October 2000.

Holmes, T.H., and Rahe, R. "The Social Readjustment Rating Scale," *Journal of Psychosomatic Research* 11(2):213-18, August 1967.

Mentgen, J.L. "Healing Touch," *Nursing Clinics of North America* 36(1):143-58, March 2001.

Slater, V.E., et al. "Journey to Holism," *Journal of Holistic Nursing* 17(4):365-83, December 1999.

Smuts, J.C. *Holism and Evolution.* New York: Macmillan Publishing Co., 1926.

Stone, J. "Using Complementary Therapies Within Nursing: Some Ethical and Legal Considerations," *Complementary Therapies in Nursing Midwifery* 5(2):46-50, April 1999.

U.S. Department of Health and Human Services. *Healthy People 2010: Understanding and Improving Health.* Washington, D.C.: U.S. Department of Health and Human Services; for sale by the Government Printing Office, November 2000.

PART THREE

Common alternative therapies

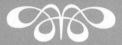

4

Alternative systems of medical practice

Many Americans and others raised in the West assume that Western allopathic medicine is the predominant system of health care in the world. In fact, only 10% to 30% of all health care worldwide is delivered by conventional biomedical practitioners, according to a 1994 report on alternative therapies prepared for the National Institutes of Health. The rest consists of everything from popular home remedies (such as drinking hot tea with honey for a sore throat) to the complex ancient healing traditions of China and India discussed in this chapter.

Western biomedicine is actually a relative newcomer in health care, even in the United States. Until the early 1900s, Americans had many health care options — herbal therapy, homeopathy, midwifery, naturopathy, and Chinese techniques, to name a few. At that time, about 1 in 5 doctors in the country was a homeopathic doctor. All of these options were gradually supplanted by the rise of the biomedical model. (See *Evolution of the biomedical approach*.)

❝All of these systems emphasize wellness — with the individual as an active participant in the healing process and in maintaining a harmonious balance of body, mind, and spirit. ❞

Evolution of the biomedical approach

Emergence of germ theory

The discovery that microscopic organisms could cause disease and that vaccines could help prevent them heralded the era of bio-medicine, the term used to describe the style of medicine prac-ticed by practitioners holding a medical doctor (MD) degree— clinical medicine based on the principles of the natural sciences.

As more and more infectious diseases were conquered, many clinicians came to believe that all disorders (even mental illness) could eventually be eliminated after the offending microbe or chemical imbalance was discovered. This germ theory of disease slowly came to dominate medical practice in the United States.

Crowding of competition

The formation of the American Medical Association (AMA) in 1847 helped lead to the decline of competing health care systems. By 1900, every state required medical practitioners to be licensed as a result of AMA lobbying. In 1910, a report titled *Medical Education in the United States and Canada* by Abraham Flexner, a U.S. educa-tor, established guidelines for the funding of medical education in the country. Flexner's report favored AMA-approved medical schools—those with a biomedical orientation. As a result, these schools received more financial funding, which eventually crippled competing schools of medicine.

Common threads

Most systems of medical care discussed in this chapter are based on a highly developed body of thought, which in turn is based on many years of experience using that system in its culture of origin. Traditional Chinese medicine and the Indian Ayurvedic system are approaches to health and illness that have endured for thousands of years. The other systems cov-ered in this chapter — homeopathy, naturopathy, osteopathy, and environmental medicine — evolved from the Western bio-medical model developed in Europe and North America over the past several hundred years.

Although each of these systems offers different explanations of disease and healing, most share a few central concepts. One is the belief in an invisible life force, or energy, at the core of each person. Disruptions in this life force are believed to cause illness, and treatments are aimed at restoring equilibrium. In addition, all of these systems focus on the need not only to halt disease but also to maintain wellness — with the individual as an active participant in the healing process and in maintaining a harmonious balance of body, mind, and spirit.

Traditional Chinese medicine

Traditional Chinese medicine is a sophisticated and complex system of health care that has been practiced for over 3,000 years and is rooted in Chinese culture; it long ago spread throughout Asia and today is used by about one-quarter of the world's population. Japan, Vietnam, and Korea have developed strong variations that also have influenced practitioners of Chinese medicine around the world.

Over the centuries, Chinese medicine has expanded to embrace many theories, methods, and approaches, an abundance that's often missed by Westerners, who assume that Chinese medicine is a monolithic structure similar to that of modern Western medicine. Some of Chinese medicine's theories are contradictory, yet none is rejected outright. Instead, all the additions and accretions have remained in the main body of knowledge, awaiting a time when they may be seen in a new light and be integrated into the living system of medicine in a new way.

In traditional Chinese medicine, diagnosis focuses on detecting the pattern of imbalances in a particular patient, rather than labeling the person's disease state.

This ancient system's approach to health and illness — from its basic understanding of human physiology to its methods of diagnosis and treatment — is very different from that of modern Western medicine. The focus of traditional Chinese medicine is prevention. According to ancient tradition, there are three levels of doctors: The lowest level cures a disease after it manifests; the middle level cures disease before it manifests; and the highest level prevents disease by curing society of its ills. The ideal doctor is thus one who teaches patients to maximize good health by living correctly.

Traditional Chinese theory holds that good health depends, to a large extent, on the patient's lifestyle, thoughts, and emotions. This means that the patient bears much responsibility for his own well-being. The doctor can serve as a guide and role model on the patient's journey to good health and long life by recommending measures to modify behavior and by offering help, when needed, in the form of herbs, needles, and massage.

Basic principles

The fundamental concepts underlying traditional Chinese medicine evolved from the metaphysical worldviews of Taoism, Confucianism, and Buddhism. They are based on 3,000 years of observation and philosophy rather than on the scientific method underlying Western medicine. Whereas Western philosophy and medicine view the body, mind, and spirit as separate entities, Eastern philosophy and medicine see them as interrelated elements that are intertwined with nature and the cosmos as a whole.

The cornerstone of Chinese theory is the concept of *qi* (pronounced *chee*). This concept, foreign to Western thought, is best described as a vital life force, or energy, that flows through the body along channels known as meridians. According to Chinese belief, *qi* is necessary to maintain life. A balance of *qi* — neither too much nor too little — is necessary to maintain health, and an imbalance or blockage of *qi* can cause disease.

Another fundamental concept in Chinese medicine is *yin-yang*, the interaction of opposing forces (such as male-female, hot-cold, light-dark). (See *Central concepts of Chinese medicine,* page 86.) All of these elements must be in balance for a person to maintain good health.

Diagnostic approach

In traditional Chinese medicine, diagnosis focuses on detecting the pattern of imbalances in a particular patient, rather than labeling the person's disease state. This approach is fundamentally different from that of Western medicine. Whereas a Western physician typically will make the same diagnosis for two patients with the same symptoms, a doctor of Chinese

Central concepts of Chinese medicine

The two most basic concepts of traditional Chinese medicine, underlying much of its theory and practice, are *qi* and *yin-yang*.

Qi

Because the concept of *qi* (pronounced *chee*) is foreign to Western medicine, its nuances are difficult to explain. Commonly translated as a form of vital energy found in the body, *qi* encompasses much more than is connoted by the English word *energy*. There are many kinds of *qi* in the body, some of which are more substantial than what we think of as energy. For example, blood is thought to be a condensed form of *qi*. It may be more useful to define *qi* by its functions in the body: activation, warming, transformation, defense, and containment.

Qi is derived from three sources: one's parents at the moment of conception ("original *qi*"), the foods one eats ("nutritional *qi*"), and the air one breathes ("air *qi*"). *Qi* flows through the body along 12 invisible, interconnected channels called meridians, which run through the entire body.

A healthy person has the right amount of *qi* flowing smoothly through his body. Illness can occur when there's an excess or deficiency of *qi* or when this vital force becomes obstructed in the meridians.

Yin-yang

According to Taoist philosophy, the principle of *yin-yang* is the basis of the entire universe. *Yin* and *yang* are the opposing yet complementary aspects of all of creation, such as cold and hot, female and male, and active and passive, to name a few. All objects, actions, and phenomena may be categorized according to these two concepts. For example, cold is *yin* and hot is *yang;* female is *yin* and male is *yang*. However, *yin* and *yang* are constantly interacting and changing in proportion to each other, and something is only *yin* or *yang* in comparison to something else. Also, there's a bit of *yin* in every *yang,* and vice versa.

The body, too, is a complex interconnected system of *yin* and *yang*. For example, solid organs are classified as *yin;* hollow organs as *yang*. Chronic diseases are *yin,* and acute diseases are *yang*. These two elements ebb and flow throughout the body and organs, affecting each other through constant motion.

Good health requires a balance of *yin* and *yang* throughout the body. Imbalances of either are thought to produce too much or too little activity in particular organs, thus resulting in illness.

medicine might arrive at two very different diagnoses (and treatment plans) based on different types of imbalances in the two patients.

To make a diagnosis, the doctor of Chinese medicine uses his own senses to gather data. By looking, questioning, listening, checking body sounds and odors, and palpating, the doctor can gather the essential information needed for a diagnosis. Laboratory tests may be useful but only to provide corroborating data. (See *Diagnostic principles in Chinese medicine*, page 88.)

Diagnostic frameworks

The doctor may use a variety of diagnostic frameworks to identify a pattern of imbalance, depending on the particular patient. In addition to assessing the patient's *qi* through the techniques mentioned above, he evaluates body functions using the following methods:

▶ Eight Principles (or Eight Parameters): These principles are hot versus cold, interior versus exterior, excessive versus deficient, and *yin* versus *yang*. Based on the patient's symptoms and the results of the physical examination, the physician detects a pattern of illness that he describes in terms of these eight parameters. For example, whereas a Western physician might diagnose pneumonia (the name of a condition), the Chinese doctor might diagnose "excessive heat in the lung and insufficient *qi.*"

▶ Pathogenic factors: These factors include the Six Evils (or Six Excesses) — wind, cold, heat, dampness, dryness, and fire (which can either invade the body from outside or be generated internally) — and the Seven Moods — joy, anger, anxiety, obsession, sorrow, horror, and fear. Disease is seen as resulting from the struggle between *qi* and these pathogenic factors. If the body has sufficient *qi,* it can resist even the most dangerous pathogenic factors; if not, even a minor pathogenic factor can lead to disease.

▶ Lifestyle factors: The idea that health is influenced by behavior and thought is fundamental to Chinese medicine. According to this philosophy, leading a balanced lifestyle can improve one's ability to prevent (or combat) illness. On the other hand, intemperate practices — such as poor diet, excessive alcohol intake, insufficient sleep, and too much or too little sexual activity — can cause alterations in the physical body or dis-

Diagnostic principles in Chinese medicine

Practitioners of traditional Chinese medicine use the following methods to develop a diagnosis, paying utmost attention to the tongue and pulse.

Looking
The doctor evaluates the patient's general appearance, demeanor, body language, posture, and gait, and then inspects the tongue, eyes, hair, and complexion.

Traditional Chinese medicine places great importance on the tongue in assessing health status because of its close relation to internal organs through the meridian system. Illness can cause the tongue to become yellow, red, swollen, cracked, or coated with mucus — changes that indicate specific body imbalances to an experienced doctor. Chinese doctors use tongue diagnosis to direct therapy and to track the patient's changing condition.

Asking
The doctor questions the patient about current symptoms, medical history, lifestyle, diet, and any previous or current therapies. He also assesses personal and environmental factors that can affect health and healing — including mood, activity, drugs, weather, and the seasons — and asks about changes in appetite, perspiration, and sensitivity to hot and cold.

Listening and smelling
The doctor evaluates the patient's breath sounds and bowel sounds and the smell of his breath, body odor, and any body excretions.

Touching
The doctor palpates the patient's pulses, abdomen, skin, and troublesome areas for temperature, moisture, pain, and swelling.

Skilled practitioners of traditional Chinese medicine can obtain a wealth of information from the pulse, but this is a very subjective form of diagnosis that requires much practice to learn. Chinese doctors palpate six pulses (three superficial and three deep) in each wrist at specific points along the radial artery. In addition to measuring frequency, they also check for rhythm, strength, and other characteristics.

Each pulse corresponds to an internal organ. By palpating these 12 pulses, practitioners can detect imbalances of *qi* in specific organs and thus diagnose medical problems.

ruptions in the *qi,* blood, body fluids, or organ systems, resulting in disease.

▶ Six Stages: This pattern, which consists of the three *yin* and three *yang,* attempts to identify the location of disease within the meridians, the 12 channels of the body along which *qi* is said to flow. Each of the 12 major organs is associated with a channel bearing the organ name. Any abnormality that appears along the pathway may indicate an imbalance in that channel.

▶ Four Levels of Disease: These levels are *qi,* defense, construction, and blood. They're used to indicate the depth at which a pathogenic factor is affecting the body and applied to infectious febrile disease (also called an attack of external wind-heat).

▶ Three Burners: This diagnostic pattern — referring to the division of the abdomen into upper, middle, and lower burners — is commonly used as a metaphor for the processes of metabolism.

▶ Five Phases theory: This diagnostic system is based on the premise that each organ either enhances or inhibits the function of another organ, just as the five elements — fire, earth, metal, water, and wood — affect each other adversely or beneficially. (See *Five Phases theory,* pages 90 and 91.)

The art and skill of the traditional Chinese doctor lie in knowing which combination of signs and symptoms should be interpreted within which of these diagnostic frameworks. In making the diagnosis, the doctor considers the presenting complaint within the context of the patient's emotional state, medical history, family and home environment, and social environment as well as other factors that may help to provide a fuller understanding of the patient.

Therapies

When a diagnosis is made, the doctor prescribes the appropriate therapy to restore the balance of elements in the patient. Therapies include herbal remedies, acupuncture, acupressure, diet, moxibustion, massage, cupping, and *qigong* (pronounced *chee-goong*).

Herbal remedies

Developed over the centuries, herbal remedies are the backbone of traditional Chinese therapy, far outweighing acupuncture and massage. The herbal formulary consists of more than 3,000 herbs as well as animal and mineral substances (such as deer antlers and oyster shells). A typical herbal preparation contains a dozen or so herbs, roots, powders, or animal substances and may be prepared for administration in a number of ways. A traditional Chinese herbalist must be able to recall thousands of combinations and know the best way to administer them.

The most common administration form is *decoction*—herbs boiled in water and then drunk as an herbal tea in several doses throughout the day. Herbs may also be prepared as powders, pills, syrups, liniments, suppositories, and enemas. Al-

Five Phases theory

According to the Five Phases theory of Chinese medicine, every aspect of nature and man, including sickness and health, can be analyzed in terms of five elements: fire, earth, metal, water, and wood. In the human body, every organ and system is associated with one of these elements—for example, the heart with fire and the lungs with metal. Just as the five elements affect each other in nature, so their corresponding organs are believed to influence each other in predetermined ways. For example, as fire melts metal, so the heart (fire) controls the lungs (metal); as metal cuts wood, so the lungs control the liver (wood).

	Fire	**Earth**
Yin organ	Heart	Spleen
Yang organ	Small intestine	Stomach
Season	Summer	Late summer
Climate	Heat	Dampness
Taste	Bitter	Sweet
Sensory organs	Tongue	Mouth
Tissues	Vessels	Muscles
Emotions	Joy	Pensiveness, anxiety

though many of the formulas are prescribed for specific diagnostic patterns, the dosages—percentages of particular herbs in the formula—are adjusted for each patient. What is appropriate for one person may be toxic for another, even though both may have the same illness by Western diagnostic criteria.

Acupuncture

Acupuncture involves the insertion of thin metal needles at specific points on the body that relate to the *qi* meridians. This therapy, commonly used to relieve pain, is discussed in more detail in chapter 7, Manual healing therapies.

Acupressure

Instead of using needles, acupressure involves the stimulation of acupuncture points by applying direct pressure on them with

Everything that's classified as *yin* or *yang* also corresponds to one of the five elements, which are themselves subdivisions of *yin* and *yang*. In addition, every element also corresponds to a specific season, color, taste, and other characteristics, as shown in the chart below. For example, the spleen and stomach are associated with the element earth and with the taste of sweetness. Thus, an excess of something sweet can harm the spleen and stomach. Conversely, something sweet could also be used to strengthen these organs.

Metal	Water	Wood
Lungs	Kidneys	Liver
Large intestine	Bladder	Gallbladder
Autumn	Winter	Spring
Dryness	Cold	Wind
Pungent	Salty	Sour
Nose	Ears	Eyes
Skin	Bones	Sinews
Sadness	Fear	Anger

the hands or fingertips. This therapy is also typically used for pain relief and during labor and delivery. (For more information, see *Relieving a headache with acupressure* in chapter 7, page 238.)

Diet

Traditional Chinese practitioners view food as a type of medicine. According to this outlook, everything one eats is primarily *yin* or *yang* by nature and consequently has an effect on various imbalances in the body. Depending on the specific patient, certain foods should be avoided, whereas others can have a therapeutic effect.

In addition, foods are organized into groups based on their energetic qualities, such as heating, cooling, and moistening. Special importance is also given to "eating in harmony with seasonal shifts and life activities."

Moxibustion

Moxibustion involves the burning of a mound of the plant moxa (*Artemisia vulgaris*) on specific points of the body near *qi* meridians. The moxa may be burned directly on the skin or on acupuncture needles, which are then implanted in the skin. The heat produced by this procedure is believed to penetrate deep into the body, stimulating or inhibiting certain target points, and thereby restoring the balance of *qi*.

Massage

Like acupuncture and moxibustion, massage and manipulation are practiced on specific parts of the body associated with meridians, to restore the balance of *qi* in areas where it's lacking, excessive, or blocked. Massage is often used in combination with other therapies, such as acupuncture. *Tui na* — a combination of massage, manipulation, and acupressure — has been practiced in China for nearly 2,000 years.

Cupping

In the cupping technique, suction is created by warming the air inside a glass jar and placing the overturned jar over the part of the body requiring treatment. The vacuum created by the heat is believed to dispel dampness, warm the *qi*, and reduce swelling. Cupping is commonly used to relieve bronchial congestion and to treat chronic conditions, such as arthritis and bronchitis.

Qigong
There are hundreds of forms of *qigong,* a therapy consisting of exercise, breathing techniques, and meditation that's also aimed at balancing *qi. Qigong* is discussed in more detail in chapter 7, page 232.

Therapeutic uses
Because traditional Chinese medicine looks at illness in an entirely different way than Western medicine, it's difficult to discuss therapeutic uses in the usual Western biomedical framework. Treatment and dosage are determined not by a specific disease but by the patient's overall pattern of signs and symptoms.

For example, in the West, a patient with an acute infectious disease is treated with a standard course of antibiotics, and two people with the same condition typically receive the same type of treatment. In Chinese medicine, the treatment varies, depending on such factors as the state of the patient's *qi* and the balance of *yin* and *yang.* For example, a patient with a severe infectious disease whose *qi* is strong is able to receive a stronger treatment than a patient with a milder case whose *qi* is impaired. That's because the person with impaired *qi* needs a gentler treatment to nourish and support his weakened physiologic and *qi* status.

RESEARCH SUMMARY At least one therapy—acupuncture for pain relief—has undergone considerable scientific testing, with positive results. However, the fundamentally different methods of diagnosis and treatment have made it difficult to prove the efficacy of Chinese medicine in treating specific diseases or conditions. Most of the studies done in China involve empirical methods—observing the results of various treatments—rather than the double-blind, placebo-controlled studies used in Western research. Traditional Chinese medicine isn't conducive to Western-style research because of the great variations in treatment for similar symptoms. Yet, despite this lack of scientifically proven evidence, Chinese medicine is used to treat the full range of human illnesses—from asthma, allergies, and headaches to cancer and infertility. ■

Nursing perspective

If your patient is receiving a traditional Chinese therapy, you can help prevent problems by taking these steps:

▶ Obtain an accurate health history, including allergies. A patient with an allergy to specific herbs obviously shouldn't take herbal remedies that contain the offending herbs.

▶ Obtain a medication history to ensure that the herbal remedy doesn't interact with previously prescribed medications or herbs.

▶ Warn the patient about the risks involved in sharing his individually prescribed remedies with others.

▶ Advise the patient that a combination of Western and Chinese medicine may be the best course when treating life-threatening illnesses, such as the use of *qigong* or tai chi, with western medicine.

▶ Instruct the patient to discontinue the therapy and notify his physician if signs or symptoms worsen.

▶ If the patient is a recovering alcoholic, tell him to make sure that herbal tinctures are mixed with water, not alcohol.

Ayurvedic medicine

India's ancient healing system, *Ayurveda* (meaning "knowledge of life" in Sanskrit), is an integrated approach to the prevention and treatment of illness that combines philosophical, spiritual, and scientific principles dating back thousands of years. Derived from the Vedas — the ancient body of literature, prayers, and teachings that forms the foundation of Hinduism and Indian culture — Ayurveda is a philosophy of living that encompasses the whole of human life, including the individual's place in the cosmos. According to the Vedic view, the living physical body is made of dual qualities — the *bhutas*, which constitute the matter and the senses of the body, and the *prana*, the life energy that's vital and holds together the physical form as an organic whole. The books of Dr. Deepak Chopra have helped to popularize Ayurvedic beliefs in the West in recent years.

In its basic concepts, Ayurvedic medicine is similar to traditional Chinese medicine. Both systems stress the interconnectedness of body, mind, and spirit and of the individual and the environment, and both espouse the need for balance and harmony among these elements. Both maintain that the cosmos is made up of five basic elements — in Ayurvedic belief, earth, air, fire, water, and space. Both also place great emphasis on the prevention of disease and on the individual's responsibility for achieving that goal primarily through proper diet, exercise, sleeping patterns, and other lifestyle interventions.

> 66 *Determining an individual's body type, or* dosha, *is the* cornerstone of Ayurvedic medicine. 99

Basic principles

Determining a person's metabolic body type, or *dosha,* is the cornerstone of Ayurvedic medicine. The three *doshas* — known as *vata, pitta,* and *kapha* — loosely correspond to the Western categories of body physique (thin, muscular, and fat), but they're believed to have more far-reaching effects on a person's health, personality, and susceptibility to illness. Each *dosha* is associated with specific body organs and with two of the five environmental elements.

Most people are a combination of *doshas,* but one type usually predominates. The predominant *dosha* is believed to determine not only the person's metabolic body type but also his personality traits and the types of illness he's likely to develop. It also serves as a guideline for the types of food he should eat, the types of exercise he should practice and, in general, how he should conduct his life.

For instance, *vata's* natural element is air, which is constantly moving, so *vata* characteristics pertain to motion, movement, lightness, and changeability. *Pitta's* element is fire, so its qualities are associated with heat, such as anger, redness, and inflammation. *Kapha's* element is earth, so its characteristics signify solidity, slowness, and strength. (See *Characteristics of the three* doshas, page 96.)

According to Ayurvedic beliefs, good health requires a balance between the three *doshas* within each individual; between body, mind, and spirit; and between the individual and the environment. Disease results from an imbalance of the *doshas,* which can be influenced by an unhealthy lifestyle, internal and external stressors, emotions, seasonal influences,

Characteristics of the three *doshas*

The three *doshas* of Ayurvedic medicine are believed to control all body functions. Each *dosha* is associated with specific body organs, personality traits, physiologic functions, and natural elements, as shown in the chart below.

	Vata	Pitta	Kapha
Body type	Slender	Medium build, well-proportioned	Heavy build
Physical characteristics	Cool, dry skin; prominent features	Fair or red hair, ruddy complexion, freckles, tendency to perspire heavily	Oily skin, thick hair, slow moving
Personality traits	Hyperactive, unpredictable, nervous, moody, energetic, intuitive, imaginative, impulsive; eats and sleeps erratically	Predictable, moderate in daily habits, intelligent, articulate, warm and loving, explosive temper; eats and sleeps regularly	Relaxed, slow to anger, slow to eat, slow to act, tolerant, affectionate, obstinate; procrastinates; sleeps long and deeply
Metabolic tendencies	Prone to nervous disorders, energy and weight fluctuations, anxiety, insomnia, constipation, and premenstrual syndrome	Prone to heartburn, ulcers, and other GI complaints; acne; and hemorrhoids	Prone to obesity, high cholesterol, allergies, and sinus problems
Associated internal organs	Large intestine, pelvic cavity, bones, ears	Stomach, small intestine, blood, skin, sweat glands, eyes	Lungs, chest, spinal cord, and spinal fluid
Associated natural elements	Air and ether (space)	Fire and water	Water and earth
Physiologic function	Breathing, blood circulation, movement	Digestion, metabolism	Nourishment and protection of the body

genetic predisposition, and an accumulation of toxic substances in the body.

When people are aware of their *dosha* type and its characteristics, they can make appropriate lifestyle changes designed to restore the balance of *doshas* and thus maintain well-being.

Indian thought also includes the concept of *chakras*, which are physically unobservable. They're described as vortices of energy. There are seven major chakras — the first, beginning at the base of the spine, known as the "root" chakra, continuing upward to the seventh, known as the "crown" chakra, at the top of the head. Through concentration, meditation, and yoga, one activates the chakras, bringing them into balance. Each chakra is connected to physiologic functioning as well as emotional and spiritual dimensions.

Diagnostic approach

Diagnosis involves determining the patient's predominant *dosha*, obtaining a detailed history (including interpersonal and family relationships and job situation), performing a physical examination, determining the illness and its causes, and establishing a prognosis. (Because the Ayurvedic doctor typically doesn't treat incurable disease, it's important to know the patient's chances of recovery.)

The Ayurvedic doctor uses observation, questioning, palpation, and auscultation (of the heart, lungs, and intestines), paying special attention to the pulse, tongue, eyes, nails, and urine. As in traditional Chinese medicine, pulse measurement is much more detailed and significant than in Western medicine. Like their Chinese counterparts, Ayurvedic doctors can distinguish 12 distinct radial pulses, which help them assess the functioning of specific body organs and the interaction of the three *doshas*. Observing the tongue surface provides insight into organ function and *dosha* imbalances. Examining the urine for unusual colors or odors can also help the doctor detect any *dosha* imbalances.

Therapies

Once the Ayurvedic doctor has determined the patient's particular *dosha* imbalance, he'll recommend an individualized treatment plan aimed at restoring equilibrium. The regimen typically includes some combination of dietary and lifestyle changes, purification therapy, and mental exercises.

Diet and lifestyle

Lifestyle interventions are prescribed according to the person's constitutional type. They may include changes in diet and eating patterns, sleeping and waking times, and sexual activity. Specific foods (and condiments) are selected not because of their nutritional value but because of their taste (sweet, sour, salty), hot- or cold-producing tendency, and other factors believed to affect *dosha*-balance. (See *Ayurvedic approach to coronary artery disease.*) The doctor may also recommend chanting or sitting in the sun for a specified period.

Purification

Purification of the body, known as *panchakarma*, is a complex series of steps undertaken to rid the body of physical impurities, or "toxins." The process, which usually takes about a week, includes herbal oil massage to loosen the excess *doshas*, steam treatments to open up the pores, therapeutic vomiting to cleanse the stomach, bowel purging and enemas to flush out the GI tract, and nasal inhalation of herbal potions to drain excess mucus. The Vedic texts recommend undergoing purification three times per year, ideally at the beginning of spring, fall, and winter.

Mental exercises

Meditation, yoga, and breathing exercises are believed to do for the mind what *panchakarma* does for the body: rid the mind of negative thoughts and emotions, such as fear, anger, greed, and doubt, and generally help the mind achieve a higher level of functioning. As with the other measures, they're recommended not only to treat various disorders but also to maintain good health and prevent disease.

Therapeutic uses

RESEARCH SUMMARY   Although many people practice meditation and yoga simply to achieve a sense of serenity and relaxation, extensive research in India and the West has discovered clear physiologic benefits from these two practices. Harvard Medical School Professor Herbert Benson's studies of people who practiced transcendental meditation in the 1970s showed that meditation decreases oxygen consumption and metabolism; lowers blood pressure, heart rate, and respirato-

PERSONAL ACCOUNT

Ayurvedic approach to coronary artery disease

Dr. Virender Sodhi, director of the American School of Ayurvedic Sciences in Bellevue, Washington, reported treating a 55-year-old Asian man who had refused emergency bypass surgery. The patient had such severe angina that he could walk no more than 10 steps without sitting down. A battery of laboratory tests showed severe coronary artery blockages: left main coronary artery, 90% blocked; anterior descending artery, 80% blocked; and right coronary artery, 30% blocked. In addition, blood tests revealed a cholesterol level of 278 with a decreased high-density lipoprotein (HDL) level of 38.

Dr. Sodhi determined that the patient was a *pitta-kapha* individual and started him on an appropriate cleansing program that included a change of diet and appropriate herbs. After 3 months of therapy, the patient's cholesterol level had decreased by more than 30%, and his HDL level had risen to 48. He was able to walk on a treadmill at a speed of 5 miles (8 km) per hour for 45 minutes without experiencing angina. Two years later, the patient was still doing fine; he was able to jog up and down hills without symptoms and his electrocardiograms showed improvement.

According to Dr. Sodhi, a hospital in Bombay has treated more than 3,000 cases of coronary artery disease using Ayurvedic methods and has achieved a success rate of 99%.

Adapted with permission from Burton Goldberg Group. *Alternative Medicine: The Definitive Guide.* Fife, Wash.: Future Medicine Publishing, Inc., 1994.

ry rate; increases the production of alpha brain waves (associated with feelings of well-being); relieves stress; and enhances overall well-being. In fact, research on meditation practice led to the development in the West of biofeedback and relaxation training. (For more information, see "Meditation" in chapter 5, page 157.)

In India, yoga has been practiced for thousands of years as part of an integrated approach to good health. In the West, it has recently been incorporated into a number of programs aimed at treating chronic diseases. An example is Dr. Dean Ornish's successful program to reverse coronary artery disease by combining yoga with dietary changes, moderate exercise, and support groups. Numerous research studies on yoga have shown that regular practice can help patients learn to control blood pressure, heart rate, respiratory function, metabolic rate, body temperature, and brain waves as well as improve circulation, flexibility, and stamina. (For more information, see "Yoga" in chapter 5, page 189.)

A 1989 Dutch study of patients using a combination of Ayurvedic therapies for certain chronic conditions (asthma, hypertension, arthritis, constipation, headaches, eczema, bronchitis, and type 2 diabetes mellitus) documented improvements in 79% of patients.

Laboratory studies of certain Ayurvedic herbal preparations have demonstrated potentially beneficial effects for certain cancers, including colon, breast, and lung cancer. The National Cancer Institute has included Ayurvedic compounds on its list of potential chemopreventive agents. The 1994 report to the National Institutes of Health entitled *Alternative Medicine: Expanding Medical Horizons* concluded: "Because of the potential of Ayurvedic therapies for treating conditions for which modern medicine has few, if any, effective treatments, this area is a fertile one for research opportunities." ■

Nursing perspective

If your patient is receiving Ayurvedic therapies, take the following steps to prevent complications:

◗ Help the patient understand that he'll need to cooperate in making recommended changes in his diet and lifestyle.

◗ Obtain the patient's medication history to ensure that herbal compounds don't interact with other prescribed herbs or drugs.

◗ Tell the patient not to share Ayurvedic compounds with others.

◗ Make sure that colonic equipment is sterilized or disposable to avoid the spread of communicable disease.

◗ Rectal insertion of hydrotherapy equipment requires caution; vagal stimulation with hypotension and bradycardia may occur.

Homeopathic medicine

The word *homeopathy* stems from the Greek words *homoios,* meaning similar, and *pathos,* meaning suffering. Homeopathic medicine, a medical system that predates the Western biomedical approach, is based on the principle that "like cures like" — that is, a small amount of the substance that *causes* a person's symptoms can actually *relieve* them.

Basic principles

Samuel Hahnemann, the German physician who founded homeopathy in the late 18th century, set out to discover a more humane approach to medical treatment than the primitive methods that were popular in his day, such as blood letting and purging. He suspected that disease resulted from an imbalance in the body's "vital force" (a concept modern homeopaths believe refers to the immune system) and that with only a small stimulus the balance could be restored, enabling the body to heal itself.

Hahnemann developed his theory while trying to understand how cinchona bark (whose active ingredient is quinine) worked as a cure for malaria. When he tested cinchona on himself, he experienced chills, fever, and weakness, the classic symptoms of malaria. When he stopped taking it, the symptoms disappeared. From this experience, he reasoned that if a substance could cause certain symptoms in a healthy person, a small amount of the same substance given to an ill person with those same symptoms might stimulate the body to fight the disease. Similar theories had been proposed by Hippocrates in the 4th century B.C. and by the Swiss alchemist Paracelsus in the 16th century.

Hahnemann studied hundreds of other substances in the same way, first getting volunteers to ingest them and then noting the symptoms — physical, mental, and emotional — that each produced. He began treating sick people with small amounts of the particular medicine whose effects most closely resembled their symptoms. Based on the results of these studies, Hahnemann formulated the principles of homeopathy:

▶ Like cures like (the Law of Similars).
▶ The more diluted a remedy is, the greater its potency (the Law of the Infinitesimal Dose).
▶ Illness is specific to the individual (the model for holistic medicine).

These hundreds of studies eventually evolved into a compilation of symptoms and corresponding homeopathic remedies that has been used ever since.

Today, homeopathy is practiced around the world by an estimated 500 million people and is endorsed by the World Health Organization. Homeopathic medicine is especially popular in Europe, its birthplace. In France, pharmacies are required to stock homeopathic remedies, which are used by more than one-third of the population; in Britain, homeopathic clinics are a part of the national health system. Homeopathy is also widely practiced in India and Russia.

In the United States, the rise of Western allopathic medicine with its antagonistic approach to disease led to the decline of homeopathy, which had been practiced by about 1 in 5 doctors until the early 1900s. However, homeopathy has seen a resurgence of interest in the past 20 years. Today, more than 3,000 health care professionals — including MDs, osteopathic doctors, dentists, veterinarians, acupuncturists, chiropractors, naturopaths, nurse practitioners, and physician assistants — are licensed to practice homeopathy. In addition, homeopathic remedies are a multimillion-dollar industry regulated by the Food and Drug Administration.

Diagnostic approach

Homeopathic practitioners view illness as a disturbance of the vital force, a disturbance that manifests as a whole pattern of physical, mental, and emotional responses that are unique to each patient. Following Hahnemann's third principle of homeopathy — illness is specific to the individual — homeopaths don't treat all patients with similar symptoms identically. Whereas a conventional physician will typically treat an ordinary headache with analgesics or anti-inflammatory drugs, a homeopathic practitioner will try to get a more complete picture of the patient, analyzing the headache's characteristics in that particular person. For example, does cold or heat affect the headache? Does it improve when the patient changes position?

Seeking not one disease but an overall pattern of symptoms, the practitioner will elicit as many symptoms as possible from the patient, even those that may not seem to be directly related to the patient's reason for seeking care. The practitioner will ask about lifestyle, diet, and family dynamics. Emotional and mental symptoms are especially relevant because they're believed to be a good indicator of how the patient generally feels.

After gathering sufficient information to identify the patient's overall symptom picture, the homeopathic practitioner will try to match that pattern to a homeopathic remedy listed in the official compendium known as the *Homeopathic Pharmacopoeia*, using an index that lists all symptoms and their corresponding remedies. This tool helps guide the practitioner to possible remedies, but he must then study the remedies to choose the appropriate one. As in the Eastern medical systems discussed earlier, it isn't unusual for two people with identical complaints to be diagnosed and treated differently.

Therapies

Homeopathic medicines are prepared from raw herbs and other natural substances derived from animal and mineral sources. These substances are crushed and dissolved in water or grain alcohol. Each compound is diluted many times, depending on the patient's symptoms. (Homeopaths believe that this process minimizes adverse effects.) After each dilution, the solution is shaken vigorously (a process known as *succussion*).

> 66 *In homeopathy, the process of healing doesn't end when the initial symptoms are resolved. Instead, the practitioner then attempts to discover and treat 'residues' of illnesses that were treated incompletely in the past.* 99

A 1:100 dilution means that 1 drop of a plant extract or other substance is placed in 99 drops of water or alcohol. After succussion, 1 drop of the new solution is diluted in another 99 drops of water or alcohol and shaken again. This process may be repeated 20 to 30 times. In the end, the remedy may contain less than one molecule of the original extract. Yet, homeopathic practitioners believe that each dilution strengthens the solution.

This use of highly diluted remedies is the most controversial aspect of homeopathic medicine. If the solution contains less than a molecule of the medicinal substance, how can it have any effect on the patient's symptoms? The answers haven't

HOW IT WORKS

⮃ Understanding homeopathy

Homeopathy's inability to provide a scientifically proven explanation of how its remedies work has been an ongoing problem for its proponents.

Electromagnetic imprint?

Of the various theories advanced to explain the therapeutic actions of homeopathic remedies, the most popular is the "memory of water" theory. This theory maintains that the active ingredient leaves an electromagnetic "imprint" in the water molecules of the homeopathic solution and that shaking (succussion) activates this "memory," stimulating the body's self-healing response.

Conventionally trained scientists say that if water had a memory, it would also "remember" all the other substances (such as minerals) removed during the purification process, some of which might have harmful effects on the patient or might cancel out the supposed beneficial effects of the original extract. However, homeopathy proponents say magnetic resonance imaging has shown subatomic activity in various homeopathic remedies.

Or placebo?

Proponents of homeopathy say that their remedies work, regardless of the exact mechanism. Western scientists say that these remedies act only as placebos and haven't been proved effective in treating serious illnesses. This controversy is likely to continue until more scientific research is done.

been found in conventional pharmacology. Proponents of homeopathy offer a number of theories. (See *Understanding homeopathy*.)

Homeopathic remedies are regulated by the Food and Drug Administration, and most are considered safe enough to be sold over the counter in many health food stores. High-potency compounds that are intended for serious conditions must be dispensed by a licensed practitioner.

In homeopathy, the process of healing doesn't end when the initial symptoms are resolved. Instead, the practitioner then attempts to discover and treat older underlying symptoms — residues of fevers, trauma, or other illnesses that were treated incompletely in the past and eventually resulted in the patient's presenting symptoms. This practice of restoring health layer by layer dates back to Dr. Constantine Hering, the founder of American homeopathy, who believed that healing should proceed in reverse chronological order, from the most recent symptoms to the oldest.

Therapeutic uses

Proponents claim that homeopathy can be used to treat a wide range of chronic conditions, such as headaches, allergies, asthma, eczema, arthritis, and digestive problems; acute infections, such as bronchitis, influenza, and strep throat; and minor problems, such as colds and rashes. Homeopathic remedies are also used to treat ordinary scrapes, strains, and sprains, and homeopathic first-aid kits are available in many health food stores. (See *Homeopathic first aid.*)

Homeopathic first aid

Homeopaths recommend that every home contain 10 basic remedies to treat everyday accidents and ailments. The following list groups them by their natural sources and supplies the specific source in parentheses.

From animal sources
▶ Apis (honeybee) — for insect bites and bee stings

From mineral sources
▶ Arsenicum (arsenic) — for upset stomach, food poisoning, vomiting, and diarrhea

From plant sources
▶ Aconite (monkshood) — for swelling or fever
▶ Arnica (leopard's bane) — for bruises and muscle soreness
▶ Belladonna (nightshade) — for sore throats, colds, coughs, headaches, earaches, and fever
▶ Gelsemium (yellow jasmine) — for colds and tension headaches
▶ Ipecacuanha (ipecac root) — for nausea and bleeding from the nose or other body parts
▶ Ledum (marsh tea) — for bites, stings, puncture wounds, eye injuries, and ankle strains
▶ Nux vomica (poison nut) — for hangovers
▶ Ruta (rue) — for sprains, tendinitis, and soreness (if arnica doesn't work)

Homeopathy isn't an appropriate self-treatment for illnesses involving advanced tissue damage, such as cancer or heart disease; for medical or surgical emergencies; or for severe infections.

RESEARCH SUMMARY As with traditional Chinese and Ayurvedic systems of medicine, the whole-person approach used in homeopathic diagnosis and treatment doesn't generally lend itself to placebo-controlled, double-blind studies. In spite of this difficulty, there have been some successful attempts to demonstrate the efficacy of specific homeopathic treatments with this kind of research as well as research that examines patient outcomes and cost-effectiveness.

The 1994 report to the National Institutes of Health entitled *Alternative Medicine: Expanding Medical Horizons* lists a number of studies published in mainstream medical journals that reported positive effects with homeopathic treatment. Clinical trials in Europe in the 1980s suggested benefits from homeopathic therapy in patients with allergic rhinitis, fibromyalgia, and influenza. A 1986 article in the British medical journal *Lancet* reported that homeopathic remedies were more effective than placebos in treating asthma and hay fever. A double-blind study comparing homeopathic treatment with a placebo for childhood diarrhea, and reported in the May 1994 issue of *Pediatrics,* found significant improvement in the children who received homeopathic remedies.

German researchers have reported success in treating bronchitis, migraines, influenza, and Parkinson's disease with homeopathic remedies. (Homeopathic practitioners have also claimed success in treating epilepsy, mental and emotional disorders, and premenstrual syndrome, but there's no scientific research to support these claims.)

Despite such studies, many in the mainstream medical community still dismiss homeopathy outright, claiming any positive results are a result of the placebo effect. ■

Nursing perspective

If your patient is receiving homeopathic remedies, take the following steps to prevent complications:

▶ Always obtain a thorough history before administering homeopathic remedies. This will help identify not only the patient's current problems but also any potential problems that the therapy could impose. For example, a patient with dia-

betes mellitus or lactose intolerance shouldn't take homeopathic remedies in tablet form because the tablets contain lactose. Advise such patients to request a liquid form of the medication.

▶ Explain the limitations of homeopathic treatment, and encourage patients with serious disorders or worsening symptoms to seek further advice from their homeopathic practitioner and their traditional health care provider.

▶ Tell recovering alcoholics to make sure the remedies they
take are mixed with water, not alcohol.

▶ Homeopathic remedies carry precautions similar to conventional medications. Advise patients to store them in a cool, dry
place away from the sun and away from mints and other
strong aromatic substances, to take nothing by mouth for 15
minutes before and after each dose, and to avoid coffee, home
remedies, mints (including mint toothpaste), and over-the-
counter drugs during the treatment period.

▶ Inform the patient that conventional medications may interfere with the actions of homeopathic remedies and should be
avoided unless the patient is seriously ill. Consult with a
homeopathic practitioner.

Naturopathic medicine

Naturopathy, a distinctly American approach to health care
that developed in the late 19th century, emphasizes health
maintenance, disease prevention, patient education, and the
patient's responsibility for his own health. More a way of life
than a system of medicine, naturopathy isn't based on a
unique view of human physiology, function, and disease, as the
Chinese and Ayurvedic systems are. Naturopathic doctors
study the same subjects that allopathic doctors do (including
anatomy and physiology, pathophysiology, cell biology, and epi-
demiology). They also use conventional diagnostic methods,
such as laboratory tests to detect pathogens, and perform minor surgeries. What differs is their approach to treatment.

Naturopathic medicine evolved from a number of 19th century health movements that emphasized the importance of
lifestyle, including good nutrition and avoidance of alcohol and
meat, in maintaining health and fighting disease. By the early
1900s, there were more than 20 naturopathic medical schools
in the United States, and naturopathic doctors were licensed

in most states. The rise of biomedicine, with its emphasis on the pharmaceutical treatment of disease, led to the decline of naturopathic practice.

However, as with many of the alternative therapies discussed in this book, interest in naturopathy has risen sharply in the past few decades, spurred largely by consumer interest in natural remedies. More than 1,000 naturopathic doctors are currently licensed to practice in 10 states and the District of Columbia as well as 4 Canadian provinces; other states allow naturopathic practice within certain limitations. The three accredited schools in the United States are the National College of Naturopathic Medicine in Portland, Oregon; Bastyr College of Natural Sciences in Seattle; and Southwest College in Scottsdale, Arizona. Some of the programs are distance learning models that don't offer clinical supervision. Educate patients to inquire about the credentials of the naturopath they choose.

As practiced today, naturopathy combines conventional diagnostic methods and standards of care with traditional and alternative natural treatments. Avoiding pharmaceuticals and surgery, naturopathic doctors rely instead on natural treatments aimed at stimulating the body's own healing functions, such as botanical, nutritional, and homeopathic remedies; acupuncture; traditional Chinese medicine; hydrotherapy; physical manipulation; and counseling.

Basic principles

The fundamental principle underlying naturopathy is the concept of *vitalism,* the belief that the body has an innate "intelligence" that strives to maximize health. Naturopathic doctors believe that symptoms aren't directly caused by a pathogen (such as a virus or bacterium) but are a manifestation of the body's effort to defend itself against the pathogen. Like Chinese doctors, they believe that pathogens must land on "fertile soil" to produce illness — that is, a person with a strong immune system may be able to fend off illness, whereas a person with a high stress level or poor nutrition may succumb. Naturopathic doctors strive to understand and support, rather than take over, the body's natural defense efforts.

In naturopathy, the absence of detectable disease doesn't equal health. Health is seen as a dynamic state of being that

Eight principles of naturopathy

The following eight basic principles form the foundation of naturo-pathic medicine:

▶ *The human body has its own inherent healing ability.* The doctor must work to restore the patient's own healing system, using medicines that are in harmony with nature.

▶ *Find and treat the cause.* The doctor must find and treat the underlying cause of illness, not just the symptoms.

▶ *Use therapies that do no harm.* Natural therapies are less likely to cause complications than stronger treatments, such as drugs and surgery.

▶ *The doctor is a teacher.* The doctor should educate the patient in how to prevent disease and maintain health.

▶ *Optimal health is the goal.* The doctor and patient aim to establish and maintain optimal health and balance, not merely to treat a particular disorder.

▶ *Treat the whole person.* An individual is a complex interaction of physical, mental, emotional, spiritual, and environmental systems; the doctor must assess all of these aspects to determine a diagnosis and treatment.

▶ *Focus on prevention.* Each individual has an inherent state of wellness, even if a disease is present. The doctor must recognize and foster the individual's wellness by encouraging a healthy lifestyle and minimizing risk factors.

▶ *Good nutrition is essential.* Good nutrition is an important tool in promoting health and fighting chronic and degenerative disorders.

allows the individual to adapt and thrive in various environments and to cope with the stresses of daily living. Naturopathy places great emphasis on disease prevention through healthful diet and lifestyle. A healthy lifestyle is believed to promote health; an unhealthy lifestyle, degeneration, disability, and early death. (See *Eight principles of naturopathy.*)

Diagnostic approach

Through questioning and physical examination, the naturopathic doctor learns as much as possible about the patient's overall state of health. He then combines the results of this thorough patient history and physical examination with the results of any necessary radiologic and laboratory tests — conventional tests as well as tests outside of conventional medicine such as a digestive stool analysis — to form a diagnosis and treatment plan.

Therapies

Treatments are aimed at mobilizing the patient's own immune system to combat the disease and to regain and maintain optimal health. The naturopathic doctor may choose from a wide range of available treatments, including nutritional therapy, homeopathic remedies, acupuncture, herbal therapy, hydrotherapy, naturopathic manipulative therapy, and counseling.

Nutritional therapy

Naturopathic doctors receive extensive training in nutrition to ensure that they can provide each patient with a healthy and nutritionally balanced diet that's appropriate to his condition. Nutritional therapy uses whole foods, nutritional supplements if needed, and controlled fasting to treat disease and maintain health.

Herbal therapy

Herbal remedies may be taken internally or applied externally to treat the internal conditions that manifest as disease. Naturopathic doctors claim that botanical medicines are safer, more effective, and cheaper than pharmaceutical drugs.

Homeopathic remedies

Homeopathic solutions are very dilute preparations of natural substances that, in large amounts, cause certain symptoms but in small amounts are believed to relieve them. (See "Homeopathic medicine," page 101.)

Acupuncture

Commonly used to relieve pain, acupuncture involves the insertion of very fine needles into designated points on the skin to stimulate the body's vital flow of energy, called *qi* in traditional Chinese medicine. (See "Acupuncture" in chapter 7, page 235.)

Hydrotherapy

Hydrotherapy involves the use of special baths and other water-based treatments to cure disease and maintain health.

In Europe, many patients are sent to spas for rest and rejuvenation. (See "Hydrotherapy" in chapter 7, page 265.)

Naturopathic manipulative therapy
Physical treatments may include manipulation of the bones and spine (in a manner similar to chiropractic) as well as massage, heat, cold, touch, electricity and sound, ultrasound, diathermy, and therapeutic exercises.

Counseling
Because naturopathic doctors believe that mental and emotional factors play a role in disease, counseling in lifestyle management is an important element of naturopathic treatment. Some naturopathic doctors are specially trained in biofeedback, stress reduction, meditation, yoga, and other techniques aimed at inducing a more balanced and natural lifestyle.

Therapeutic uses
Naturopathic doctors claim to be able to treat a wide range of illnesses, including minor, self-limiting conditions, such as the common cold and allergies, and — in combination with conventional medical treatments — life-threatening diseases, such as cancer and acquired immunodeficiency syndrome. However, they commonly make referrals to conventional specialists for emergency cases or patients with serious or complicated illnesses.

RESEARCH SUMMARY Showing an interest in women's health problems, naturopathic medical researchers have reported positive results using natural (botanical) remedies for cervical dysplasia and as an alternative to estrogen replacement therapy. In a 1993 study on cervical dysplasia, 38 of the 43 women treated naturopathically returned to a normal Papanicolaou test and a normal tissue biopsy. In another 1993 study on a substitute for estrogen, 100% of the women treated with the botanical formula showed a significant reduction of symptoms compared with 17% of the placebo group.

The effectiveness of acupuncture for pain and dietary changes to reduce the risk of heart disease has been well documented. ∎

Nursing perspective

If your patient is receiving naturopathic treatment, take the following steps to help prevent complications:

▶ Educate the patient about the need to take responsibility for his own health, which may require lifestyle changes. Teach him ways to improve his health through diet changes and safe exercises.

▶ Inform the patient that naturopathic doctors don't perform major surgery or provide emergency care.

▶ Obtain a medication history from the patient to ensure that prescribed botanical remedies don't interact with already prescribed conventional medications.

▶ Warn the patient about the risks involved in sharing his prescribed remedies with others.

▶ If the patient is a recovering alcoholic, tell him to make sure that the remedies he takes are mixed with water, not alcohol.

Osteopathic medicine

Developed in the United States in the late 19th century, osteopathy (derived from the Greek words *osteon*, meaning bone, and *pathos*, meaning suffering) is a health care system that views structural and mechanical problems as the source of disease. Based on the belief that structure directly influences function, osteopathic doctors use various forms of physical manipulation to correct structural anomalies, thereby stimulating the body's own self-healing mechanisms. However, osteopathy is closely intertwined with conventional medicine; it's more a healing system that uses alternative therapies than an actual alternative medicine system.

Basic principles

Andrew Taylor Still (1828-1917), the founder of osteopathy, was a medical doctor who became disillusioned with orthodox medicine after his father and three of his children died of infectious diseases against which the medicine of the time was ineffective. Still believed that the human body contained the ability to heal itself and that physicians should take steps to elicit that self-healing power. How he came to believe that physical manipulation was the way to unleash that power is unclear; however, he began practicing his new system, which started as a combination of bone setting and the magnetic healing system of Franz Mesmer, in the 1870s.

In 1892, Still founded the American School of Osteopathy in Missouri, based on the belief that manually restoring structural integrity could improve physiologic function. Eventually, Still and his colleagues developed interventions to assist in labor and delivery and to treat specific disorders, such as neck and back pain, migraines, asthma, otitis media, hypertension, coronary artery disease, and diabetes.

> ❝ *Osteopaths receive the same training as MDs and must pass the same medical board examinations to become licensed. But their education emphasizes osteopathic philosophy and principles, including 'structural diagnosis' and 'manipulative treatment.'* ❞

As currently practiced, osteopathy blends conventional medical and obstetric practices with osteopathic manipulation. Today, there are more than 33,000 licensed Doctors of Osteopathy in the United States, providing all aspects of medical care. Osteopaths receive the same training as conventional medical practitioners, must pass the same medical board examinations to become licensed, and have the same ability to prescribe medications. However, their education places considerable emphasis on osteopathic philosophy and principles, including "structural diagnosis" and "manipulative treatment." (See *Four principles of osteopathy,* page 114.)

Diagnostic approach

Osteopaths believe that any restriction in the spine or other bony structures can impair the function of entire organs and body systems. Thus, the musculoskeletal system is the focus of diagnosis and therapy.

Using palpation and inspection, the osteopath will evaluate the patient's posture and gait (assessing how he holds himself while sitting, standing, and walking), mobility of moving parts (looking for restricted movements during bending, side bending, extension, and rotation), symmetry of body parts (checking for overuse of one side and for abnormal curvature of the spine), and soft tissues (looking for tenderness, hardening, skin or temperature changes, and signs of fluid retention).

Four principles of osteopathy

The following four principles form the foundation of osteopathic medicine:

▶ *Each person is an integrated unit consisting of body, mind, and spirit.* Because physical, mental, emotional, and spiritual factors are inseparably linked within each person, any stress or alteration in one area will affect all the others. Thus, the doctor must take into account the whole person in diagnosis and treatment.

▶ *The body is capable of healing itself.* Under ideal conditions, the body, mind, and spirit work together to maintain health and to heal. Disease begins when one or more body systems are overwhelmed. The doctor's role is to enhance the patient's own healing process as much as possible.

▶ *Body structure can't be separated from function.* Abnormal structure leads to abnormal function and vice versa. When the mechanical structure of the body is corrected, its functioning will also improve.

▶ *Treatment must be based on the preceding three principles.* The key to effective care is the recognition that disease isn't the invasion of a host by some external entity but a breakdown of the body's capacity for self-maintenance.

Therapies

Like practitioners of other complementary therapies, osteopaths take a holistic approach to health care, treating the patient as an integrated whole rather than focusing on a specific symptom or complaint. They believe that given a favorable environment, adequate nutrition, and properly functioning body structures, the body is capable of healing itself. The doctor's task is to assist the body in this process of self-healing.

The osteopath can choose from a number of manipulation techniques. Some require the patient to be passive as the doctor performs the technique; others require the patient to actively perform the technique while the doctor guides and assists him. Some are used alone; others are combined with conventional allopathic treatments. Specific techniques include:

▶ *Gentle mobilization* involves moving a joint slowly through its range of motion while gradually increasing the motion to eliminate restrictions.

▶ *Articulation* consists of performing a quick thrust (similar to a chiropractic maneuver) to restore joint mobility.

▶ *Muscle energy technique* involves gently tensing and releasing certain muscles to induce relaxation.

▶ *Positional release method* involves placing the patient in a specific position to release muscle spasms.

▶ *Cranial techniques* (also known as cranial manipulation), consist of very gentle manipulation of the cranial and sacral bones, and is used to treat headaches, spinal injuries, and temporomandibular joint syndrome. (For more information, see "Craniosacral therapy" in chapter 7, page 259.)

In addition, osteopaths teach their patients various self-care practices designed to keep their bodies functioning properly. These may include relaxation techniques, specially designed exercises and stretches, breathing exercises, postural changes, and proper nutrition. All of these practices are aimed at reducing stress on joints and muscles, maintaining structural and functional integrity, and teaching the patient how to use his body more efficiently.

Therapeutic uses

Osteopathic doctors claim that they can successfully treat nearly any health problem, including some that have failed to respond to conventional medical treatment or surgery. Osteopathic manipulation is commonly used to treat alterations in musculoskeletal structure, such as whiplash injuries, scoliosis, and neck and lower back pain. Other disorders that reportedly respond to osteopathic treatment are arthritis, digestive problems, menstrual problems, chronic pain, cardiac and pulmonary diseases, chronic fatigue, high blood pressure, headaches, sciatica, and various neural disorders.

How does one treat a cardiac or respiratory disease by adjusting musculoskeletal structures? According to osteopathic practitioners, diseases of the internal organs are commonly manifested as musculoskeletal pain. For example, musculoskeletal misalignment over a long period can compromise a coronary artery, leading to angina or myocardial infarction. Detecting and correcting the musculoskeletal dysfunction before major tissue damage has occurred can increase oxygen delivery and decrease venous congestion, thereby preventing a serious cardiac event.

RESEARCH SUMMARY According to the 1994 report to the National Institutes of Health (NIH) entitled *Alternative Medicine: Expanding Medical Horizons,* extensive research done by the osteopathic profession supports the contention that osteopathic techniques can affect physiologic functioning. The report finds "of particular interest" studies dealing with interactions between neuromuscular structures and internal organs, alterations in reflex thresholds, and effects of manipulation on disease processes and physiologic functioning.

Among the studies showing physiologic effects from manipulation techniques are two reporting changes in postoperative pulmonary flow rates and electromyographic tests. Studies have also documented effects on visceral and neuromuscular function, including lower back pain, carpal tunnel syndrome, neurologic development in children, collapsed lung, and burning pain in an extremity. Other studies have supported the usefulness of palpation of musculoskeletal structures to help diagnose visceral disorders — for example, a 1994 report found that diagnoses based on palpation were backed up by X-ray and autopsy results.

Noting that federally funded research into osteopathic medicine has historically been controlled by "traditionally defined disciplines and their expert panels," the report urges the NIH to ensure that experts with osteopathic experience serve on peer review panels to enhance understanding of this field. ■

Nursing perspective

If your patient is under the care of an osteopathic doctor, take the following steps to help prevent adverse effects:

▶ Caution a patient at risk for injury, such as a pregnant woman or a patient with a prosthetic joint, to inform the doctor of the condition before undergoing osteopathic manipulation.

▶ Teach the patient self-care techniques, such as breathing and stretching techniques, to maintain proper body function and alignment. Reeducation is the final step of osteopathic treatment. Teach the patient how to keep his body optimally functioning in a relaxed state to reduce anxiety and tension.

Energy medicine

The human body is an electromagnetic unit. Electricity makes the heart beat and muscles expand and contract, and fires impulses across tiny fibers in the nervous system to make possible our every thought, mood, and physical reaction. Energy medicine, or vibrational medicine, is a form of therapy in which the patient's own electromagnetic, or energy, field is used to promote wellness or healing. Energy medicine consists of various therapeutic modalities, each of which has its own healing frequency, or energetic waveband. Some of these healing practices include healing touch, Therapeutic Touch, *qigong*, Reiki, tai chi, acupuncture, acupressure, and gem therapy.

Basic principles

Throughout history, the peoples of many nations have used various forms of vibrational energy for healing. Most traditional cultures identify some form of a basic life force flowing from a universal creator. In China it's called *chi*; in ancient Greece, *pneuma*; in India, *prana*; in Japan, *qi*. To the natives of North America, this force is known as the *flow of spirit*. To all these peoples, the life force is the basis of physical, psychological, and spiritual health. These subtle, unseen energies are incorporated in the therapeutic vibrational methods of the different modalities, as healers work to enhance or rebalance this life force, strengthening it where it's weak and modulating it where it's excessive.

One popular form of energy medicine works with the patient's aura, or energy field. The aura, or auric field, reflects how one's life is being lived at that moment. The vibration, color, and sound of the aura are all interrelated and represent a means of determining the frequency of energy in the auric field. A healer channeling energy to a patient will often experience reactions in his own body — for example, he may feel a vibration, "see" the color of the energy, or "hear" a sound he associates with a particular color or feeling (a phenomenon known as clairaudience). There are seven layers of the auric field.

▶ The etheric body or layer is joined directly to the physical body, from which it extends outward 2″ to 6″ (5 to 15 cm); it's referred to as "etheric double" because it contains a blueprint as well as replications of all the organs in the physical form.

▶ The emotional body is the wellspring from which all our emotions, desires, joys, pain, suffering, and passions emerge. Beliefs, perceptions, attitudes, and emotions — particularly fear — affect the body through the nervous, endocrine, muscular, and immune systems; they can change the field or cause it to shut down.

▶ The mental body is responsible for rational, clear, and intellectual functions. It's responsible for the conscious (what we are aware of) and unconscious (what has been repressed or forgotten and exists just beneath the surface of consciousness) mind as well as memories.

▶ The astral body bridges dimensions of matter and spirit and is transitional between the first and last auric bodies. The astral body contains the entire personality and contains all the extraordinary abilities — intuition, extrasensory perception, image projection, spiritual sight, and clairvoyance — as well as compassion for others.

▶ The causal, or second etheric, body is the first layer of the spiritual realm, which contains the knowledge of the individual's purpose in life, his talents, and the lessons he must learn during the course of his lifetime.

▶ The celestial body is the site of clear vision, in the spiritual sense of individual future, and is believed to contain a love that surpasses human love. It influences sight and other manifestations of visualization — insight, foresight, inspiration, clairvoyance, and physical manifestation. It's sometimes erroneously called the third eye.

▶ The spiritual and cosmic consciousness, also called the ketheric layer or body, is said to be in direct contact with the divine universe; it's the body's energy blueprint. It's also a center of knowing without thought or reason. Our spiritual life resides here.

The auric fields are created and controlled by the chakras. *Chakra* is a Sanskrit word meaning "wheel" or "circle of movement." The chakras are spirals of concentrated life force or vortices of energy. They're arrayed in a straight line at the center of the body, with the energy vortices of the second through the sixth extending out the front and back. The root chakra points downward, and the crown chakra points upward. In the northern hemisphere, healthy chakras spin in a clockwise direction, facing the front of a person. South of the equator, chakras spin in a counterclockwise direction. The direction of radiation, shape, and diameter of a chakra indicate the state of its energy and the health of the corresponding or adjacent physical organs. (See *Characteristics of the seven primary chakras*, page 120.)

There are 6 secondary chakras located in the palms of the hands, backs of the knees, and soles of the feet near the arches and 20 smaller tertiary chakras located on the tips of the fingers and toes. The second and third chakras in the hands are used to direct energy during healing practices; the second and third chakras in the feet, to ground the healer while performing healing activities. Additionally, minor chakras are designated anteriorly over both hip joints, tips of the shoulder, and elbows.

Another type of energy medicine is nonlocal healing, in which the practitioner may be at some distance from the person to be healed. Nonlocal healing includes prayer, empathetic concern, and distant intentionality, in which healing thoughts and vibrations are sent to the person in need.

Diagnostic approach

Diagnosis is done through assessment. The practitioner assesses, manipulates, and evaluates the patient's energy field based on the type of energy medicine to be used. Treatment is based on the results of this assessment. For example, an acupuncturist will assess the balance of *qi* flow in the network of channels, known as meridians, and will assess the patient's symptoms in relation to the meridians.

Therapies

The healing practitioner begins by "centering" — that is, focusing his creative or healing intention by directing it inward — to ready himself for assessing and treating the patient. The practitioner draws energy into himself through his crown chakra and sends it to his own heart (to ensure that no harm is done), and then out through his hands to the patient. The energy may go through both hands, or through only the left hand, with the right hand drawing negative energy away from the patient. The practitioner may envision a desire and commitment to creating a specific outcome for the patient — for example, fulfilling a personal goal or aspiration, or he may simply facilitate the energy to be used for the patient's best interest. This creative, healing intention aligns the conscious, subconscious, and su-

Characteristics of the seven primary chakras

Chakra	Location	Glands	Color	Issues
7. Crown	Slightly above the top of the head; 2″ to 3″ (5 to 7.5 cm) in diameter	Pituitary, pineal	Violet	Worthiness, trusting God
6. Brow	Just above the eyebrow line; 1″ to 2″ (2.5 to 5 cm) in diameter	Pituitary, hypothalamus	Indigo	Seeing and admitting what is or what has happened
5. Throat	Larynx, just above the junction of the collarbones; 1½″ to 3″ (4 to 7.5 cm) in diameter	Thyroid, parathyroids	Blue	Safety in speaking out
4. Heart	One inch above where the ribs meet on the lower chest; 1½″ to 4″ (4 to 10 cm) in diameter	Thymus	Green	Trust and love
3. Solar plexus	Centered in the pit of the stomach, 2″ below the joining of the ribs; 1½″ to 4″ in diameter	Pancreas	Yellow	Self-image, self-esteem
2. Sacral	A few inches below the navel and above the pubic bone; 2″ to 4″ in diameter	Adrenals	Orange	Power
1. Root	Perineum; 1″ to 3″ in diameter	Gonads	Red	Survival, safety, basic instincts, sexuality

per conscious aspects of the mind; sets energy forces in motion; and may create instantaneous healings or other manifestations.

Therapeutic uses

Energy medicine may be used with a more traditional regimen to treat anemias, cancer, arthritis, colitis, Alzheimer's disease, inflammatory diseases, hypertension and heart disease, cellular diseases, viral diseases, overdoses, and fractures. Energy therapy isn't effective with genetic diseases.

RESEARCH SUMMARY Numerous studies support the efficacy of vibrational or energy medicine. However, further study regarding its efficacy is necessary. ■

Nursing perspective

If your patient is receiving energy medicine treatment, take the following steps to help make the process easier:

▶ Consult the patient about cultural issues or rituals that are important to him, and incorporate them into the healing session in the manner agreed upon.

▶ Instruct your patient that although no adverse effects arising from energy medicine have been identified, some patients may express discomfort with the intensified energy. At that point, the therapist may move to another location or end the treatment depending on the type of energy medicine being used.

▶ Explain that the use of vibrational toxins may impede the success of energy therapy. Such toxins include alcohol (loosens and misaligns the subtle anatomy), cigarette smoke (clouds and weakens the subtle anatomy), and caffeine (disturbs the flow of energy). These affect the acupuncture meridian system that affects the etheric body, which in turn causes energy leaks in the emotional and mental bodies.

Environmental medicine

Environmental medicine identifies and treats toxicity in the body that results from exposure to and accumulation of environmental chemicals or toxins. More and more health care providers — including both conventional biomedical doctors and alternative therapy practitioners — are recognizing that such substances as chemicals, dust, molds, and certain foods can cause allergic reactions that may result in or exacerbate a wide range of disorders, such as immune dysregulation, autoimmunity, asthma, allergies, cancers, cognitive deficits, mood changes, neurologic illnesses, changes in libido, reproductive dysfunc-

> ❝Chemical sensitivity to foods, allergens, and other environmental substances may help explain many signs and symptoms that have been difficult to diagnose and treat. ❞

tion, and glucose dysregulation in susceptible persons. These disorders may manifest as a complex assortment of chronic or cyclic signs and symptoms, usually involving more than one organ system and typically mediated by the immune system.

Chemical sensitivity to foods, allergens, and other substances in the environment appears to be a growing problem among wide segments of the population and may help to explain many signs and symptoms that have been difficult to diagnose and treat. Many experts attribute this increased incidence to the huge growth of the petrochemical industry since the end of World War II. Countless chemical products are produced worldwide today, including thousands that are used in food processing. Many of these substances — for example, petroleum products, insecticides, and household cleaners — can't be properly broken down by the body. According to specialists in environmental medicine, toxins from these products accumulate in the body, eventually resulting in a host of disorders ranging from neurologic and GI disturbances to mental problems and cancer.

Food allergies are considered a form of environmental illness. In this type of allergy, a specific food triggers an adverse reaction of the immune system. Other potential environmental challenges include chemicals in food, water, and air; inhaled materials, such as pollens, molds, and dust; electromagnetic fields; ionizing and nonionizing radiation; medical and nonmedical drugs; noise pollution; and temperature and humidity.

Individual sensitivity to chemicals varies widely. For example, 90% of the population is apparently unaffected by small amounts of formaldehyde in the environment (emitted by many building and furnishing materials such as new carpet); 10% is highly sensitive to it. Until recently, people in the 10% group were labeled as hypochondriacal, with psychosomatic symptoms, because no one else seemed to be affected as they were.

Specialists in environmental medicine classify ecological illness into two categories: differentiated and undifferentiated disease. Differentiated disease includes recognized clinical diagnoses that can be attributed wholly or partly to an ecological cause, such as hay fever and other seasonal allergies, asthma, eczema, and anaphylactic food allergies. Undifferentiated disease includes symptoms (many of which are apparently unrelated) that don't fit a standard diagnosis and that are often attributed to psychological causes but may have an underlying ecological cause. Illnesses in this category may include arthritis, colitis, depression, general malaise, fatigue, headaches, and aches and pains with no ascertainable cause.

Primary care physicians are commonly the first contact for persons suffering from environmental sensitivities, although a growing number of physicians in the United States, Canada, and Europe are entering this specialty field. Nurses have a special opportunity to identify possible environmental influences on their patients' illnesses by being aware of the wide range of effects that environmental toxins can have on complex disease states.

Historical background

Allergies have been studied since the 19th century, but only in the past 30 years has the field of environmental medicine become widely recognized. The pioneer in this field was Dr. Theron Randolph, a Chicago allergy specialist who believed that in certain people sensitivity to many common foods (such as wheat, milk, and eggs) could cause a wide range of medical problems. By withholding the suspect food for 4 days and then giving the patient a challenge dose, Randolph was able to identify foods that triggered assorted symptoms, including fatigue, headaches, skin conditions, arthritis, asthma, GI disorders, and depression. He later discovered that chemicals could also cause serious problems in susceptible people.

In attempting to understand how environmental substances can ultimately cause disease, environmental medicine has used Hans Selye's general adaptation syndrome model. This model describes how continued exposure to stressors, such as environmental toxins, can develop into a maladaptive response. (See *Selye's general adaptation syndrome,* page 124.)

Selye's general adaptation syndrome

Canadian physiologist Hans Selye, a pioneering researcher on stress, developed his general adaptation syndrome model to explain how chronic exposure to stressors can eventually lead to illness. According to his theory, the body responds to stress through a built-in series of physiologic responses that both protect the body and help it adapt to the stressor.

However, chronic activation of this stress response (commonly known as the fight-or-flight response) leads to strain on an organ system over time and impairs its ability to adapt. Eventually, the system breaks down and organ damage and illness result. According to Selye, this process occurs in three stages (shown below): the alarm reaction (fight-or-flight response), the stage of resistance, and the stage of exhaustion.

**Physical, psychological,
or environmental stressor**

STAGE 1

ALARM REACTION
▶ Stress stimulates the sympathetic nervous system, which constricts the blood vessels and activates the release of certain hormones from the endocrine glands.
▶ Stimulation of the endocrine glands results in an increase in heart rate, force of cardiac contractions, oxygen consumption, and glucose metabolism.

STAGE 2

RESISTANCE
▶ The body marshals internal resources and adapts to the stressor, attempting to return to homeostasis.

STAGE 3

RECOVERY OR EXHAUSTION
▶ If stress comes to an end, the body should be able to return to a normal state and recover.
▶ If stress continues, the body proceeds to the exhaustion stage. Internal resources are depleted, and the body can no longer adapt to the stress. Organ damage begins, marking the onset of disease.

However, each individual's reaction to a particular toxin or combination of toxins is also affected by other factors, including heredity, history, psychological stressors, and nutritional status. In addition, a particular environmental challenge may have a greater or lesser effect on an individual from day to day, depending on his physical and mental condition as well as the presence of other challenges in the environment.

Diagnostic approach

Because the response to a particular environmental stressor varies greatly from person to person, identifying the cause of a patient's symptom pattern can be very difficult. The first step is to obtain a detailed chronological history targeting exposure to possible environmental stressors over time and relating exposures to the appearance of symptoms. The history should include any possible influences on the development or course of the patient's symptoms.

A detailed description of the patient's home and work environments along with the effects of seasons or activity should be obtained to detect exposure to toxins. Laboratory tests and a physical examination are performed to identify nutritional problems, organ system dysfunction, or problems with the body's detoxification process.

Allergy and hypersensitivity tests are an important aspect of the assessment process. These tests may include both traditional allergy tests, such as scratch tests for allergies to pollen, and newer antigen tests, such as serial end-point titration, provocative neutralization, and bronchoprovocation. Complex symptom patterns may require inpatient hospitalization in an environmental control unit, which is free from all common chemical exposures. The patient consumes only water until all symptoms disappear; then he's challenged by foods and inhaled chemicals to assess his responses. These units are available in several hospitals in the United States and Canada.

For suspected food allergies, the doctor may propose an elimination diet in which the suspected food is eliminated from the patient's diet for at least 10 days to see if his symptoms disappear. Among the most common food allergens are dairy products, wheat, corn, eggs, soy products, peanuts, potatoes, tomatoes, and sugar.

Therapies

Once the causative environmental toxin or food allergen has been identified, the primary treatment is avoiding exposure to it. For persons with multiple sensitivities, avoidance can be problematic. For example, a person sensitive to perfume would theoretically need to stay away from enclosed spaces where people are wearing perfume. This could severely restrict the patient's social life as well as limit his ability to work in many work environments.

Patient education is essential. Patients must understand the factors that contribute to their illness to ensure long-term improvement. Environmental controls in the home and workplace to reduce exposure to the causative agents are essential. Immunotherapy may be used to reduce the patient's sensitivity to the offending substance.

Therapeutic uses

Environmental medicine has been found effective in the treatment of mold and pollen allergies, food allergies, chemical sensitivity, and assorted disorders.

RESEARCH SUMMARY Studies have supported an environmental link to numerous disorders, including arthritis, asthma, eczema, urticaria, migraines, colitis, fatigue, depression, hyperactivity, vascular problems, and psychological problems. Other studies have been done on the diagnostic techniques used in environmental medicine, including a 1993 study that supported the effectiveness of provocation-neutralization testing. ■

Nursing perspective

You can play an important part in helping the patient with an environmental illness learn new ways to adjust to a life that may seem extremely constricted. Education of family, coworkers, and friends is essential to help the patient participate in life as fully as possible. The following measures may help make the process easier for the patient:

▶ Teach the patient and his family as much as possible about his illness, its cause (if known), and the need to avoid the causative food or substance.

▶ If the patient must keep a diary of his symptoms (or a food diary) to aid in diagnosis, show him how to do so correctly.

◗ Warn the patient that trial-and-error testing may be necessary to determine the cause of his symptoms.

◗ If testing determines that the patient has a food allergy, make sure he understands that he'll have to eliminate the food from his diet or undergo immunotherapy to decrease his sensitivity to it. Some environmental practitioners recommend eating only organic foods; if this is the case, recommend local sources the patient can use.

Selected references

Benson, H. *The Relaxation Response.* New York: William Morrow & Co., 2000.

Cassidy, C. *Contemporary Chinese Medicine and Acupuncture.* New York: Churchill Livingstone, Inc., 2001.

Freeman, L.W., and Lawles, G.F. *Mosby's Complementary and Alternative Therapy: A Research-Based Approach.* St. Louis: Mosby–Year Book, Inc., 2001.

Gallagher, R. *Osteopathic Medicine: A Reformation in Progress.* New York: Churchill Livingstone, Inc., 2001.

Gerson, S. *Ayurveda: The Ancient Indian Healing Art,* 2nd ed. Colfax, Wash.: Cougar Graphics, 2001.

Goldsmith, S. "Homeopathic Family Diagnosis: The Fifth Dimension," *Journal of the American Institute of Homeopathy* 93(3) Autumn 2000.

Hershoff, A. and Rotelli A. *Herbal Remedies: A Quick and Easy Guide to Common Disorders and their Herbal Treatments.* New York: Avery, 2001.

Johnson, S.M., and Kurtz, M.E. "Diminished Use of Osteopathic Manipulative Treatment and Its Impact on the Uniqueness of the Osteopathic Profession," *Academic Medicine* 76(8):821-28, August 2001.

Lee, A.C., and Kemper K.J. "Homeopathy and Naturopathy: Practice Characteristics and Pediatric Cases," *Archives of Pediatric and Adolescent Medicine* 154(1):75-80, January 2000.

Licciardone, J.C., and Herron, K.M. "Characteristics, Satisfactions, and Perceptions of Patients Receiving Ambulatory Healthcare from Osteopathic Physicians: A Comparative National Survey," *Journal of the American Osteopathic Association* 101(7):374-85, July 2001.

Micozzi, M.S., ed. *Fundamentals of Complementary and Alternative Medicine,* 2nd ed. New York: Churchill Livingstone, Inc., 2001.

Parkman, C.A. "A Look at Naturopathic Medicine," *Case Manager* 12(5):29-31, September-October 2001.

Yang, Y. *Chinese Herbal Medicines: Comparisons and Characteristics.* New York: Churchill Livingstone, Inc., 2001.

5

Mind-body
therapies

The idea that the mind plays an important role in health isn't new. In fact, it's a central concept of most ancient healing systems, such as traditional Chinese and Ayurvedic medicine. However, Western medicine has largely ignored the mind-body connection for the past 3 centuries, since the philosopher Descartes separated the transcendent mind from the material and mechanical body.

This scientific distinction between body and mind allowed science to focus on the biology and chemistry of the body while letting theologians, philosophers, and mental health professionals concentrate on the mind. Exciting scientific discoveries about the physical causes of many diseases, such as viral and bacterial diseases, led researchers to focus even more narrowly on the body's myriad minute components in an effort to understand the nature of disease. The result has been a tendency to view the body as a complex machine and disease as primarily a breakdown of mechanical parts.

The mind-body link

Today, researchers and health care practitioners are reexamining the complex relationship between mind and body in an attempt to understand how thoughts and emotions influence health. An increasing body of evidence is demonstrating that the mind — feelings, thoughts, fears, and outlook — can indeed affect all body systems and contribute to physical disease.

Much of the recent research has focused on the relationship between stress and the immune system.

Effects of stress

When confronted with a real or perceived threat, human beings react with the *fight-or-flight response,* an autonomic nervous system reaction in which adrenaline and other hormones mobilize the body into action to either fight the stressor or flee from it. This response is normal in situations of extreme stress or danger. However, scientists believe that when the fight-or-flight response is mobilized too often in reaction to minor everyday stressors, it can strain the immune system and other physiologic functions, making the body more prone to illness. Any event that requires us to change can cause stress. Even positive events—such as marriage, a vacation, or a job promotion—are considered stressors.

> *Research in the new medical discipline known as psychoneuroimmunology may eventually explain how patients with serious illnesses sometimes experience a spontaneous remission for no apparent medical reason.*

Pioneering research in psychology and immunology in the 1970s led to the development of a new medical discipline known as *psychoneuroimmunology,* which studies the complex interactions between the mind and the neurologic and immune systems. Numerous studies since then have shown that stress appears to contribute to heart disease and various other conditions, such as chronic pain, arthritis, skin disorders, and even the common cold. Research in this field may eventually explain how patients with serious illnesses sometimes experience a spontaneous remission for no apparent medical reason.

The mind-body therapies discussed in this chapter are all based on the theory that if stress can lead to illness, stress reduction can help restore health. All of the approaches mentioned require the active participation of the patient and assume that the individual can affect—and sometimes even regulate—his own body functions. This active involvement in the healing process not only helps the patient reduce stress but also increases his sense of control over his own life, which can further boost the immune system and promote healing.

Nursing's role

Whether at the bedside in an acute care hospital, in the patient's home, or in an outpatient setting, more and more nurses are learning about and using mind-body therapies. Because of their pivotal role in teaching patients about prevention and wellness, preparing them for diagnostic procedures and surgeries, and helping them recover from illness or trauma, nurses are in an excellent position to teach patients the basics of stress reduction and to offer support to patients who choose to use mind-body interventions.

The nurse's role in mind-body therapy is to objectively inform the patient, to offer empathetic support, to deliver medical interventions when necessary, and to use the nursing process to deliver interventions in accordance with the patient's changing responses and needs.

Art therapy

Art therapists believe that the release of creative energy associated with artistic expression can lead to physical, emotional, and spiritual healing. They believe that the act of drawing, painting, or sculpting helps patients by promoting self-awareness, reducing loneliness, and allowing patients to express feelings that they can't verbalize. Art therapy by itself can't cure disease; rather, it's used to complement the overall health care plan.

Art therapy can use any artistic medium and can occur in any setting, from a hospital bed to the patient's home or an artist's studio. Patients who are unable to create art may benefit by looking at the art of others.

In addition to providing the patient with a means of self-expression and a pleasant diversion, art therapy also helps nurses and other health care providers understand the patient. A patient's drawings may reveal his state of mind, including his feelings about his health problem and his subconscious concerns. Such insight can help the nurse or art therapist develop or refine a diagnosis and formulate a plan to help the patient with his specific health problem.

The concept of using art as therapy began in the 1800s in mental institutions. The art of mental patients was seen as valuable, not only in assisting with a diagnosis but also in rehabilitating the patient. In the 1940s, art and psychoanalysis were combined as a method of helping patients release thoughts and feelings buried in the subconscious.

With the formation of the American Art Therapy Association (AATA) and the Art Therapy Credentials Board (ATCB) in 1969, a code of ethics and standards for the profession were developed. The AATA approves educational programs and works to educate the public about the field. The ATCB offers two levels of credentials. A registered art therapist (ATR) must have a master's degree in art therapy, complete a supervised internship, and meet contact hour requirements. Once registered, an ATR has the option of becoming board-certified in art therapy by sitting for a certification examination.

Most art therapists practice in psychiatric centers, drug and alcohol rehabilitation programs, prisons, day care treatment centers, children's hospitals, schools for people with mental retardation, residences for the developmentally delayed, geriatric centers, and hospices.

Therapeutic uses

Art therapy can be used in various clinical situations. (See *Indications for art therapy*, page 132.)

66 *Art therapy is especially useful in dealing with children and survivors of physical or sexual abuse, who often have difficulty expressing themselves verbally.* 99

RESEARCH SUMMARY Little scientific research has been done on this form of therapy, but some studies have reported benefits for patients with psychiatric illnesses, spinal cord injury and other disabilities, chronic stress disorders, and Alzheimer's disease. ∎

Art therapy is especially useful in dealing with children, who often can't express their feelings or physical sensations verbally. Many survivors of physical or sexual abuse also benefit from art therapy. These patients commonly have feelings

Indications for art therapy

Art therapy can be used for the following types of conditions:

- age-related role changes
- Alzheimer's disease
- attention deficit hyperactivity disorder
- catastrophic illness (such as cancer or acquired immunodeficiency syndrome)
- chronic disease
- chronic fatigue syndrome
- chronic pain
- chronic stress disorders
- couples and family therapy
- extensive surgery
- learning disabilities
- loss of voice
- posttraumatic stress disorder
- prolonged hospitalization or treatment
- psychiatric disorders
- spinal cord injuries
- substance abuse and addiction
- terminal illness.

Art therapy is also effective in treating children who have been abused or neglected or who come from homes with drug abusers.

of anger, rage, shame, guilt, and fear that they have difficulty expressing verbally. Art therapy provides them with a safe means of expressing those feelings.

Art therapy is also useful as a follow-up to other image-evoking mind-body therapies, such as relaxation, guided imagery, and hypnotherapy. It allows the patient to externalize mental images and emotions that form during the session and helps to ground his experience. Progress in life-threatening illnesses can be accurately tracked by reviewing a patient's drawings.

Equipment
The art supplies used should match the patient's abilities and the financial resources of the facility. Almost any medium the patient can physically manage can be used for art therapy: paints, pens, pencils, felt markers, chalks, clay, or crayons. Flowers, grasses, seeds, shells, nuts, stones, feathers, or bones may also be used. The artwork can range from two-dimensional drawings, paintings, or collages to three-dimensional sculptures. Wood or soap carving, papier-mâché, metal sculptures, and plaster of paris are other possibilities.

If an art therapist isn't present, you'll need to assess the patient's abilities yourself before starting a project so you can prepare and have the appropriate materials on hand. Young children and patients with impaired fine motor skills may work better with larger crayons and markers, finger paints, or modeling clay. Small shells or seeds and projects involving scissors aren't a good choice for very young patients. Make sure you provide the patient with a variety of colors regardless of the medium he's using. He should be able to choose just the right color to express his mood, feeling, or memory.

Mask making is another powerful and popular form of art therapy used for both individuals and groups. Masks can be made from many materials, including paper bags, cardboard, Styrofoam, leather, wood, plaster, papier-mâché, and metal. Ready-made masks can be purchased and decorated. Masks may be used to mark a life passage (such as adolescence, adulthood, or elderhood) or to celebrate the successful completion of a healing process (such as a substance abuse program, a chemotherapy regimen, or an organ transplant).

Another form of art therapy, puppetry, can be as simple as creating hand puppets from socks or as involved as constructing marionettes, a stage, scenery, and a puppet theater. Cameras and computers are also being used as art therapy expands into photography, videography, and computer-generated art.

Procedure

Structuring the environment is an important component of art therapy. The patient should be as comfortable as possible, and the surroundings should be free from distractions. It's important to offer supportive feedback, not criticism or judgment. Only when the patient feels safe will he allow his hidden feelings to surface in his artwork.

Art therapy sessions are usually run by a facilitator. The AATA recommends that the facilitator be someone who is sensitive to human needs and expressions, emotionally stable, and patient. The facilitator should also have insight into the psychological process, attentive listening skills, keen observation skills, flexibility, a sense of humor, and an understanding of art media. Many nurses possess the skills necessary to act as a facilitator.

If you'll be acting as an art therapy facilitator, begin by explaining the procedure to the patient and asking his permission. Assess his need for special equipment, and ask him whether he prefers a particular art medium. Assemble the necessary materials, and provide a quiet, comfortable work area. Ideally, the work surface should be large and flat, but you may need to adapt the space around the patient, using an overbed table or a large clipboard. Reassure the patient that he doesn't need any special drawing talent and that stick figures can convey a message effectively. Praise all efforts the patient makes, and be careful not to make suggestions about colors. Remain nonjudgmental and supportive.

One approach is to encourage the patient to draw a picture representing himself in relation to his disease. For example, you can ask him to draw himself in the past (before the disease), now (with the disease), and in the future (after treatment). Another approach is to ask him to draw the disease. This method is commonly used with cancer patients to help them visually express the way they see their disease.

Allow the patient to complete the drawing to his satisfaction. Some patients may need to draw every minor detail and search for just the right color. When the drawing is finished, allow the patient to show it, and ask him to tell you about it. Listen attentively and reflect back to the patient what he has said to validate the meaning. Be supportive of his efforts, and summarize the experience for him.

When you look at the drawing, be alert for clues to the patient's feelings. Note how he represents himself in relation to other figures or objects in the drawing. Is the size proportional? Has he drawn his entire body? Does his face have a smile or a frown? Note the overall mood of the drawing. Even without formal training in art therapy, you can gain a great deal of insight from a drawing.

Document the outcome of your session and the patient's response. If appropriate, offer the patient an opportunity to draw again.

Complications
Before you begin a project, make sure the patient is physically capable of carrying it out. Some medications, a weakened condition, or inflamed or painful hand joints can interfere with the patient's ability to perform or complete an artistic task. Although no patient should be discouraged from trying, the inability to finish an art project may diminish the patient's self-esteem.

Strong emotions may surface as the patient explores his feelings about an illness through his artwork. If the patient shows signs of agitation or uncontrolled emotion, end the session, stay with the patient, and be empathetic. Reassure him that it's normal to have strong feelings and that it's all right to express them. Involve the appropriate member of the health care team: physician, social worker, or psychotherapist. If you make any referrals, document them in the patient's record.

Nursing perspective

▶ If the patient doesn't want to participate in an art session, don't insist; instead, work on building a trusting therapeutic relationship. The patient may be open to participating in the future.

▶ Patients who are physically unable to manipulate a crayon or paintbrush may be able to put together a collage or to finger paint. Allow them to choose pictures, words, colors, and placement to help them express their feelings.

▶ Although art therapy can be used with individuals, couples, families, and groups, it's particularly valuable with children, who often can't talk about their most painful and important concerns. Remember to get permission from the child's parents before beginning any art sessions. You may also want to provide young patients with art supplies so they can choose to draw on their own.

▶ Use art supplies that are age-specific — for example, nontoxic crayons and markers for young children prone to putting objects in the mouth.

▶ Be aware that the patient's images may change over time. Initially, they may be dark, strong, or heavy, with hard geometric shapes. As healing begins and the patient establishes trust with the therapist and the environment, the images typically become softer and more rounded, with less severe boundaries. The colors become lighter, and the drawings may contain representations of hope, freedom, or release, such as suns or rainbows.

▶ If the patient is especially proud of a piece of art, arrange to have it displayed so that others may admire it. Displaying the work is another source of acknowledgment for the patient.

▶ Teach the patient to keep a journal or log of daily, weekly, or periodic drawings as a useful personal coping mechanism. The log also helps voice negative or positive thoughts and feelings and serves as a personal diary or record of significant events.

Biofeedback

Biofeedback teaches people how to exert conscious control over various autonomic functions with the help of physiologic feedback. Monitoring of physiologic functioning can be simple or complex, depending on whether electronic machines are used. By observing the fluctuations of a particular bodily function — such as breathing, heart rate, or blood pressure — patients eventually learn how to adjust their reaction and thoughts in order to alter that autonomic response. By learning to modify vital functions at will, patients develop the ability to control certain conditions — such as high blood pressure — without the use of medications or other conventional medical treatments.

> 66 *In the early 1960s, an experimental psychologist showed that patients could learn how to control physiologic processes that were previously thought to be beyond voluntary control, such as heart rate, blood pressure, and GI function.* 99

The idea that people can control vital body processes voluntarily has been accepted in the West for only a few decades, but it has been practiced in the East, through meditation and yoga, for thousands of years. Today, biofeedback is widely used and approved by both conventional and alternative practitioners. It is popular with patients because it gives them a sense of control over their health problem and helps to lower health care costs; after 8 to 10 training sessions, the patient can usually learn to regulate the desired body process without the help of the monitoring device.

The most common forms of biofeedback are electromyographic (to measure muscle tension), thermal (to measure skin temperature), electrodermal (to measure the skin's electrical conductance), electroencephalographic (to measure brain wave activity), and respiration (to measure breathing rate). Although simple monitoring devices — such as a thermometer or blood pressure monitor — or basic pulse taking can be used, increasingly sophisticated devices are continually expanding the applications for biofeedback. For example, sensors can now monitor the action of the internal and external rectal sphincters, allowing treatment of fecal incontinence; the activity of the bladder's detrusor muscle, allowing treatment of urinary incontinence; as well as esophageal motility and stomach acidity, providing information on ulcers and esophageal reflux.

The origins of biofeedback date back to the early 1960s, when Neil Miller, an experimental psychologist, suggested that the autonomic nervous system could be "trained." In a series of experiments, he showed that patients could learn how to control physiologic processes that were previously thought to be beyond voluntary control, such as heart rate, blood pressure, and GI function.

Biofeedback began attracting widespread attention in the late 1960s, when researchers at the Menninger Foundation in Topeka, Kansas, discovered that elevating the temperature of the hands by biofeedback could alleviate migraine headaches. Since then, extensive research has led to numerous new applications for biofeedback as well as increasing acceptance by traditional health care providers, including medical doctors, physical therapists, psychiatrists, psychologists, and dentists.

Biofeedback practitioners need a firm grasp of both physiology and psychology. (In fact, many biofeedback therapists are trained psychologists.) The Biofeedback Certification Institute of America runs the major certification program for biofeedback practitioners and provides information about certified local practitioners.

Therapeutic uses

Biofeedback has more than 150 applications for disease prevention and health restoration. However, it's used most often for stress-related disorders, such as insomnia, anxiety, headaches, hypertension, asthma, GI disorders (ulcers, irritable bowel syndrome), temporomandibular joint syndrome, and hyperactivity in children. The American Medical Association has even endorsed electromyographic biofeedback for the treatment of muscle contraction headaches.

RESEARCH SUMMARY According to the 1994 report *Alternative Medicine: Expanding Medical Horizons,* extensive research (including about 3,000 articles and 100 books) has demonstrated biofeedback's effectiveness in treating alcoholism, drug abuse, tension and migraine headaches, chronic pain syndromes, cardiac arrhythmias, essential hypertension, irritable bowel syndrome, bronchial asthma, hyperactivity, attention deficit disorder, epilepsy, and hot flashes. Biofeedback is also effective in muscle reeducation and is the preferred treatment for Raynaud's disease and certain types of fecal and urinary incontinence.

Improvement has also been seen in patients with chronic pain, heart disease, difficulty swallowing, esophageal dysfunction, tinnitus, twitching of the eyelids, fatigue, and cerebral palsy. Biofeedback isn't recommended for severe structural problems, such as broken bones or slipped discs. ■

Equipment

The equipment needed for biofeedback training varies, depending on the targeted body function. Biofeedback machines are variations of common diagnostic monitoring systems that have been modified to produce a continuous flow of specific information to the patient. For instance, a biofeedback machine geared toward helping the patient lower his heart rate might be a cardiac monitor with a light that flashes each time the heart beats. For biofeedback training involving muscle control or activity, a modified electromyelograph might be used. Relaxation and emotional stress can be monitored using a modified electroencephalograph. Muscle tension can be monitored using an electromyograph.

Modified temperature probes are used in biofeedback training to treat migraines, hypertension, anxiety, and Raynaud's disease; lung volume measurements are used to train asthmatic patients to control their breathing; and modified sphygmomanometers are used to train patients to control hypertension. Some biofeedback machines require the use of special goggles to eliminate distractions, allowing the patient to focus on the feedback, which is projected on the inside of the goggle.

Electrodermal feedback (electrical conduction or resistance of the skin) allows an examiner to monitor changes in perspiration. Specialized motility sensors, which pick up movement of the GI tract, are used in the treatment of GI disorders. To treat curvature of the spine, a specialized biofeedback unit worn by the patient emits a soft beep if the patient slouches forward. If the patient doesn't straighten his posture, the device sounds a louder alarm.

Procedure

In a typical session, electrodes are attached to the area of the body being monitored, such as the head (for brain wave activity), the fingers (for pulse rate), or the muscles (for muscle tension). The electrodes feed information into a small monitoring box, which registers the results by a sound or light that varies in pitch or brightness as the body function fluctuates. A biofeedback practitioner interprets the signals and guides the patient in mental and physical exercises designed to help him achieve the desired result. The patient eventually trains himself to control his body's physiologic functions by altering thoughts, breathing, posture, or muscle tension. (See *Understanding biofeedback.*)

If you'll be helping in a biofeedback session, make sure the patient understands the procedure and has had his questions answered. Reassure him that biofeedback isn't a test he has to pass but is a learning experience. Depending on the body function that will be monitored, you may be asked to clean and prepare the patient's skin and attach the electrodes according to the manufacturer's instructions.

HOW IT WORKS

⟷ Understanding biofeedback

In biofeedback, the patient learns to change a specific body function, such as heart rate or skin temperature, by changing his thoughts, breathing pattern, posture, or muscle tension. To treat a patient with migraine headaches, for example, a special temperature probe monitors skin temperature, which reflects the amount of blood flowing beneath the skin. Temperature changes, reflecting vasoconstriction and vasodilation, are indicators of the stress response.

As the skin temperature fluctuates, lights on the monitor indicate the patient's response: black if he's tense, blue if he's relaxed. (Environmental conditions must be constant when monitoring skin temperature.) The therapist helps the patient interpret the signals and teaches him relaxation and imagery techniques designed to maintain a blue light. The patient repeats this process until he achieves the desired response—relief of his headaches.

At the end of the session, disconnect the monitor and remove the electrodes if the practitioner hasn't done so. Clean the patient's skin as needed. Document the length of the session, the patient's baseline measurement, and his best result. Also document the techniques used, identifying those that were successful and those that weren't as well as the patient's response to the session. If appropriate, arrange for a follow-up session for the patient. Assign homework practice of the behavioral technique used such as relaxation procedures.

Complications
Patients may experience local skin irritation from the electrodes used in biofeedback monitoring. Wash the skin well with soap and water to remove any remaining irritants, and pat it dry. Notify the physician, and document your findings and interventions.

Nursing perspective
▶ Biofeedback is contraindicated in patients with low blood pressure, psychiatric disorders (including severe depression), impaired attention or memory, or mental disabilities such as dementia.

▶ Make sure the patient continues to take prescribed medications, such as antihypertensives, while receiving biofeedback training.

▶ Minimize distractions during the biofeedback session; they can prevent the patient from focusing and achieving optimum results.

▶ Clean electrodes properly between patients, and alternate electrode placement sites to reduce associated skin irritation.

Dance therapy

A major movement therapy, dance therapy (also known as dance movement therapy) capitalizes on the direct relationship between body movement and the mind. The music, rhythm, and synchronous movement associated with dance are believed to promote healing by improving mood, reducing social isolation, awakening old memories and feelings, and enhancing overall well-being. (See *Understanding dance therapy.*)

HOW IT WORKS

↶ Understanding dance therapy

In dance therapy, visible movement is thought to represent personality. Practitioners of this therapy believe that in changing the way a person moves, dance therapy changes the way the total person functions. For instance, in a patient with a disorganized personality who has fragmented movement, moving toward integrated or graceful movements theoretically will also integrate and organize the personality.

The physical activity entailed in dance therapy increases levels of endorphins, naturally occurring proteins in the brain that inhibit the transmission of pain impulses. The result is a naturally induced state of well-being. Movement of the whole body stimulates the circulatory, respiratory, skeletal, and neuromuscular systems. Additionally, the activation of muscles and joints reduces body tension. Practitioners believe that these physical effects, together with the relationship between physical movement and personality, bring about dance therapy's therapeutic effects.

Used throughout history to celebrate major events and heal the sick, dance was first adopted as a medical therapy in the United States in 1942. Dance teacher Marian Chace was asked to work with psychiatric patients at a Washington, D.C., hospital after psychiatrists found that her dance classes seemed to benefit patients who were considered too disturbed to join in other group activities. Chace's work paralleled the work of Trudi Schoop, a dancer and mime who worked with noncommunicative patients in California.

Today, dance therapists typically work with people who have emotional, social, cognitive, or physical problems. Depending on the goal, dance therapy can be done alone, with a partner, or in a group. Range-of-motion exercises set to music or formal dance routines may be used in individual dance therapy. Group dance, probably the most common form of dance therapy, allows people of different physical abilities to participate. By tapping their feet or patting their thighs in time to the music, patients can feel as if they're part of the session. Dance routines range from simple clapping and swaying to intricate aerobic sessions.

Founded in 1956, the American Dance Therapy Association (ADTA) promotes research, monitors standards for professional practice, and develops guidelines for graduate education. It also publishes the *American Journal of Dance Therapy* and maintains a registry of therapists. The ADTA offers a registered dance therapist certification to professionals who have a master's degree and complete a supervised clinical internship. After an extended period of supervised work, the therapist is awarded the Academy of Dance Therapists Registered certification, which qualifies her to teach, supervise, and engage in private practice.

Therapeutic uses
Dance therapy has been shown to improve the condition of patients with emotional, cognitive, or physical problems as well as elderly people suffering from impaired mobility and social isolation. For emotionally disturbed patients, dance can help reduce depression and anxiety, lead to greater self-awareness, and provide a means of expressing feelings and developing relationships. For cognitively impaired patients, including those with mental retardation, dance is used to motivate learning, increase body awareness, and develop social and communication skills. For physically disabled patients, dance improves movement and circulation, enhances self-esteem, and provides a creative outlet that is fun. For elderly patients, dance can help maintain or improve physical mobility; enhance flexibility, circulation, and respiratory function; improve vitality and self-esteem; reduce isolation; and assist with the expression of fear and grief.

Dance therapy is also used to reduce stress for patients with cancer, acquired immunodeficiency syndrome, or Alzheimer's disease and for their caregivers. Healthy people use dance therapy to help prevent disease and maintain well-being because it promotes flexibility, strengthens muscles, and improves cardiovascular and pulmonary function. As an added benefit, the interaction with others provides socialization, touch, and a sense of connectedness.

Equipment
Adequate space and enjoyable music are the only types of "equipment" needed for dance therapy. The music should be appropriate to the population, both in its pace and aesthetic

appeal. A group of agile senior citizens probably wouldn't enjoy fast-moving rock and roll as much as a fast polka. Faster music can be used to stimulate the group; slower music, to provide a calming effect.

Arrange the space to accommodate free movement of the participants. Arrange chairs around the periphery for those who can't participate while standing or who become tired during the session.

Procedure

If you'll be assisting in a dance session, begin by assessing the group for risk factors. The presence of one or more risk factors doesn't preclude group members from participating but may influence the type of dance and the length of the session. Risk factors to consider include poor cardiovascular status and a history of chronic obstructive pulmonary disease or degenerative musculoskeletal problems. Muscle atrophy or obesity and the participant's exercise history should also be considered along with the use of tobacco or alcohol.

After the dance therapist chooses appropriate music and dance, arrange the room and introduce the participants. Explain the purpose of the session, and encourage everyone to participate according to ability. Circulate through the group during the dance, providing encouragement and motivation to those who are hesitant. Always praise the participants' efforts.

After the session, document the type of activity and the group's response. Encourage the participants to discuss the feelings they experienced while dancing.

Complications

Because dancing is an aerobic activity, patients may experience signs and symptoms of cardiovascular compromise, such as dizziness, flushing, profuse sweating, and disorientation. Dizziness may also be a result of rapid motion. Group members who exercise strenuously may experience muscle soreness or strain.

Nursing perspective

▶ If your patient experiences signs of cardiovascular compromise, help him to a seated position and obtain his vital signs.

Compare the readings to the patient's baseline, and notify the physician of any changes.

▶ If your patient experiences muscle soreness, immobilize the affected body part, notify the physician, and apply cold or heat therapy as ordered.

RESEARCH SUMMARY   The concepts behind dance therapy and the claims made haven't been scientifically proven. ■

Gem therapy

Since ancient times, people have believed that crystals have supernatural powers. Throughout history, people have worn crystals in amulets, as love tokens, and for simple decoration in jewelry. Wearing crystals often brought a sense of peace to the wearer, and over time healers began to use crystals to affect healing of various illnesses.

Renewed awareness of the various uses for crystals began in the late 1970s, with the increasing use of crystals as tools to help people focus energy. Human problems are seen as a result of blockages, congestion, and depletion of energy, and the universe as a field of energy with different levels that flow into one another. Crystals are used to detect and clear blockages in the body's energy flow, bringing it back into alignment and harmony with the universal energy flow.

Crystals are said to increase the effects of other healing modalities — for example, acupuncture is believed to be 10% to 12% more successful when the needles are coated with quartz crystal. Proponents believe that crystals can enhance muscle testing and protect wearers from some radiation. It has been shown that simply wearing or putting a crystal in the home or workspace has positive effects. People occasionally experience feelings of discomfort when wearing a particular piece of jewelry; it's believed that the feeling is caused by the energy level of the crystals in the jewelry.

In general, the colors of crystals correspond to the seven main colors of the visible spectrum and each, in turn, resonates with one of the seven primary chakras. (See *Gemstones and the seven primary chakras*.)

Therapeutic uses

Crystalline structures can collect, focus, and emit electromagnetic energy; they transmit and receive radio waves, power

Gemstones and the seven primary chakras

Chakra	Color	Crystals
Root chakra	Red	Ruby and garnet
Sacral	Orange	Carnelian and orange jasper
Solar plexus	Yellow	Amber, citrine, and yellow topaz
Heart	Green	Emerald and malachite
Throat	Blue	Sapphire and lapis lazuli
Brow	Violet	Amethyst and violet fluorite
Crown	Magenta	Rose quartz

quartz watches, set timers on computers, and release the sound recorded on records. Crystals are believed to affect the body by influencing the etheric layer, located 2″ to 4″ (5 to 10 cm) from the body and just outside our visual range. Crystals are used as guides to help focus energies and put us in touch with the universal forces around us. Crystals aren't forces themselves, but merely reflect energy, amplify it, and tune it for our use. Crystals are used as guides into the world of spiritual awareness.

Combinations of crystals can be used to treat various disorders. For example, allergies may be treated with blue lace agate, picture jasper, and rhodonite; blocks and resistances may respond to amethyst, aqua aura, and rainbow fluorite or sugilite, diamond, and bustamite; hyperthyroidism may be treated with rhyolite, emerald, and any brown stone. Crystals may also be used to obtain positive results — for example, a person seeking business success may use amber, azeztulite, turquoise, picture jasper, or topaz. Citrine is used for those most resistant to treatment; herkimer is useful to affect dreams; smoky quartz is a grounding tool that helps the wearer regain contact with reality; aquamarine is used for reconciliation, phobias, paralyzing fears, and human relations in general; and red coral is used to promote the growth of bone cells.

RESEARCH SUMMARY The concepts behind the use of gem therapy and the claims made regarding its effects haven't been scientifically proven. ■

Equipment

Various crystals are used for different purposes, and the place of therapy may also change depending on the area to be treated. For example, amethysts are related to transformation and travel and may therefore be kept in the car to enhance safety. They're also used to treat addictions and other excesses — for example, it's believed that placing a small piece of amethyst under the tongue for 10 minutes will help the patient stop smoking.

Procedure

Crystals are typically "programmed" before they're used — that is, they're charged and empowered with the intended use. Fundamental laws for programming a crystal include:

▶ compassion — the desire to relieve the patient's suffering
▶ nonattachment — objectivity regarding results, awareness of the patient's responsibility to heal himself
▶ intention — the end result or outcome.

With these feelings in mind, the practitioner cups the crystal in his hands and gently breathes on it, thereby charging it with the intended purpose. A charged crystal may be used for up to 28 days.

Crystals are used in various ways. Practitioners of Reiki, a Japanese method that uses the laying on of hands to facilitate healing, may select nine crystals in different colors and lay one on each of the seven main chakras, one between the feet, and one in the practitioner's hand. People react very strongly to colors, both visually and through the chakras. Each chakra is stimulated and supported by the color energy of the crystals. Red garnet may be used to activate joy, orange amber to facilitate success in life, and dark blue lapis lazuli to strengthen faith and peace. Alternatively, the practitioner may select seven crystals of the same type to stimulate the same aspect of all the chakras. Crystals may be placed directly on the chakra for 20 to 45 minutes.

A technique used by Ayurvedic and gemstone therapists in India for many years calls for gemstone powders to be ingested after being burned to ash. Crystals may also be ingested in the form of gem elixirs, which are prepared in a manner similar to flower essences — the gem is placed in a clear bowl of water and the bowl set in bright morning sunlight for several hours. It's believed that the magnetic influence of solar power energetically imprints some of the subtle energy pattern of the gem into the water. The resulting elixir is then placed, several drops at a time, under the tongue. Two unique gem elixirs are prepared from the magnetic materials of lodestone and magnetite. Lodestone is said to align our physical body's biomagnetic field with the earth's magnetic field. It's also a general tonic for the endocrine system and may also be valuable in stimulating tissue regeneration, balancing the acupuncture meridians and the opposing forces of yin and yang, and helping with detoxifying the body after exposure to radiation. The elixir of magnetite is said to enhance blood circulation as well as energize and align the chakras, meridians, and subtle or spiritual bodies.

To protect the crystal, it should be wrapped in leather or 100% cotton, silk, wool, or linen fabric, which is always red in color. (It's believed that red has the slowest rate of absorption of luminous vibrations.) If the crystal is worn, it should be placed between the heart and solar plexus chakras, with the point down; if double pointed, both points should be left unwrapped.

Complications
No adverse effects are associated with the use of most crystals. However, amethysts shouldn't be used by those with hyperactivity, schizophrenia, or mental retardation.

Nursing perspective
▶ Consider having a cleaned crystal in the office to enhance a healing environment.
▶ Using crystals for healing requires reading and training with a knowledgeable practitioner.

Hypnosis
Used to manage numerous medical and psychological problems, hypnosis applies the power of suggestion and altered

levels of consciousness to effect positive changes in behavior and treat a range of health conditions. Under hypnosis, the patient can experience relaxation and changes in respiration, which can lead to a positive shift in behavior and an enhanced sense of well-being. Physiologically, the hypnotic state can give the patient greater control over his autonomic nervous system, functions that would ordinarily be considered beyond his control.

> ❝ Under hypnosis, a person is very susceptible to suggestion. However, the person must be willing to follow the suggestions offered: he can't be hypnotized to follow suggestions that go against his wishes. ❞

Defined as a state of attentive and focused concentration, *hypnosis* leaves people relatively unaware of their surroundings. In this state of concentration, a person is very susceptible to suggestion. However, the person must be *willing* to follow the suggestions offered; he can't be hypnotized to follow suggestions that go against his wishes.

The three major components of hypnosis are absorption, dissociation, and responsiveness. *Absorption* refers to the rapt attention that the subject pays to the words or images that the hypnotherapist presents. The subject then begins to *dissociate* from his ordinary consciousness and surroundings and becomes *responsive* to the therapist's suggestions. To bring the subject to a hypnotic state, the therapist leads him through relaxation, mental imagery, and suggestions. The subject can also be taught to hypnotize himself. The therapist may provide the patient with audiotapes to enable him to practice the therapy at home.

There are actually two states of hypnosis: the superficial state and the deeper somnambulistic state. In the superficial hypnotic state, the patient accepts suggestions but doesn't necessarily carry them out. In the somnambulistic state, the patient is better able to carry out suggestions made during the trance once the session has ended. Although an estimated 90% of the population can be hypnotized, only 20% to 30% are susceptible enough to enter the somnambulistic state, making them good candidates for treatment. (See *Understanding hypnosis*.)

A part of healing since ancient times, hypnosis was a central feature of early Greek healing temples. Modern applications date back to the 18th century, when Viennese physician Franz Anton Mesmer used what he called "animal magnetism" to treat various psychological and physiologic disorders, such as hysterical blindness, paralysis, headaches, and joint pain. Using iron rods along with soothing words and gestures, Mesmer claimed he could realign his patients' "magnetic fluids." Although his magnetism theory was disproved, Mesmer's practices laid the foundation for hypnotherapy by demonstrating that medical conditions could be affected by the power of suggestion. Sigmund Freud also used hypnosis until he became uncomfortable with the powerful emotions it evoked in his patients.

The American Medical Association recognized hypnotism as a legitimate practice in 1958. Although it still isn't completely understood, hypnosis has become accepted and has been used by a growing number of physicians, dentists, psychologists, and other mental health professionals in recent years.

The American Society of Clinical Hypnosis is the professional organization for physicians and dentists in the field. Training and certification are provided by the American Institute of Hypnotherapy for hypnotherapists and by the International Medical and Dental Hypnotherapy Association for physicians,

---

HOW IT WORKS

⮂ Understanding hypnosis

Under hypnosis, the patient experiences a general decrease in sympathetic nervous system activity, a decrease in oxygen consumption and carbon dioxide elimination, a decrease in blood pressure and heart rate, and an increase in certain types of brain wave activity. These physiologic effects resemble those associated with other forms of deep relaxation.

Exactly how this state of relaxation makes the subject more receptive to suggestion isn't known. One theory, based on the results of a 1978 study, is that the left side of the brain (the center for verbalization) is less active under hypnosis and that the right side then "hears" messages that can be used to transform the body.

dentists, and hypnotherapists. The National Guild of Hypno-
tists is the oldest certifying guild in the United States.

Therapeutic uses

Hypnotherapy has therapeutic application for both psychological and physical disorders. A competent hypnotherapist can
facilitate the patient with profound changes in respiration and
relaxation, so that positive shifts in behavior and enhanced
physiologic well-being can occur. Almost any ailment that the
mind can affect lends itself to hypnosis. Hypnosis has been
shown to be effective in managing pain (including pain associated with dentistry and childbirth), reducing anxiety, and enhancing immune system function. As a method of pain management, hypnosis helps patients gain control over the fear and
anxiety typically associated with pain, thereby also reducing
the pain. In dentistry, hypnotherapy is used to replace or supplement anesthesia, to reduce anxiety and postprocedural discomfort, and to control bleeding.

Pregnant women who receive hypnosis before delivery have
reported having shorter, less painful labor and delivery. People
with phobias, such as fear of flying or stage fright, can learn to
establish a new response to the trigger activity through hypnosis. Hypnosis has even been used to help people stop smoking
and to reduce bleeding in hemophiliacs. (See *Indications for
hypnosis.*)

RESEARCH SUMMARY Controlled studies have shown that hypnosis effectively treats childhood migraine headaches. A 1989
study of pain in chronically ill patients showed that those who
underwent hypnosis increased their pain tolerance by 113%.
Studies have also shown positive effects on the immune system, including increased immunoglobulin levels in children and
increased white blood cell activity. Other reports have noted
success in treating hay fever, asthma, warts, and allergic reactions.

One of the most unusual uses of hypnosis is in the treatment of a genetic skin disorder known as ichthyosis, in which
the skin is covered with a hard, wartlike crust. This condition
was considered incurable until an anesthesiologist used hypnosis on a teenager he thought had warts. After the hypnosis,
the scaly crust fell off, and within 10 days, normal skin replaced it. Since then, hypnosis has often been used to treat

Indications for hypnosis

Hypnotherapy can be used to treat the following conditions:

- behavioral problems
- childbirth
- chronic pain
- depression
- facial neuralgia
- headaches
- ichthyosis
- low self-esteem
- menstrual pain
- osteoarthritis
- pain and anxiety associated with dental procedures
- phobias
- reflex sympathetic dystrophy
- rheumatoid arthritis
- sciatica
- surgical anesthesia
- tennis elbow
- traumatic memories
- whiplash.

this condition, usually resulting in a major improvement, if not a complete cure.

Research has demonstrated that a person's body chemistry actually changes during a hypnotic trance. In one experiment, a young girl was unable to hold her hand in a bucket of ice water for more than 30 seconds. Testing showed that blood cortisol levels were high, which indicated that she was experiencing severe stress. Under hypnosis, however, she was indeed able to keep her hand in ice water for 30 minutes with no rise in blood cortisol levels. ■

Equipment

Hypnosis requires a quiet, private environment that's free from distractions and has a comfortable place for the patient to recline. It also requires the subject's willingness and desire to be hypnotized.

Procedure

Hypnotherapy should be performed only by a qualified practitioner. The hypnotherapist will begin by addressing any concerns the patient has and illustrating how suggestion works in everyday life. The hypnotherapist will also explain what to expect while in the trance — namely, physical relaxation, distraction of the conscious mind, a narrowed focus of attention, increased sensory awareness, reduced awareness of physical surroundings, and increased awareness of internal sensations.

The therapist may test the subject for suggestibility. The therapist will then ask the patient to concentrate on an object or the sound of his voice as he guides the patient into a state of relaxation. The therapist may express suggestions, such as "your eyelids are growing heavy," to help induce the hypnotic state. The sessions usually last from 60 to 90 minutes, depending on the goal and the patient's receptivity.

After the session, document any changes in behavior or answers to questions the patient provided while in the hypnotic state. Include the patient's response to the session.

Complications
Because it deals with subconscious areas of the mind, hypnosis may elicit disturbing emotions or memories. If the patient becomes upset or aggressive or exhibits strong negative emotions, the hypnotherapist should redirect him to a safe memory and terminate the session, staying with him until another qualified professional arrives.

Nursing perspective
▶ According to the World Health Organization, patients with psychosis, organic psychiatric conditions, or antisocial personality disorders shouldn't be treated with hypnosis.
▶ Although hypnosis sessions usually involve only the therapist and the subject, if they're of the opposite sex, it may be prudent to have a nurse or assistant attend sessions as a safeguard against liability.
▶ Be aware that some patients experience light-headedness or psychological reactions after hypnosis. Be prepared to deal with these effects if they arise.

Imagery
Imagery is a mind-body technique in which patients use the imagination to promote relaxation, relieve symptoms (or better cope with them), and heal disease. It doesn't always involve *visualization*—the act of picturing something in one's mind; it can involve mentally hearing, feeling, smelling, or tasting as well. Like other alternative therapies—such as biofeedback, hypnosis, and meditation—imagery is based on the principle that the mind and body are dramatically interconnected and can work together to encourage healing.

Imagery has been used for therapeutic
least the Middle Ages, when Tibetan monks
visualize the Buddha healing diseases. Today, i
cessfully used to control pain in various settings,
immune function in elderly patients, and as an adjun
apy for a number of diseases, including diabetes mellit
agery is widely used in cancer patients to help mobilize th
mune system, to alleviate the nausea and vomiting associate
with chemotherapy, to relieve pain and stress, and to promote
weight gain. It's also used in many cardiac rehabilitation programs and centers specializing in chronic pain.

According to imagery advocates, people with strong imagi-
nations — those who can literally "worry themselves sick," —
are excellent candidates for using imagery to positively affect
their health. Like other relaxation techniques, imagery has
documented physiologic effects: It can lower blood pressure,
decrease heart rate, affect brain wave activity, increase oxygen supply to the tissues, promote vascular dilation, increase
salivation, and alter skin temperature, cochlear and pupillary
reflexes, galvanic skin response, and GI activity. Advocates believe imagery enhances the effectiveness of conventional medical treatments by allowing them to work in less time and by
minimizing their adverse effects. (See *Understanding imagery*,
page 154.)

Palming and guided imagery are two of the more popular
imaging techniques. In *palming*, the patient places the palms
over his closed eyes and tries to fill the entire field of vision
with only the color black. The patient then tries to picture the
black changing to a color associated with stress, such as red,
and then mentally replaces that color with one found to be
soothing, such as pale blue. In *guided imagery*, the patient is
asked to visualize a desired goal and then picture taking action
to achieve it. An example is the pioneering technique developed by radiation oncologist O. Carl Simonton in the 1970s,
which calls for cancer patients to visualize their white blood
cells destroying cancer cells, much like the video Pac-Man
characters swallowing their victims. This type of therapy is intended to complement traditional cancer treatments, not replace them.

The Academy for Guided Imagery in Mill Valley, California,
trains health professionals in the use of interactive guided imagery, publishes a directory of imagery professionals, and pro-

purposes since at
reportedly tried to
magery is suc-
to enhance
ctive ther-
s. Im-
e im-

gery

y that messages can be sent
here images are located, to
gic functions (such as
d pressure, digestion, im-
arise from unconscious
ved to be located in the
ed to smell or feelings may
primitive brain centers. The regulation of wak-
ing and sleeping rhythms, hunger, thirst, and sexual function may
also be affected through imagery.

Picturing brain activity

Using positron emission tomography scanners, scientists have
been able to visualize the areas of the brain that are active as a
person performs certain tasks. For example, the optic cortex,
which is active when a person is looking at something, is also active when a person visualizes. The auditory cortex is active when a
person imagines hearing things, and the sensory cortex is active
when a person imagines feeling things.

Practitioners of guided imagery believe that if the cortex can
create these imaginary realities, the lower centers of the nervous
system—in the absence of conflicting information—can respond
to them. This theory is the basis of *sensory recruitment,* an imagery
approach that uses as many senses as possible. By stimulating various senses, this form of imagery increases the amount of information sent through the lower brain centers and autonomic nervous
system, increasing the likelihood of achieving the desired response.

vides educational materials and tapes for professionals and
laypeople. Practitioners who complete a 150-hour program
can obtain certification in guided imagery.

Therapeutic uses

In addition to its documented effectiveness in reducing pain
and inducing relaxation, imagery can also be an effective tool
for reducing adverse effects of conventional treatments, stimulating the body's healing response, and helping patients tolerate medical procedures. Imagery also facilitates recovery and

can strengthen coping skills in patients with acute or chronic illness. It has also been used to help patients clarify attitudes, emotions, behaviors, and lifestyle patterns that may be central to an illness. As an active means of relaxation, imagery is a central part of almost all stress-reduction techniques. (See *Indications for imagery,* page 156.)

Imagery can benefit almost any medical situation in which problem solving, decision making, relaxation, or symptom relief is useful. It has even been used successfully to help people prepare for surgery and to speed postsurgical recovery. Additionally, imagery is a useful self-care tool. With proper instruction, patients can use imagery to relieve stress, enhance immune function to fight a cold virus, and improve their sense of well-being.

RESEARCH SUMMARY Numerous studies have documented imagery's ability to produce the physiologic and biochemical changes listed above. Although most of the research evidence is based on small, unreplicated studies, the 1994 report to the National Institutes of Health concludes that "there is a relationship between imagery of bodily change and actual bodily change. Without question, imagery calls for further and more precise investigation." ■

Equipment

For imagery to be successful, the patient will need a private, quiet environment that's free from distractions and has a comfortable place in which to lie down. If a taped imagery sequence will be used, make sure the tape player is working and that the room has an electrical outlet.

Procedure

Imagery can be practiced by an individual alone or led by a trained practitioner. Sessions with a therapist usually last 20 to 30 minutes. A variety of imagery techniques and paths can be used. The sample path described below, which focuses on relaxation, is one that most nurses could conduct in almost any health care setting. For sessions that focus on altering specific disease states, the nurse should consult with a professional trained in imagery techniques.

Gather any supplies you'll need, and wash your hands. Help the patient into a comfortable position, and explain the exercise. Reassure the patient that he doesn't have to participate,

Indications for imagery

Imagery may facilitate smoking cessation as well as help treat the following conditions:

- allergies
- anxiety
- asthma
- cancer
- cardiac arrhythmias (benign)
- chronic fatigue syndrome
- chronic pain
- cold symptoms
- dysmenorrhea
- excessive uterine bleeding
- fibromyalgia
- flu symptoms
- functional urinary complaints
- GI symptoms related to stress
- headaches
- hypertension
- menstrual irregularity
- multiple sclerosis
- premenstrual syndrome
- sprains and strains
- surgical recovery.

and answer any questions he may have. When the patient is comfortable, instruct him to close his eyes. If possible, lower the lights.

Use a steady, soothing, low voice throughout the exercise. Instruct the patient to take a few deep breaths and to imagine that with each breath, he's taking in calmness and peacefulness and releasing tension, discomfort, and worry. Tell the patient to let his breath find its own natural rate and rhythm and to continue to breathe in calmness and peacefulness and breathe out tension and worry.

Help the patient to relax his body. Instruct him to imagine that he's breathing calmness into his feet and legs and releasing tension with each exhalation. Continue this sequence, moving from feet to head, having the patient breathe calmness into each successive body part. Remind him not to make any effort during this process but to let it happen in its own natural way. As you complete this portion of the exercise, remind the patient to let his whole body sink into a peaceful, relaxed state.

Next, tell the patient to imagine himself being in a place that's peaceful and beautiful. Suggest that he choose a place he has visited or imagined or a special place where he would like to be. Encourage the patient to notice the details in this place — the colors, shapes, and living things found there. Have him think about the sounds and smells of the place and pay attention to any feelings of peacefulness and relaxation.

Allow the patient to spend as long as desired in this place; tell him that when he's ready, he should allow the images to fade and should slowly bring himself back to the outer world. Remain quiet until the patient opens his eyes. If he's willing, discuss the experience with him, concentrating on the positive feelings of relaxation and peace. Document the length of the session, the imagery path used, and the patient's response.

Complications

One of the benefits of imagery is the relative absence of complications. Occasionally, an imagery session may lead a person to remember an unpleasant period or event in his life. If that occurs, stop the session and encourage the patient to tell you what he was seeing and feeling. If the patient becomes upset, stay with him. When possible, notify the health care provider.

Nursing perspective

▶ Imagery is contraindicated in psychotic patients.

▶ To enhance the effects of imagery, consider adding a smell to trigger the image that the patient is trying to experience.

▶ Be aware that patients with breathing problems may have difficulty controlling their breathing.

▶ Taking the patient's pulse and blood pressure before and after guided imagery helps the patient understand the physiologic benefits of guided imagery.

Meditation

The ancient art of meditation — focusing one's attention on a single sound or image or simply on the rhythm of one's own breathing — has been found to have positive effects on health. By directing attention away from worries about the future or preoccupation with the past, meditation reduces stress, a major contributing factor in many health problems. Stress reduction in turn results in a wide range of physiologic and mental health benefits, from decreased oxygen consumption, heart rate, and respiratory rate to improved mood, spiritual calm, and heightened awareness.

Most meditation approaches fall into one of two techniques: concentrative meditation or mindful meditation. *Concentrative meditation* involves focusing on an image, a sound (called a mantra), or one's own breathing. For example, by concentrating on the continuous rhythm of inhalation and exhalation, the meditating person slows and deepens breathing—a physiologic benefit—and achieves a state of calm and heightened awareness. *Transcendental meditation,* a form of concentrative meditation that became popular in the 1960s, arose out of the practice of yoga (discussed later in this chapter). In this form of meditation, the individual repeats a mantra over and over again while sitting in a comfortable position. When other thoughts enter his mind, he's instructed to notice them and return to the mantra. Concentrating on the mantra prevents any distracting thoughts.

Mindful meditation takes the opposite approach. Instead of focusing on a single sensation or sound, the individual is aware of all sensations, feelings, images, thoughts, sounds, and smells that pass through his mind without actually thinking about them. The goal is a calmer, clearer, nonreactive state of mind.

> **❝The National Institutes of Health now recommends meditation as a first-line treatment for mild hypertension. ❞**

Although meditation is primarily associated with Eastern religions, variations can be found in nearly all cultures and religions. For example, saying the Christian rosary or "Hail Mary" can be considered a form of meditation. The Chinese practice of tai chi chuan (discussed later in this chapter), Japanese aikido, and Zen Buddhist walking meditation are forms of moving meditation. Yoga is also considered a form of meditation.

The health benefits of meditation have long been recognized in the East; however, only in the past 2 decades has meditation become widely accepted in the West, largely as a result of Harvard professor Herbert Benson's pioneering research in the 1970s on the physiologic effects of transcendental meditation. (See *Relaxation response,* pages 160 and 161.) Since that time, instruction in meditation has been added to the curriculum of hundreds of universities and medical schools (including Harvard, whose Mind-Body Medical Institute is run by Benson), and the National Institutes of Health (NIH) now recommends meditation as a first-line treatment for mild hypertension.

Patients interested in learning meditation can get help from many kinds of health care providers, including mental health practitioners, stress-reduction experts, and yoga teachers. Numerous hospitals and clinics offer classes in meditation as part of stress-reduction programs. The Institute of Noetic Sciences in Sausalito, California, is an information resource.

Therapeutic uses

Meditation has a wide variety of indications. It's used to enhance immune function in patients with cancer, acquired immunodeficiency syndrome, and autoimmune disorders and has been successful in treating drug and alcohol addiction as well as posttraumatic stress disorder. Anxiety disorders, pain, and stress are also commonly treated with meditation. Many mainstream medical practitioners recommend meditation in conjunction with dietary and lifestyle changes for patients with hypertension or heart disease.

Because meditation is so suited to self-care, an increasing number of healthy people are incorporating it into an overall wellness strategy. According to the 1994 report to the NIH *Alternative Medicine: Expanding Medical Horizons,* "If practiced regularly, meditation develops habitual, unconscious microbehaviors that produce widespread positive effects on physical and psychological functioning. Meditating for even 15 minutes twice a day seems to bring beneficial results."

RESEARCH SUMMARY   Since Dr. Herbert Benson's studies on transcendental meditation in the 1970s, numerous other research centers have published studies documenting meditation's effectiveness in reducing anxiety, chronic pain, serum cholesterol levels, high blood pressure (in the population at large and in blacks specifically), and substance abuse; cutting health care costs; and enhancing quality of life. Over the past 25 years, Benson and his colleagues also have continued to produce volumes of research on the benefits of the relaxation response.

Despite this evidence, most mainstream medical practitioners still regard meditation as an unconventional practice and overlook it as a potential therapy. The NIH report urges them

Relaxation response

In 1968, a group of transcendental meditation (TM) practitioners came to Dr. Herbert Benson at his laboratory at Harvard Medical School and asked if he would study them because they believed that TM could lower their blood pressure. After initially dismissing the idea, Benson changed his mind and began a study of volunteers who had been practicing TM for less than 1 month to more than 9 years.

The volunteers were studied for 20- to 30-minute periods before, during, and after meditation. The results were startling. Benson found that during meditation:

▶ oxygen consumption decreased markedly
▶ metabolism decreased
▶ heart and respiratory rates decreased
▶ alpha waves (associated with a feeling of well-being) increased in intensity and frequency
▶ levels of blood lactate (a substance produced by skeletal muscle metabolism and associated with anxiety) decreased.

All of these physiologic changes were similar to feats observed in highly trained yoga and Zen masters with 15 to 20 years of experience in meditation. The one measurement that was unchanged during meditation was blood pressure. That value was low before, during, *and* after meditation. Benson reasoned that perhaps the volunteers had low blood pressure because of their practice of meditation. He con-

Technique	Oxygen consumption	Respiratoy rate
Transcendental meditation	Decreases	Decreases
Zen and yoga	Decreases	Decreases
Autogenic training	Not measured	Decreases
Progressive relaxation	Not measured	Not measured
Hypnosis with suggested deep relaxation	Decreases	Decreases

Adapted with permission from Benson, H. *The Relaxation Response.* New York: William Morrow & Co., 1975.

to reconsider, concluding that "given their low cost and demonstrated health benefits, [meditation techniques] may be some of the best candidates among the alternative therapies cluded that if this was true, people with hypertension might be able to lower their blood pressure through meditation.

Protective response to stress

Further experiments over several years led Benson to conclude that the various hypometabolic changes that accompanied TM were part of an integrated response opposite to the fight-or-flight response and that they were in no way unique to TM. Just as humans have an innate way of reacting to stress—the fight-or-flight response—they also have a natural protective mechanism against overstress, which Benson called the *relaxation response.*

By learning to consciously activate the relaxation response through such techniques as TM and yoga, Benson theorized, humans could off-set the negative physiologic effects caused by stress and ultimately prevent ravaging diseases, such as hypertension, strokes, and heart attacks. Benson's work ultimately played a large part in changing the attitudes of conventional medicine toward meditation—from regarding it as a dubious practice to viewing it as a technique that could indeed have a positive effect on health. The chart below outlines the practices that produced the physical changes of the relaxation response in Benson's studies.

Heart rate	Alpha waves	Blood pressure	Muscle tension
Decreases	Increase	May decrease in hypertension	Not measured
Decreases	Increase	May decrease in hypertension	Not measured
Decreases	Increase	Inconclusive	Decreases
Not measured	Not measured	Inconclusive	Decreases
Decreases	Not measured	Inconclusive	Not measured

for widespread inclusion in medical practice and for investment of medical resources." ■

Equipment

To assist your patient with meditation, you'll need a private, quiet environment that's free from distractions and offers a comfortable place for your patient to sit or recline.

Procedure

Nurses and other health professionals can obtain the same benefits from meditation as patients. If you learn how to meditate and find it relaxes you or provides some other therapeutic benefit, you can then teach interested patients the techniques you've learned. (See *Basic requirements for relaxation*.) The simple meditation exercise described here can be used in most settings.

If you'll be helping a patient with meditation, begin by explaining the procedure and answering any questions. Tell the patient that he can stop the exercise at any time if he becomes uncomfortable. Help the patient into a comfortable position. If he's in a sitting position, ask him to keep his back straight and let his shoulders drop.

Using a calm, soothing, low voice, instruct the patient to close his eyes, if doing so feels comfortable. Tell him to focus on the abdomen, feeling it rise with each inhalation and fall with each exhalation. Tell him to concentrate on his breathing. Explain that if his mind wanders off his breathing, he should simply bring it back, regardless of what the thought was. Have the patient practice this exercise for 15 minutes every day for a week; then evaluate its benefits. Remember to document the session, the instructions you gave the patient, and his response. You may want to record the patient's heart rate, respiratory rate, and blood pressure before and after a meditation session. You may also want to note any changes in pain or anxiety levels at the end of a session and document those changes.

Complications

Occasionally, meditation may elicit negative emotions, disorientation, or memories of early childhood abuses and other traumas. Although this is more common with imagery, be prepared to deal with an upset patient. If possible, find out what the feeling or memory concerns and direct the patient to a safer, more pleasant thought or memory. If this isn't possible,

Basic requirements for relaxation

According to Dr. Herbert Benson, the Harvard professor who first described the relaxation response, four basic elements are needed to elicit this response:

▶ quiet environment (absence of external distractions)
▶ object to dwell upon (such as the pattern of one's own breathing or the mantra used in transcendental meditation)
▶ passive attitude (emptying the mind of all thoughts and distractions; if thoughts or images enter the consciousness, one should let them pass and return to the object being dwelled upon; possibly the most important element in eliciting the relaxation response)
▶ comfortable position (a posture that will allow the person to stay in the same position for at least 20 minutes; usually sitting, kneeling, or squatting).

stop the session and notify the health care provider. Stay with the patient until he's calm and controlled.

Nursing perspective
▶ Meditation should be used cautiously in schizophrenic patients and those with attention deficit disorder.
▶ Remind your patient that meditation isn't a substitute for medical treatment. If your patient is taking prescribed medications such as antihypertensives, tell him to keep taking them.
▶ Be aware that patients with respiratory problems may have difficulty with meditation techniques that focus on breathing.

Music therapy

Music therapy, a form of sound therapy (discussed later in this chapter), uses the universal appeal of rhythmic sound to communicate, relax, encourage healing, and create a general feeling of well-being. It can take the form of creating music, singing, moving to music, or just listening.

Music as a healing technique dates back to Aristotle, who touted the power of the flute, and Pythagoras, who taught his students that singing and playing musical instruments could erase negative emotions, such as worry, fear, sorrow, and anger. Documents from the Renaissance era describe the influence of music on breathing, blood pressure, digestion, and muscular activity.

In 1896, physicians discovered that a young boy's brain, partially exposed from an accident, responded differently when different types of music were played. Cerebral and peripheral circulation increased in response to some music; mental lucidity increased with other types. (See *Understanding music therapy*.) In the 1940s, Veterans Administration hospitals incorporated music into rehabilitation programs for disabled soldiers returning from World War II.

Music therapy today is used to ameliorate physical, psychological, and cognitive problems in patients with illnesses or disabilities. It's offered in various settings, including general and psychiatric hospitals, rehabilitation facilities, mental health centers, senior centers and nursing homes, hospices, halfway houses, and substance abuse clinics. More than 5,000 registered music therapists practice in the United States today.

The National Association for Music Therapy (NAMT) was established in 1950, around the time that degree programs for professional music therapists were developed. The NAMT maintains curricular programs and training internships, a scientific database, standards of practice, and a code of ethics. It offers a board-certification examination for registered music therapist to professionals with a bachelor's degree in music therapy who have completed a 6-month internship. The NAMT also sponsors two publications: *Journal of Music Therapy* and *Music Therapy Perspectives*.

Therapeutic uses

As a complementary therapy, music therapy benefits patients with such developmental disabilities as mental retardation and such mental health disorders as anxiety. It also helps reduce chronic pain and is used as adjunctive therapy for patients with burns, cancer, cerebral palsy, stroke and other brain injuries, Parkinson's disease, and substance abuse problems.

RESEARCH SUMMARY Numerous studies conducted in the past 30 years have shown that music can be an effective complementary therapy for various medical conditions. Music has successfully reduced anxiety in children undergoing surgery,

HOW IT WORKS

Understanding music therapy

Many different theories exist about why music affects the body. One theory holds that the resonance emitted by sound waves restores the body's natural rhythm and encourages healing. Another theory proposes that the brain reacts to sound waves by sending out directions to control the heart rate, respiratory rate, and other body functions, which can result in lower blood pressure and decreased muscle tension. Endorphins, which alleviate pain and elevate the mood, may also be released in response to the sound impulses. This combination of factors can create a state of total relaxation, possibly allowing the body to heal itself.

In some cases, music therapy may work simply by conjuring up happy memories in the listener. These memories produce positive emotions, which may work to reduce stress and enhance feelings of well-being.

The Ayurvedic theory

In the Ayurvedic system of medicine, sound waves are believed to balance energy centers known as *chakras* within the body. According to this philosophy, the body has seven chakras, which vibrate at different frequencies, similar to the notes on a scale. When stress or disease disrupts the chakras, the frequencies are thrown off. Music is one way to reharmonize the chakras, allowing the body to heal itself.

decreased pain associated with dental and medical procedures, and improved the rehabilitation of patients with stroke and Parkinson's disease. Patients who listened to classical music before surgery and again in the recovery room reported minimal postoperative disorientation.

Music has also been used successfully to communicate with Alzheimer's patients, autistic persons, and head trauma victims when other approaches failed. Patients who can't communicate verbally or initiate purposeful movement need increased sensory and environmental stimulation, especially stimulation that can tap into their remote memory. Music provides both psychological comfort and a means of communication for withdrawn or depressed institutionalized patients. A study of Alzheimer's patients showed that those who listened to big band music during the day were more alert and happier and had better long-term recollection than the control group. In some cases, music is the only thing that elicits any type of response from these patients.

> 66 *Therapists say music can reduce depression, anxiety, and pain and improve the overall quality of life for terminally ill patients.* 99

Music thanatology, a new branch of sound therapy focused on psychological mechanisms for coping with death and dying, uses music to ease the emotional and physical pain of terminally ill patients. Therapists say music can reduce depression, anxiety, and pain and improve the overall quality of life for these patients. Music thanatology is used in a wide variety of settings, including homes, hospitals, and hospices.

At the other end of the spectrum, music therapy is used in delivery rooms to enhance the mother's feeling of comfort and security, to reduce the need for medication, and to promote a feeling of personal control over the situation. Studies have shown that premature infants who hear music in the intensive care unit are discharged earlier than infants who aren't exposed to music. In addition, relaxing music played to a fetus still in the womb is believed to improve the newborn's developmental capabilities. ■

Equipment

A comfortable environment and enjoyable music are the two necessary ingredients for music therapy. The music should be appropriate for the patient and the goal of the session. Faster music will stimulate the patient; slower music will have a calming effect. Calming music is usually slower than the patient's pulse (ideally less than 60 beats/minute). Music selection can also be based on the patient's ethnic background. Whatever the choice, the music should be meaningful to the patient.

If the session will involve making music, appropriate instruments will be needed. Tambourines, drums, kazoos, and banjos are usually adaptable to even the most nonmusical participant.

Simple adaptations can also be fun to use, such as utensils and pots (for cymbals), plastic jars or tin cans containing paper-clips (for maracas), or upside-down plastic food tubs (for drums). For patients with physical disabilities, a music-making tool can be adapted to fit their needs. Even keeping time by hitting a spoon against a table will enable a person to participate.

For sessions involving singing, the therapist will usually choose music that's familiar to the patient (or group). This is easier to do if all of the participants belong to the same generation. He'll provide words for the songs, either by repeating them to the group or in a written format. Large chalkboards or projections of overhead transparencies are another way to communicate song lyrics to a large group.

Procedure

A music therapy session can involve playing musical instruments, singing, or simply listening to music. It can be directed at a single patient or a group and can be conducted by a music therapist or a trained nurse. The facilitator may perform, listen with the patients, compose songs, or join in improvisation.

If you'll be facilitating the session yourself, choose appropriate music, gather your equipment (if applicable), arrange the room, and introduce the participants. Explain the purpose of the session, and encourage all patients to participate as they feel able. When the group is ready, start the music and position yourself so you're facing the group. If the group will be listening to music, watch the reactions of the participants. If they're making the music, circulate among the participants and offer support individually. Always praise the participants' efforts.

After the session, document the type of activity and the members' responses. Encourage the participants to discuss the feelings they experienced while listening to the music.

Complications

Complications are rarely associated with music therapy. As with other mind-body therapies, there's a chance that a musical selection will bring back an unpleasant memory or experience. However, in most sessions, the experience will be enjoyable for both the participants and the facilitator.

Nursing perspective

▶ Music therapy is especially effective as a means of reminiscence therapy for elderly people. Very few radio stations play songs from their era, and few elderly patients enjoy modern music, such as rock and roll or rap. Patients of similar ethnic backgrounds may enjoy ethnic music. For children, music therapy is an excellent form of play therapy.

▶ If the music evokes an unpleasant memory in a patient, comfort the patient and help him change his focus to more pleasant thoughts.

▶ Inform relatives of a patient with Alzheimer's disease that they can use music as a tool to improve communication, especially in the middle phases of the disease. Also, simple acts—such as tapping the patient's hand in rhythm to speech, reading poetry to music, and playing slow music with language-based phrasing—are often effective.

Prayer and mental healing

Humans have used prayer and mental healing throughout the ages to seek assistance from a higher being for a wide range of problems, including illness. The earliest faith healers were shamans, priests, and medicine men who used chants and ritual dances to try to influence evil spirits they believed were responsible for disease. However, seeking divine intervention to heal the sick isn't limited to ancient or primitive cultures. In the United States, the Christian Science Church uses prayer instead of conventional medical treatments. And the hundreds of thousands of pilgrims who flock to Lourdes, France, every year in search of miraculous cures are proof that prayer is still viewed as a powerful tool in healing.

The underlying beliefs of those who use prayer for healing are the same for all religions. They include the belief that a higher power exists, that humans can communicate with this higher being through prayer, and that this deity can hear human prayers and intervene in human affairs, including healing the sick. Today, science is exploring whether prayer and mental healing can indeed influence health and illness.

In prayer, the person communicates directly with the divine being, asking him to intervene to heal the patient. In mental healing, the power of the divine being is channeled through a healer. Prayer can take the form of silent meditation or be spoken aloud, either by individuals or a group; the person engaging in prayer may seek assistance for himself or for others (intercessory prayer). Most people who use prayer for healing view it as an adjunct to conventional medical treatment.

There are two main categories of mental healing. In type 1 healing, the healer enters into a spiritual level of consciousness in which he views himself and the patient as a single being. The healer doesn't have any physical contact with the patient, and the two don't even need to be in the same part of the country. The healer doesn't really attempt to "do anything"; he merely tries to achieve a spiritual unity with the patient and God in the hope that love, empathy, and unity will lead to healing. In type 2 mental healing, the healer does touch the patient, attempting to transfer energy from the healer's hands to the diseased parts of the patient's body. Both the healer and the patient commonly report a feeling of heat during this process.

Therapeutic uses

Although the therapeutic uses of prayer and mental healing are limitless, the reliability of these practices still needs to be established. Proponents of prayer argue that even if prayer can't cure disease, it can at least relieve some of its effects, enhance the effectiveness of conventional medical treatments, and provide meaning and comfort to the patient.

RESEARCH SUMMARY The history of medicine is full of stories of supposedly incurable patients who were miraculously cured through the power of prayer, but these anecdotal accounts contain little scientifically valid evidence. The first scientific study of the connection between prayer and longevity, conducted in the 1870s, showed no demonstrable effect. However, since then, a large body of scientific literature has accumulated showing intriguing results.

According to a 1994 report to the National Institutes of Health (NIH), there have been numerous published reports on studies in which people were able to influence various biological and cellular systems through mental techniques. The "target systems" included bacteria, yeast, fungi, plants, insects, chicks, mice, cats, and dogs as well as blood cells and cancer cells. In human subjects, eye and muscle movements, respiration, and brain rhythms have reportedly been affected through mental means.

On a more practical level, recent studies have shown tangible health benefits in people with strong religious faith. Statistics show an increased survival rate after open-heart surgery for patients who draw comfort and strength from religion, lower blood pressure in patients who attend religious services, and a lower incidence of depression and anxiety among the religiously committed. Such data are causing physicians and

66 Statistics show an increased survival rate after open-heart surgery for patients who draw comfort and strength from religion, lower blood pressure in patients who attend religious services, and a lower incidence of depression and anxiety among the religiously committed. Such data are causing physicians and laypeople to explore further the relationship between prayer and mental powers and healing. 99

laypeople to explore further the relationship between prayer and mental powers and healing.

Although modern science has no explanation for type 1 mental healing, the NIH report says the lack of a known mechanism shouldn't lead scientists to dismiss the phenomenon. Pointing out that scientists had no explanation for sunlight until the development of nuclear physics in the 20th century, the report concludes that "mental healing may be valid in the absence of a validating theory." (See *Understanding prayer and mental healing.*) ■

Equipment
No special equipment is needed for prayer or mental healing. If possible, provide the patient with privacy in a quiet, distraction-free environment.

Procedure
Nurses and other health care providers can facilitate the use of prayer and mental healing by asking patients a few simple questions, such as "Is religion important to you?" and "Is religion important in how you cope with your illness?"

If the patient answers yes, explore his religious practices to identify ways to incorporate them into the present situation.

HOW IT WORKS

❧ Understanding prayer and mental healing

Opinions differ on why prayer and mental healing affect health. The more scientific explanation is that these practices lower the levels of epinephrine and corticosteroids (stress hormones) in the body, resulting in decreased blood pressure, heart rate, and respiratory rate. These hormones have also been shown to affect the immune system.

To explain the connection between prayer and altered hormone levels, researchers are also looking at the brain's limbic system. This system — made up of the amygdala (a small, almond-shaped organ), hippocampus, and hypothalamus — is the center of emotions, sexual pleasure, strong memories, and spirituality. Electrical stimulation of the limbic system during surgery has been associated with religious visions. In addition, many patients whose limbic system is chronically stimulated by drug abuse or a tumor experience some type of religious fanaticism. These discoveries have led researchers to believe that religious experiences have a neurophysiologic basis.

Science, faith, and universal consciousness

The nonscientific explanation for the power of prayer is that there's a higher being who answers the prayers of the faithful. Although scientists admit there's no compelling body of research to support this explanation, most aren't ready to totally dismiss it. In one study, open-heart surgery patients were divided into two groups. One group was prayed for, while the other group acted as a control. None of the patients knew the experiment was being conducted. The patients who received prayers were less likely to need antibiotics or develop complications. In a similar study with alcoholics, however, no benefit was seen.

Modern science has no explanation for mental healing in which the healer is far removed from the patient. However, Dr. Larry Dossey, the author of popular books on healing and spirituality, has proposed his own theory. Dossey believes the human mind isn't limited to the brain but, rather, is connected to the minds of all people in a kind of joined consciousness that transcends such physical constraints as time and place. This phenomenon, he believes, might explain how "long-distance" healing works.

Ask the patient whether he would like to discuss his faith with the facility chaplain or another member of the clergy. Remain nonjudgmental, and offer to assist with any arrangements for spiritual intervention.

Complications
One of the benefits of prayer and mental healing is the lack of complications. However, patients who have attempted prayer and not seen the results they expected may express a sense of disappointment when the topic of spirituality is discussed. If possible, arrange for a member of the clergy to explore the patient's feelings with him.

Nursing perspective
▶ The prayer rituals associated with some religions may be more than your health care facility can handle. Rites involving incense, large groups, or loud music and dance can stress even the most tolerant facility. Although you should be sensitive to the patient's culture, sometimes a compromise is in order. For example, you could suggest that the patient be wheeled to an outside area of the facility if incense is involved or to a conference room off the unit during off-hours if noise is an issue or a prayer vigil involves a large number of people.
▶ Be aware that ethical questions arise if prayer and mental healing are used without the subject's knowledge. Additionally, some are concerned that prayer and mental healing may be used to harm an individual instead of healing him.
▶ Advise your patient to consider prayer a complementary therapy, not a substitute for conventional medical care.
▶ If you have a patient whose religion advocates the use of prayer as the sole form of treatment, make sure he understands the consequences of forgoing conventional medical treatment, so that he can make an informed decision.

Psychotherapy
Although the inclusion of psychotherapy in the category of alternative medicine is sometimes debated, psychotherapy is at the root of all mind-body therapies. Derived from the Greek words meaning "healing of the soul," psychotherapy is a method of treating disease by exploring its emotional and behavioral components. The goal of psychotherapy is to enable

an individual to satisfy his need for affection, recognition, and achievement by helping him correct negative attitudes, emotions, and behaviors that interfere with some aspect of functioning in his life. When used in the treatment of physically ill patients, psychotherapy can improve their coping ability and reduce depression and anxiety.

Types of psychotherapy

There are a number of different schools of psychotherapy:

▶ *Psychodynamic (or insight) therapy* focuses on the individual and views distress as the result of unresolved unconscious conflicts. The focus of this form of therapy is to make the unconscious conscious — and thereby modify behavior.

▶ *Psychoanalysis,* a form of insight therapy, sees these unconscious conflicts as the result of critical factors in early childhood development. Again, the focus of therapy is to bring these conflicts into the open.

▶ *Behavioral therapy* focuses on making very specific behavioral changes such as learning not to be afraid of flying.

▶ *Modeling (or operant conditioning) behavioral therapy,* rather than looking into the patient's past, focuses on the patient's interactions with his current social environment.

▶ *Existential therapy* focuses on the future, working to help the patient see new potential for personal satisfaction and growth.

▶ *Systems (or family) therapy* looks at relationship patterns among family members and tries to activate the family group as a therapeutic force.

▶ *Body-oriented therapy* hypothesizes that emotions are expressed as tension and restriction in any part of the body. Using breathing techniques, movement, and manual pressure and probing, the therapist helps the patient release emotions located in his tissues.

> 66 *By helping patients acknowledge their emotions, psychotherapy diminishes the negative effects of the emotions and enhances recovery.* 99

Any of these therapies can be used either alone or in combination. For patients with a physical illness, psychotherapy typically focuses on short-term treatment to deal with the emotions that the disorder evokes. For example, many patients with a serious illness experience depression and anxiety, emotions that can make the illness worse. By helping patients acknowledge their emotions, psychotherapy diminishes the negative effects of the emotions and enhances recovery.

Therapeutic uses

Psychotherapy is generally used to treat people with mental or behavioral problems. It can help psychotic patients recognize and deal effectively with daily stressors and help neurotic patients deal with life's unpredictable changes. For patients who are temporarily overwhelmed by daily stressors, psychotherapy can restore their emotional equilibrium. Additionally, patients with behavioral problems can be treated with psychotherapy in an attempt to modify their behavior. However, for psychotherapy to be successful, the patient must be motivated to change.

RESEARCH SUMMARY Studies show that psychotherapy can speed recovery from a medical crisis. In a 1993 study of patients with broken hips, those receiving psychotherapy had a 2-day shorter hospital stay, fewer rehospitalizations, and shorter rehabilitation times. By allowing patients to verbalize their feelings about their health, psychotherapy helps sick people cope with their fears, improve their mood, and sometimes even improve their outcome. Studies have shown that patients with a medical problem who are also depressed have a much higher mortality rate than those who aren't depressed.

Psychotherapy also benefits people with somatic illnesses — those for which no discernible organic cause for the symptoms can be found. Practitioners believe that these patients are unable to accept an emotional problem and transform it into a physical ailment. In such patients, psychotherapy has been shown to decrease the number of physician visits for physical complaints. ■

Equipment

A quiet environment, free from distractions, is essential for psychotherapy. If possible, the room should have a door that can remain closed during the entire session. Adequate seating should be available for the patient, the psychotherapist, and any other participants. Some therapists prefer to have a desk or table separating them from the patient. Lighting should be even so that the patient doesn't feel as if he's being interrogated under a spotlight.

Procedure

Although psychotherapy sessions should be conducted only by a trained psychotherapist, many health care professionals, including nurses, routinely use psychotherapeutic interventions, consciously or unconsciously, in dealing with patients. You use them when you quietly say to a patient "It must be scary here in the ICU" to try to draw him out; when you try to reassure the patient by saying "You aren't alone: We're all around you"; when you listen supportively to the patient's worries or complaints; and when you take the patient's hand in yours to provide comfort.

Good listening skills are a key to success in using psychotherapeutic interventions. It's also important to pay close attention to the patient's nonverbal behavior, looking for clues to his underlying emotions. *Reflection* — repeating to the patient what he has told you — is another useful tool. In addition to verifying what the patient said, reflection tells the patient that you're listening and not passing judgment on what he told you.

If your patient has a session with a psychotherapist, document the patient's response to the session and discuss arrangements for follow-up sessions, if appropriate.

Complications

Because psychotherapy typically deals with buried emotions, the patient may be upset or angry after a session. If so, let him discuss his feelings. If you detect signs of agitation or impending violence, keep a safe distance between you and the patient. Consider asking someone else to be present with you until the patient has vented his feelings and is once again calm. Document his responses and any actions taken.

Nursing perspective

▶ Be prepared to supply the names and numbers of support groups that deal with the patient's specific problem. Support groups can provide needed emotional and practical support for patients with chronic or life-threatening illnesses. Positive effects have been seen in patients with cancer, heart disease, asthma, and stroke. Studies have shown that breast cancer patients who participate in a support group survive longer.

▶ If your patient is severely depressed, be alert for suicide warning signs.

▶ Make sure your patient continues to take prescribed psychotropic drugs even if he's also receiving psychotherapy.

▶ Always maintain patient confidentiality.

Sound therapy

Sound therapy is based on the theory that certain sounds can have a therapeutic effect on the mind and body. Sound is created by the vibration of objects and travels from one source to another as waves. It enters the body not only through the ears but also as vibrations through other body parts such as the skull.

Pleasant, soothing sounds — such as a babbling brook, birds chirping, or a Mozart sonata — can relax a person and make him feel better. However, sound therapy goes beyond this accepted fact. Practitioners have developed techniques that focus sound waves on targeted areas of the body to achieve specific therapeutic goals. Sound therapists believe that even sounds that aren't loud enough to be heard can still cause a response in the body.

Types of sound therapy

Music therapy, probably the most commonly used form of sound therapy, is discussed earlier in this chapter. Other forms of sound therapy include the following:

▶ *Auditory integration training,* a technique developed in the 1950s, uses simulations of the stages of listening development to repattern the hearing range and attention span. The Electronic Ear, developed by French physician Alfred Tomatis, exercises the muscles of the middle ear, allowing a person to hear a wider range of frequencies. Using this device, patients with dyslexia, autism, learning disabilities, and attention deficit hyperactivity disorder (ADHD) have learned how to listen more effectively. Creativity, musical ability, foreign language learning ability, and organizational abilities are also said to have improved.

Another form of auditory integration training uses a device called the Ears Education and Retraining System (EERS) to desensitize patients who are hypersensitive to high-frequency sounds. This device was developed by another French physician, Guy Berard, who believed that certain behavioral and cognitive disorders could be traced to distorted perception of sound frequencies. In this technique, sounds — usually music — are filtered to eliminate the frequencies to which the patient is sensitive. The EERS then electronically modulates these frequencies and returns them through headphones to the patient's ears. After listening to the processed sounds, the listener is often able to accept that frequency. This type of training has been successful with autistic children who suffer from hypersensitivity.

▌ *Toning* is a technique in which a person tries to release stress by making elongated vowel sounds that are believed to resonate throughout the body. Practitioners claim that toning also improves the speaking and singing voice. Toning is thought to be more beneficial than singing because it moves the vocal chords more slowly, allowing the vibrations to perform their internal massage. Gregorian chant, performed by Benedictine monks as part of their religious ritual, is similar to toning.

▌ *Cymatic therapy* involves the use of a computerized instrument to transmit sound waves directly through the skin. This technique, an acupressure-like action, is based on the theory that illness is a form of resonant disequilibrium. Practitioners claim that cymatic therapy reestablishes healthy resonance in unhealthy tissues. They explain that cymatic therapy doesn't heal directly but, rather, places the body in the proper condition for healing itself.

Cymatic therapy is said to help children with learning disorders, such as dyslexia and ADHD. This technique has been used in the United States since the late 1960s, mainly by nurses, chiropractors, osteopaths, and acupuncturists. Training is necessary to become a cymatic practitioner.

▌ The *Infratonic QGM* is a machine that uses sound frequencies to reduce pain and headaches, increase circulatory function, relax muscles, and increase the brain's production of alpha waves. This device, invented by a Chinese scientist, simulates the high-level secondary sound waves emitted from the hands of Chinese *qigong* masters. Recognized as a pain management tool in China, the Infratonic QGM is now 510(K) listed with the Food and Drug

Administration in the United States and is covered by many insurance companies. (See *Understanding sound therapy*.)

> ❝ *Sound therapy may be most effective for autistic patients. Before sound therapy, treatment options for autism were limited and rarely successful.* ❞

Therapeutic uses

Muscle tension and stress are the health problems that sound therapy is most commonly used to relieve. Proponents say that it can also reduce pain, ease anxiety, stimulate the immune system, lower blood pressure, and improve communication in patients with autism, learning disabilities, and Alzheimer's disease. Sound therapy may be most effective for autistic patients. Before sound therapy, treatment options for autism were limited and rarely successful.

RESEARCH SUMMARY The concepts behind most sound therapies (except for music therapy) and the claims made for them haven't been scientifically proven. ■

Equipment

Sound therapy can be performed in almost any setting, as long as the environmental needs can be met. The session should take place in a quiet, private room that's free from distractions and has a comfortable place for the patient to sit or recline. The specific equipment needed will depend on the form of sound therapy being used.

Procedure

Most of the more advanced sound therapy techniques will be performed by a trained sound therapist. However, you can assist your patient with toning, a simple technique involving only the vocal cords. Begin by explaining the procedure to the patient and answering any questions. Inform him that the vibrations from the elongated vowel sounds, or tones, may help with relaxation and ease stress.

When the patient is ready to start, help him into a comfortable position. Ask him to close his eyes and focus on listening. With his eyes closed, have him take a deep, easy breath and

HOW IT WORKS

↪ Understanding sound therapy

How does sound therapy affect the body? Sound therapists believe that people primarily respond to sound vibrations in two ways: through resonance and entrainment. *Resonance* is the process by which particular sound frequencies produce sympathetic vibrations in various parts of the body. Low-pitched sounds are believed to resonate in lower parts of the body; high-pitched sounds, in the higher regions. *Entrainment* is the phenomenon in which bodily processes — such as heart rate, respiratory rate, and even brain wave activity — become synchronized with external rhythmic stimuli, such as the beat of a drum or the sound of ocean waves.

Healing's pathways

Some scientists believe sound's effects are related to how sound impulses are transmitted within the body. The 8th and 10th cranial nerves carry sound impulses through the ear and skull to the brain. From there, the vagus nerve — which helps regulate heart rate, respiration, and speech — carries motor and sensory impulses to the throat, larynx, heart, and diaphragm. Sound therapy experts believe that the vagus nerve and the limbic system (the parts of the brain responsible for emotions) may be the connecting link between the ear, brain, and autonomic nervous system that explains how sound works to treat physical and emotional disorders.

Good vibrations

Sound therapy has been a component of India's ancient system of Ayurvedic medicine for centuries. Ayurvedic practitioners believe that the effect of stress or disease on the body's seven energy centers *(chakras)* disrupts the frequencies at which the chakras vibrate. They rely on specific sounds to restore the patterns of the chakras, allowing the body to heal itself.

start humming a soft, resonant tone. Explain that the type of sound — high, low, or pretty — doesn't matter. Tell the patient to continue humming and to concentrate on the vibrations the sound is making in his chest and head. Instruct him to let the sound rise and fall naturally, without effort. After a few minutes, have the patient place his hands on his cheeks and feel the sound. Tell him to feel the sound in his face and skull as he continues to hum the tone for another 5 minutes. Then have him relax his hands and finish by making another sound, such as "ah," for another 5 minutes.

When the patient is finished, ask whether his body, mind, and breathing are more relaxed. Document the session and the patient's response.

Complications

Simple sound therapy, such as toning, isn't associated with any complications. The patient may experience an unpleasant sensation — similar to the reaction some people have to fingernails scratching a blackboard — from the more complex forms, such as auditory integration training or cymatic therapy. If the patient has an unpleasant reaction, stop the therapy immediately and notify the physician. Document the patient's reaction, clinical condition, and response to any interventions you initiate.

Nursing perspective

▶ Cymatic therapy isn't recommended for patients with pacemakers because the resonance of the sound waves may interfere with the pacemaker function. It's also contraindicated for patients with a heart condition, because the stimuli can affect the heart rate, and for patients who can't tolerate loud or jarring sounds.

▶ Make sure that all equipment is cleaned between patients.

▶ Check the volume on all equipment before treatment.

Tai chi chuan

A form of exercise built upon the mind-body connection, tai chi chuan (or tai chi) combines physical movement, meditation, and breathing to induce relaxation and tranquillity of mind and improve balance, posture, coordination, endurance, strength, and flexibility. Practiced in China for centuries as an ancient form of slow graceful and rhythmic exercise and a martial art, tai chi allows the individual to assume an active role in health promotion and disease prevention. Proponents believe that regular practice of these exercises can result in long life, good health, physical and mental vigor, and enhanced creativity. The name *tai chi* means "ultimate fist" or "poetry in motion."

There are numerous forms of tai chi, involving up to 108 different postures and controlled movements. Most of the forms have been passed down from generation to generation and have assumed the name of a particular family (such as Wu style or Yang style). Although each style is distinctive, they all follow the same basic principles.

Tai chi can be practiced by people of all ages, sizes, and physical abilities because it relies more on technique than strength. Participants learn a series of rhythmic and coordinated movement patterns that they perform slowly and methodically, with one leading into the next. The movements have descriptive names, such as Grasp the Bird's Tail and White Crane Spreads Its Wings. While they practice the movements, participants also pay close attention to their breathing, which is focused in the diaphragm rather than the chest. Abdominal breathing is believed to enhance the flow of energy, or *qi*, throughout the body. Qi is the flow of energy, and tai chi aims to restore balance so that qi flows freely.

Like acupuncture, *qigong*, and other components of traditional Chinese medicine, tai chi is based on the Taoist principle of *yin-yang*, which is the basis for the Chinese understanding of health and sickness. *Yin-yang* refers to the opposing forces in nature, such as positive and negative, active and passive, light and dark. Good health, in the Taoist view, requires a balance of these opposing forces within the body. If one or the other predominates, the result is sickness.

Tai chi movements are carried out in pairs of opposites to balance negative *(yin)* forces and positive *(yang)* forces. For example, a movement that begins on the left will typically end with a move to the right. The movements themselves are simple, involving the bending and unbending of the knees while raising or lowering the arms. The coordination of movement and breathing pattern are what constitute tai chi. The ultimate goal is to achieve harmony between body, mind, and spirit. (See *Understanding tai chi chuan*, page 182.)

Therapeutic uses

Tai chi can be used to complement physical therapy programs aimed at improving balance, posture, coordination, flexibility, and endurance. Cardiovascular indications include heart disease, hypertension, and deconditioning. Tai chi can also bene-

HOW IT WORKS

✎ Understanding tai chi chuan

According to traditional Chinese belief, tai chi's unique combination of breathing, meditation, and slow, rhythmic exercise allows the body to take in essential elements—such as oxygen, iron, copper, zinc, fluorite, quartz, and magnesium—and rid itself of wastes and poisons. In addition, the abdominal breathing techniques are thought to facilitate the flow of energy *(qi)* throughout the vital channels of the body.

Breathing, movement, and concentration
Proponents believe that as the body inhales, the mind lifts the energy from the solar plexus region, considered the central energy source of the body. During exhalation, the energy is directed from the solar plexus to the lower abdomen. The techniques of breathing and arm and leg movements alone aren't enough to move the *qi* throughout the body; they must be combined with the power of concentration. The external movements of the body are used to aid and guide internal concentration.

Scientific studies have shown that the slow movements of tai chi strengthen the muscles and enhance balance and coordination. Circulation increases, respiration deepens, and the slow, deliberate pace provides a focal point similar to that used in meditation. As with meditation, the physiologic markers of stress also decrease.

fit patients who suffer from anxiety, stress, restlessness, and depression.

> ❝Tai chi is especially well suited for elderly and frail people because its movements are slow and controlled and don't involve impact. ❞

However, tai chi's greatest benefit may be the promotion of health and wellness. It's especially well suited for elderly and frail people because its movements are slow and controlled and don't involve impact. By incorporating all of the motions that typically become restricted with aging, tai chi improves respiratory status, trunk control, balance, and coordination. Done in a group setting, tai chi also provides an opportunity for socialization.

RESEARCH SUMMARY A patient can benefit from the physical elements of tai chi without understanding its spiritual dimension. Studies printed in major medical journals have shown that this exercise program can improve stamina, agility, muscle tone, and flexibility. In elderly people, it can improve physical balance and decrease the risk of falls. ■

Equipment

No extra equipment is necessary. To engage in tai chi, you'll need a carpeted room with adequate floor space to permit participants to move their arms and bodies without interfering with one another. The room should be well lit to allow participants to see the leader. Participants should wear loose-fitting clothing and aerobic sneakers or bare feet.

Procedure

Although the guidance of a knowledgeable teacher is needed to master tai chi, careful practice of the basic steps still provides many of the benefits. Before your patients begin a session, assess their physical health, looking for endurance, balance, and mobility. Explain the purpose of the session, emphasizing that movements should be slow and nonstressful. Encourage the group members to participate to the extent that they feel comfortable, not to the point of pain.

The teacher will face the group and lead them through some simple stretching exercises to loosen their muscles and prevent injury. Then he'll begin with the first posture, demonstrating it as he describes it. For the first session, you may want the patients to learn only the first few postures. New movements as well as breathing instructions can be added with each session. Remind the group that they can skip any movement they find too difficult. (See *Basic tai chi movements,* pages 184 to 187.)

Most routines take about 20 minutes. Close the session with additional stretching exercises to allow the patients' muscles to cool down. Document the session and the participants' responses.

(Text continues on page 189.)

Basic tai chi movements

Shown below are the basic double-stance positions of tai chi, in which both legs are on the floor. There are also single-stance positions and double-stance stretching positions.

Salutation
Standing erect, turn the right foot out 45 degrees and sink down slightly on your right leg. Shift all your weight onto the right leg and extend your left leg, flexing your foot and crossing your hands in front of your chest.

hands to waist level as you shift your weight to the left leg.

Next, swing your arms to the right and press forward, shifting some of your weight to the right leg.

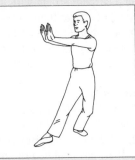

Single Whip
Pivot to the left, shifting your weight to your right leg, and bring your left foot around and open your arms.

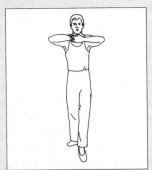

Grasp the Bird's Tail
Step back onto your left foot, turning it out, and move your

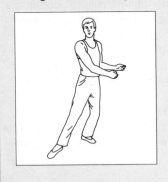

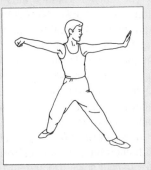

Basic tai chi movements *(continued)*

White Crane Spreads Its Wings

Step forward, leading with your right leg. Your right hand, elbow, knee, and toes should be in alignment.

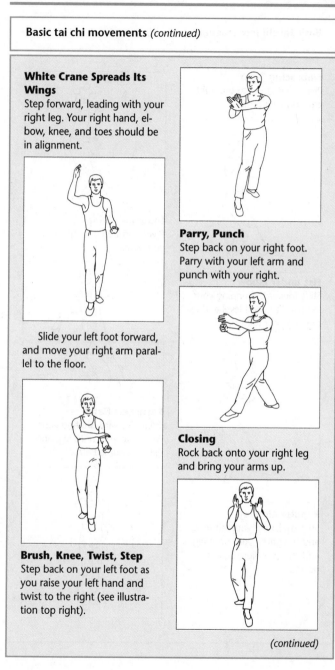

Slide your left foot forward, and move your right arm parallel to the floor.

Brush, Knee, Twist, Step

Step back on your left foot as you raise your left hand and twist to the right (see illustration top right).

Parry, Punch

Step back on your right foot. Parry with your left arm and punch with your right.

Closing

Rock back onto your right leg and bring your arms up.

(continued)

Basic tai chi movements (continued)

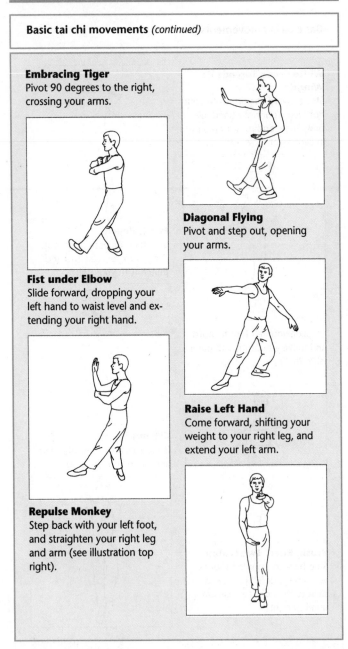

Embracing Tiger
Pivot 90 degrees to the right, crossing your arms.

Fist under Elbow
Slide forward, dropping your left hand to waist level and extending your right hand.

Repulse Monkey
Step back with your left foot, and straighten your right leg and arm (see illustration top right).

Diagonal Flying
Pivot and step out, opening your arms.

Raise Left Hand
Come forward, shifting your weight to your right leg, and extend your left arm.

Basic tai chi movements *(continued)*

Fan through the Arms
Pivot to the left and step out with your left foot, moving your right hand up to your temple.

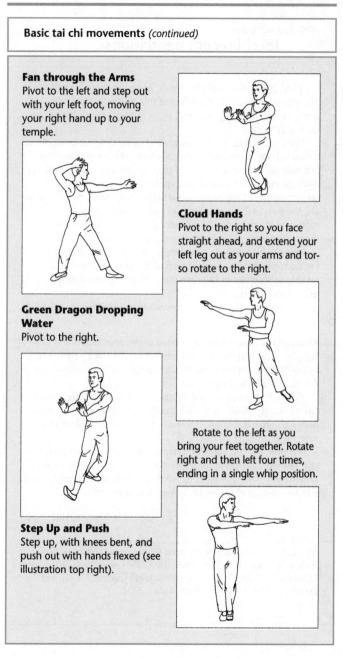

Green Dragon Dropping Water
Pivot to the right.

Step Up and Push
Step up, with knees bent, and push out with hands flexed (see illustration top right).

Cloud Hands
Pivot to the right so you face straight ahead, and extend your left leg out as your arms and torso rotate to the right.

Rotate to the left as you bring your feet together. Rotate right and then left four times, ending in a single whip position.

PERSONAL ACCOUNT

Tai chi recommendations

I've been practicing tai chi for a year, and since then I've had the opportunity to evaluate the effect of this gentle "martial art"—as stress management therapy and, more impressively, as total physical health therapy.

I had suffered for years with chronic neck pain, stemming from a whiplash injury, and with limited motion of the right shoulder, but after unsuccessful sessions of physical therapy—including mobilization, ultrasounds, and heat application—I wanted to try something new. Despite my initial skepticism, after 2 months of tai chi, the pain in the cervical region disappeared, and the range of motion of my right shoulder returned to the normal. This achievement has remained unchanged, even up to now.

I wouldn't hesitate to recommend tai chi to individuals suffering from my same ailments as well as to older persons who are seeking to maintain or improve their health and free themselves from chronic pain.

—Loredana Brizio-Molteni, M.D., F.A.C.S.

Although I've always been interested in the oriental arts and philosophy, including the "martial arts," it took my wife's persistence in July 1997 to persuade me to sign up for a tai chi course—and I've been studying it ever since.

Before I began taking the course, I suffered from symptoms related to osteoarthritis of the left coxofemoral joint and from neck pain with limited motion. However, the symptoms disappeared with my practice of tai chi.

My physician's recommendation is to continue doing tai chi—and I would pass the same recommendation to individuals with a sedentary lifestyle as well as to individuals with active lifestyles that require exertion of the musculoskeletal system.

—Agostino Molteni, M.D., Ph.D.

Adapted with permission from Stress Management and Relaxation Technology (SMART), (913) 648-CALM (2256), *www.SMARTAICHI.com.* Excerpt from Douglas, B. *The Complete Idiot's Guide to T'ai Chi and QiGong,* 2nd ed. New York: Alpha Books, 2002.

Complications

As with any physical exercise, patients performing tai chi can experience sprains or strains. Stretching before and after the session and changing positions slowly can prevent most injuries. If a patient injures a muscle, isolate the body part to restrict movement, and try to elevate it to reduce swelling. Notify the physician, and administer cold or heat therapy as ordered. Document the incident, your assessment, the patient's condition, any interventions, and the patient's response.

Falls and fractures are another possible complication, especially while performing single-stance postures. Again, proper use of stretching and slow movements should lessen the risk. If a patient falls, perform your assessment while he's still lying on the ground. Ask him to remain lying for a moment, and ascertain whether he has any pain. Ask him to move all of his extremities, saving a painful one for last. If you didn't see him fall, ask him what he hit as he fell. Check his head for any cuts or bumps. If he can move without pain, gently assist him to a chair. Notify the physician and document the incident, your assessment, the patient's condition, any interventions, and the patient's response. (See *Tai chi recommendations.*)

Nursing perspective

▶ Instruct your patients to stop exercising if they experience pain or shortness of breath.

▶ Make sure your patients are wearing appropriate footwear to reduce the risk of slipping and falling.

Yoga

One of the oldest known health practices, yoga (which means "union" in Sanskrit) is the integration of physical, mental, and spiritual energies to promote health and wellness. Yoga is based on the Hindu principle of mind-body unity: that a chronically restless or agitated mind will result in poor health and decreased mental clarity. Practitioners believe that practicing yoga techniques can combat these effects and restore good mental and physical health.

The basic components of yoga are proper breathing, movement, meditation, and posture. While practicing specific postures, the practitioner pays close attention to his breathing, exhaling at certain times and inhaling at others. The breathing techniques are believed to help maintain the postures as well as promote relaxation and enhance the flow of vital energy known as *prana*, similar to the Chinese concept of *qi*. (See *Understanding yoga*.)

As with tai chi chuan, there are a variety of styles of yoga. The type most widely taught in the West today is hatha yoga. A unique combination of physical postures and exercises (known as *asanas*), breathing techniques (known as *pranayamas*), relaxation, diet, and proper thinking, hatha yoga aims to cleanse the body of toxins, clear the mind, energize and realign the

---

HOW IT WORKS

⮑ Understanding yoga

Yoga practitioners believe that the *prana,* or life force, circulates throughout the body in a system of 72,000 subtle nerves. Improper diet, stress, or toxins can interrupt the flow of *prana,* affecting the individual's physical or mental health. Chronic blockages can lead to illness. By promoting an even flow of *prana* and removing blockages, the breathing exercises of yoga are believed to maintain and restore health.

Other yoga practices are believed to stimulate the endocrine and nervous systems specifically. Body positions and contraction of select muscles during certain postures is thought to increase circulation to the glands. The breathing exercises manipulate the respiratory system, which is believed to benefit the nervous system.

Inducing the relaxation response
Numerous scientific studies have shown that regular practice of yoga can produce the same physiologic changes as meditation. Known as the relaxation response, these changes include decreased heart and respiratory rates, improved cardiac and respiratory function, decreased blood pressure, decreased oxygen consumption, increased alpha wave activity, and EEG synchronicity (a change in brain wave activity found only in deep meditation).

body, release muscle tension, and increase flexibility and strength.

> 66 *Yoga in the West is more often practiced for its physical and psychological benefits, such as improving strength and flexibility, maintaining physical fitness, and inducing relaxation.* 99

Asanas, meaning "ease" in Sanskrit, fall into two categories: meditative and therapeutic. Meditative asanas align the head and spine to promote relaxation, concentration, and proper blood flow through the body. They're also believed to keep the heart, glands, and lungs properly energized. The therapeutic asanas are commonly prescribed to treat specific ailments, such as neck, back, and joint pain.

According to Hindu belief, the goal of a properly executed asana is to create a balance between movement and still-ness, which is the state of a healthy body. Although many of these postures require little movement, they all require the participation of the mind to concentrate on the body's pos-tures and movements. Eventually, as with meditation, practi-tioners say they can learn to regulate their autonomic func-tions, such as heartbeat and respiratory rate, while reducing physical tensions.

Although it was originally developed as part of a spiritual belief system whose purpose is achievement of a higher state of consciousness (known as *samadhi*), yoga in the West is more often practiced for its physical and psychological benefits, such as improving strength and flexibility, maintaining physical fit-ness, and inducing relaxation.

Therapeutic uses

Aside from promoting relaxation and enhancing feelings of well-being, yoga is also widely used as a complementary ther-apy to relieve the pain and anxiety that commonly accompany certain chronic illnesses, such as heart disease (as in Dr. Dean Ornish's program to reverse cardiovascular disease), di-abetes, migraine headaches, hypertension, and arthritis. (See *Indications for yoga,* page 192.)

Indications for yoga

Many studies have demonstrated yoga's effectiveness as a complementary therapy for:

- alcoholism
- anxiety
- arthritis and rheumatism
- asthma
- back and neck pain
- bronchitis
- cancer
- diabetes
- duodenal ulcers
- heart disease
- hemorrhoids
- hypertension
- insomnia
- menopause
- menstrual problems
- migraines
- nerve or muscle disease
- obesity
- premenstrual tension
- tobacco addiction.

Yoga has also been credited with decreasing serum cholesterol levels and increasing histamine levels to fight allergies. Its ability to help the user regulate blood flow is being studied for possible use in cancer therapy. Scientists are eager to see whether restricted blood flow to the tumor region will slow tumor growth.

Yoga techniques can fit the needs of people in any physical condition from age 5 up. Individuals who can't perform some of the more physically demanding postures can still benefit from the breathing or meditation techniques.

RESEARCH SUMMARY Numerous studies have demonstrated yoga's effectiveness in alleviating stress and anxiety, lowering blood pressure and respiratory rate, relieving pain, improving motor skills, increasing auditory and visual perception, improving metabolic and respiratory function, and producing brain wave activity associated with relaxation. The breath control aspect has also been shown to aid digestion, regulate cardiac function, and reduce the frequency of asthma attacks. ■

Equipment

Minimal supplies are needed to practice yoga. The most important element is a private, quiet environment that's free from distractions. Participants should have enough room to move without touching or distracting one another; they'll also need a small blanket or large towel to use for some of the postures. Have the participants wear loose clothing and sneakers or bare feet.

Procedure

Yoga programs vary with the teacher, the experience of the participants, and the goal of the treatment. A balanced program of postures will help most participants achieve positive effects on their overall health.

If your patients will be having a yoga class, explain the purpose of the session and describe the planned exercises and their benefits. Answer any questions, and remind the participants that they don't have to engage in any posture that may be uncomfortable.

The yoga teacher will talk the group through the positions and breathing techniques, demonstrating each one. After they have all assumed the position or begun the breathing pattern, the teacher will probably circulate among the members to adjust their technique as needed. At the end of the session, the teacher will have everyone take a few slow, deep breaths. Document the session, the techniques used, and the patients' responses.

Complications

Some of the more physical aspects of yoga can cause muscle injury if they aren't properly performed or if the individual tries to force his body into position.

Nursing perspective

▶ Yoga's effects are cumulative.

▶ Because some of the postures used in yoga can be stressful to people with certain health problems, advise your patients to consult their physician before undertaking a yoga program.

▶ Remind patients that yoga is a complementary therapy, not a cure for disease. They'll still need to continue their conventional medical treatments.

▶ Advise patients to attempt the different postures cautiously, and remind them that very few people can perform all of the movements in the beginning.

▶ Inform patients that yoga requires regular practice to be effective. Repetition and practicing the postures promotes the positions.

Selected references

Basmajian, J.V., ed. *Biofeedback: Principles and Practice for Clinicians,* 3rd ed. Baltimore: Williams & Wilkins Co., 1989.

Benjamin, S.A., et al. "Mind-Body Medicine: Expanding the Health Model," *Patient Care* 31(14):126-45, September 1997.

Benson, H. *The Relaxation Response.* New York: William Morrow & Co., updated and expanded edition 2000. Original edition 1975.

Burton Goldberg Group. *Alternative Medicine: The Definitive Guide.* Puyallup, Wash.: Future Medicine Pub., 1993.

Cassileth, B.R. *The Alternative Medicine Handbook: The Complete Reference Guide to Alternative and Complementary Therapies.* New York: W.W. Norton & Co., 1998.

Cohen, S., et al. "Psychological Stress and Susceptibility to the Common Cold," *New England Journal of Medicine* 325(9):606-12, August 1991.

Davis, C.M. *Complementary Therapies in Rehabilitation: Holistic Approaches for Prevention and Wellness.* Thorofare, N.J.: Slack Inc., 1997.

DeBenedittis, G., et al. "Effects of Hypnotic Analgesia and Hypnotizability on Experimental Ischemic Pain," *International Journal of Clinical and Experimental Hypnosis* 37(1):55-69, January 1989.

Dossey, L. *Healing Words: The Power of Prayer and the Practice of Medicine.* San Francisco: HarperSanFrancisco, 1993.

Eisenberg, D., et al. "Complementary and Alternative Medicine: An Annals Series," *Annals of Internal Medicine* 135(5):208, August 2001.

Fetrow, C.W., and Avila, J.R. *Professional's Handbook of Complementary and Alternative Medicines,* 2nd ed. Springhouse, Pa.: Springhouse Corp., 2001.

Gecsedi, R., and Decker G. "Incorporating Alternative Therapies into Pain Management," *AJN Supplement* 101(1):35, April 2001.

Goldberg, B. "Hypnosis and the Immune Response," *International Journal of Psychosomatics* 32(3):34-36, 1985.

Goleman, D.J., and Gurin, J. *Mind & Body Medicine: How To Use Your Mind for Better Health.* Yonkers, N.Y.: Consumer Reports Books, 1993.

Kabat-Zinn, J. *Wherever You Go, There You Are: Mindfulness Meditation in Everyday Life.* New York: Hyperion, 1994.

Lawrence, R., et al. *Magnet Therapy: The Pain Cure Alternative.* Roseville, Calif.: Prima Publishing, 1998.

National Institutes of Health. *Alternative Medicine: Expanding Medical Horizons. A Report to the National Institutes of Health on Alternative Medical Systems and Practices in the United States prepared under the auspices of the Workshop on Alternative Medicine, Chantilly, Virginia, September 14-16, 1992.* NIH pub. 94-066. Washington, D.C.: U.S. Government Printing Office, 1994.

Novey, D. *Clinician's Complete Reference to Complementary Alternative Medicine.* St. Louis: Mosby–Year Book, Inc., 2000.

Owen, L. *Pain-free with Magnet Therapy.* Roseville, Calif.: Prima Publishing, 2000.

Rosenfeld, I. *Dr. Rosenfeld's Guide to Alternative Medicine: What Works, What Doesn't, and What's Right for You.* New York: Random House, 1996.

Spencer, J., and Jacobs, J. *Complementary Alternative Medicine: An Evidence-Based Approach.* Mosby–Year Book, Inc., 1999.

Vishnudevananda, S. *The Complete Illustrated Book of Yoga.* New York: Random House, 1995, reprint of 1960 edition.

Weil, A. *Spontaneous Healing: How to Discover and Enhance Your Body's Natural Ability to Maintain and Heal Itself.* New York: Knopf, 1995.

Internet resources

www.healthweb.org
www.holistic-online.com
www.nccam.nih.gov
www.pitt.edu/~cbw/internet.html

6

Bioelectromagnetic therapies

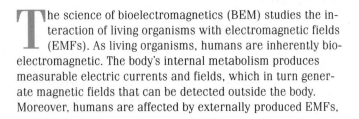

The science of bioelectromagnetics (BEM) studies the interaction of living organisms with electromagnetic fields (EMFs). As living organisms, humans are inherently bioelectromagnetic. The body's internal metabolism produces measurable electric currents and fields, which in turn generate magnetic fields that can be detected outside the body. Moreover, humans are affected by externally produced EMFs,

> ❝ *The influence of external electromagnetic fields — which include the earth's magnetic field as well as human-made electromagnetic emissions — may alter the body's own bioelectromagnetic activity sufficiently to cause physical and behavioral changes.* ❞

which include the earth's magnetic field as well as human-made electromagnetic emissions. The influence of these external fields may alter the body's own bioelectromagnetic activity sufficiently to cause physical and behavioral changes. This potential influence is the motivation for therapeutic BEM interventions. It's also the basis for concerns about the adverse physical and mental effects of continual exposure to human-made EMFs.

Electricity, radio waves, microwaves, and infrared waves are integral to our everyday lives. In addition to their positive applications, they're considered to cause possible negative effects as well, called *electropollution*. Electric current comes to our homes, schools, and workplaces over a complex grid of high-voltage transmission lines and household wiring. These wires emit extremely low-frequency EMFs. Added to this mix are radio, television, and microwave emissions as well as the influence of the earth's natural magnetic field. We're constantly exposed to electromagnetic waves of different frequencies and intensities.

In the patient care setting, nurses typically encounter such electromagnetic devices as infusion pumps, diathermy machines, and diagnostic equipment, including X-ray and magnetic resonance imaging (MRI) units. Treatments are documented on computers. Telephones and monitors enhance communication and facilitate documentation. Although we've harnessed and domesticated electrical and magnetic forces for many vital needs, they warrant careful handling to minimize the risk of harmful effects.

Ironically, the same electromagnetism that in high ranges may produce harmful biological effects may prove beneficial in lower ranges. Researchers have discovered that not only can certain extremely low-frequency magnetic fields produce strong positive effects in the body but certain frequencies can exert very specific effects on specific tissues, just as drug therapies do. This finding is the basis for BEM therapies.

Electrical and magnetic fields

Bioelectromagnetic interventions apply the principles of electromagnetism to diagnose and treat various medical conditions. Although electricity and magnetism are two forms of the same basic force — the electromagnetic force — they interact with each other in different ways and can be examined as separate phenomena. Basically, whenever electricity moves, magnetism is produced; whenever a magnetic field changes, electricity is produced.

Electricity begins with the atom, the fundamental unit of matter, which has a positively charged nucleus orbited by negatively charged electrons. Atoms form molecules by sharing electrons. When electrons become chemically or electrically excited, they can spin free from their atoms and move from orbit to orbit within a molecule. This electron movement produces electricity, and an electric current is produced when the electrons travel through a wire.

Whenever electrical charges are present, electrical fields are also present, created by the separation of positive (nucleus) and negative (electron) charges. Contact with metal or another conductive object allows the separated electrical charges to complete a circuit and return to a balanced neutral state; when a person is the "conductive object," the person feels an electric shock. The degree of separation of the charges dictates the potential strength of the electrical field, which is expressed in *volts*. The flow rate per second of the charge passing through a wire is expressed in *amperes*.

When an electric current moving through a wire produces an electrical field, it also creates a magnetic field around the wire. Energy from both of these fields interacts to form electromagnetic waves.

Magnetic fields are also created by fixed magnets, which are made from strongly magnetic materials such as iron. Such fields arise from the spinning of electrons around the nuclei of the iron atoms. The atoms all align in the same direction, and their individual magnetic fields combine to form one large magnetic field.

Positive and negative energy

The magnetic field is strongest at the magnet's ends, the "north" and "south" poles. Biomagnetic researchers call a magnet's south pole the *positive, biomagnetic south,* or *biosouth* pole, and a magnet's north pole the *negative, biomagnetic north,* or *bionorth* pole. This is because the south pole of a bar magnet causes the needle of a magnetometer to move to the positive end of the scale, and vice versa. In the context of magnet therapy, biosouth (+) and bionorth (−) are used to describe magnet placement for treatment.

Magnetic fields are similar to electrical fields in that they have direction and strength. The strength of a magnetic field is measured in units called *gauss* or *tesla*; 10,000 gauss equal one tesla. Magnets rated at a strength of 850 gauss or less are believed to reflect more nearly the strength of the earth's natural magnetic field. For this reason, practitioners consider them safe — no matter which polarity is used, even for prolonged periods. Practitioners who use stronger magnets (with field strengths of 2,000 to 4,000 gauss) maintain that prolonged application of the biosouth (+) pole can be overly stimulating and may exacerbate pain and infection symptoms. (See *Therapeutic effects of biomagnetic poles,* page 200.)

Other practitioners recommend almost exclusive application of the bionorth (−) pole for therapeutic treatment regardless of magnet strength, agreeing on the dangers of using only the biosouth (+) pole for extended periods. Biomagnetic researcher William Philpott, MD, recommends using the biosouth (+) pole for treatment periods of only 5 to 30 minutes, followed by bionorth (−) pole treatment to balance the entire body. Again, the effectiveness of this treatment hasn't yet been scientifically proven.

One application of low-gauss magnets uses a "bipolar" approach. Small magnets are arranged in a spatial pattern, such as concentric circles or a checkerboard, which places negative and positive poles close together so that both magnetic influences are applied to the body part to be treated. This approach is thought to stimulate vasodilation, which allows more oxygen and nutrients to reach tissues.

Currents and wavelengths

Magnetic fields differ in quality, depending on whether they're generated by direct or alternating electric currents. Direct current (DC), produced by storage devices such as car batteries, travels in only one direction, thus creating a steady magnetic field. Alternating current, the kind that powers our homes, continually reverses direction, so it creates a fluctuating magnetic field. Its frequency is measured in *hertz* (Hz). One complete fluctuation equals one Hz. For example, household electricity, which has a frequency of 60 Hz, fluctuates (reverses direction) 120 times (or 60 cycles) per second.

Electromagnetic fields travel through space as waves of energy. This wave motion, or wavelength, is measured from the crest of one wave to the crest of the next. The length of a wave is inversely proportional to its frequency: the greater the frequency, the shorter the wavelength. For example, household electricity falls within the extremely low-frequency range and has a very long wavelength (3,000 miles). In contrast, X-rays have extremely high frequencies but have extremely short wavelengths (less than one-billionth of a meter).

Therapeutic effects of biomagnetic poles

According to the science of bioelectromagnetics, each pole has a different function. The bionorth (–) pole of the magnet is considered akin to *yin* in traditional Chinese medicine—cooling, sedating, and dispersing. In biomagnetic theory, the bionorth pole is used for detoxifying, eliminating, and clearing. The biosouth (+) pole is considered *yang*, which practitioners claim yields a more heating, stimulating, and accumulating effect. Practitioners use this pole for strengthening and building.

Below are the indications and contraindications of the therapeutic applications of a magnet's bionorth and biosouth poles. To achieve a harmonizing effect, practitioners may recommend using both poles; they may alternate bionorth and biosouth or use them both simultaneously. They claim that using both poles is especially helpful for patients in extensive pain or with chronic disease.

Static magnetic field	Indications	Contraindications
Negative (north)	▶ Pain caused by weakness, coldness, or deficiency (chronic pain or achiness) ▶ Hypometabolic conditions associated with low energy, weak digestion, and weak immune system such as hypothyroidism	▶ Acute inflammatory conditions such as allergic reaction ▶ Bacterial, viral, or fungal infections ▶ Conditions resulting from "excess *yang*" ▶ Neoplasms
Positive (south)	▶ Inflammation, edema ▶ Hypermetabolic conditions such as fever ▶ Hypertensive conditions ▶ Insomnia or nervousness ▶ Infection	▶ Deficiency conditions ▶ Coldness ▶ Low metabolism ▶ Weakness, fatigue

Adapted with permission from Tierra, M. *Biomagnetic and Herbal Therapy.* Twin Lakes, Wis.: Lotus Press, 1997.

All electromagnetic fields carry energy through space, traveling outward from their source at the speed of light (about 186,000 miles/second). Although their strength diminishes with increasing distance from the source, they're capable of producing various effects. Many high-frequency wavelengths are classified as "ionizing radiation" because they can dislodge electrons from atoms and molecules in objects they strike. Strong ionization can damage biological tissues. X-rays and gamma rays are potent ionizers, whereas lower frequencies of the electromagnetic spectrum, from visible light down to direct current, are considered nonionizing. Because they're considered benign, some extremely low frequencies are often used in magnetic therapy. (See *Comparing electromagnetic wavelengths and effects,* pages 202 and 203.)

Earth's magnetic field

The earth, too, has a magnetic field, consisting of lines of magnetic force that surround the globe. They're thought to result from electric currents generated by the earth's molten iron core as it slowly revolves in place within the surrounding rocky mantle. The field is strongest at the earth's poles, just as it is at the poles of a simple bar magnet.

As they travel from one pole to the other, the lines of magnetic force curve far out into space, creating what is called the *magnetosphere.* The presence of the magnetosphere is strikingly demonstrated by the aurora borealis, or "northern lights," which appear in the upper atmosphere as shimmering curtains or beams of luminous particles. Besides providing us with a breathtaking light show at certain seasons, the magnetosphere protects the earth from deadly ultraviolet emissions coming from the sun.

Humans and animals alike have long used the earth's magnetic field in practical ways. Navigators have depended on a magnetized compass needle to direct their ships. Migrating fish and birds rely, at least in part, on some sort of internal compass thought to be activated by magnetic properties of magnetite, a metallic compound produced by all living organisms.

Over the past 75 to 100 years, so many electrical changes have occurred in our environment that some concerned researchers question the biological effects of living with electro-

Comparing electromagnetic wavelengths and effects

This chart shows the relative position of various types of natural and human-made radiation in the electromagnetic spectrum. It also indicates their biological strength and their wavelength patterns.

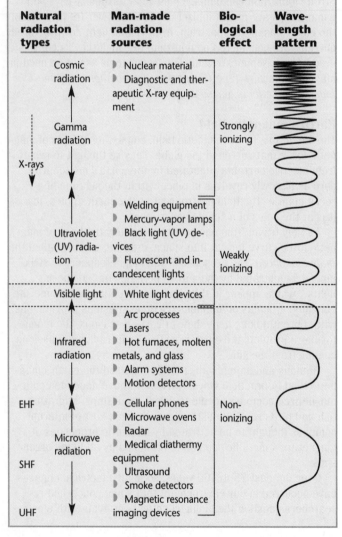

Natural radiation types	Man-made radiation sources	Biological effect	Wavelength pattern
Cosmic radiation	▶ Nuclear material ▶ Diagnostic and therapeutic X-ray equipment	Strongly ionizing	
Gamma radiation			
X-rays			
Ultraviolet (UV) radiation	▶ Welding equipment ▶ Mercury-vapor lamps ▶ Black light (UV) devices ▶ Fluorescent and incandescent lights	Weakly ionizing	
Visible light	▶ White light devices		
Infrared radiation	▶ Arc processes ▶ Lasers ▶ Hot furnaces, molten metals, and glass ▶ Alarm systems ▶ Motion detectors	Non-ionizing	
EHF	▶ Cellular phones ▶ Microwave ovens ▶ Radar ▶ Medical diathermy equipment ▶ Ultrasound ▶ Smoke detectors ▶ Magnetic resonance imaging devices		
Microwave radiation			
SHF			
UHF			

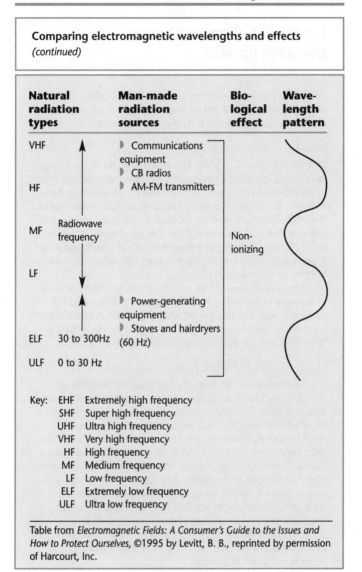

Comparing electromagnetic wavelengths and effects
(continued)

Natural radiation types	Man-made radiation sources	Biological effect	Wavelength pattern
VHF	Communications equipment		
	CB radios		
HF	AM-FM transmitters		
MF Radiowave frequency		Nonionizing	
LF			
	Power-generating equipment		
	Stoves and hairdryers		
ELF 30 to 300Hz	(60 Hz)		
ULF 0 to 30 Hz			

Key: EHF Extremely high frequency
SHF Super high frequency
UHF Ultra high frequency
VHF Very high frequency
HF High frequency
MF Medium frequency
LF Low frequency
ELF Extremely low frequency
ULF Ultra low frequency

Table from *Electromagnetic Fields: A Consumer's Guide to the Issues and How to Protect Ourselves,* ©1995 by Levitt, B. B., reprinted by permission of Harcourt, Inc.

Over the past 75 to 100 years, so many electrical changes have occurred in our environment that some concerned researchers question the biological effects of living with electromagnetic "pollution." Do the extremely low frequency EMFs around us cause ill effects? What are the effects of the thou-

(Text continues on page 206.)

Looking at electromagnetic pollution hazards

Bioelectromagnetic researchers and practitioners believe that numerous adverse medical effects may relate to changes in environmental electromagnetic fields (EMFs) and frequencies.

Magnetic field deficiency syndrome

Over 20 years ago, Dr. Kyoichi Nakagawa, director of Isuzu Hospital in Tokyo, identified a pattern of symptoms that appeared in patients without an apparent cause: stiffness of the shoulders, back, and neck; lumbago; chest pains; constant headache; heaviness of the head; dizziness; insomnia; habitual constipation; and general lassitude. Although these symptoms may accompany certain diseases, they appeared without other evidence of disease and they improved after low-level exposure to magnetic fields that resembled the earth's magnetic field.

Nakagawa postulated that the symptoms stemmed from lack of exposure to the earth's natural magnetic fields as a result of working in buildings that are artificially lit, insulated, often located hundreds of feet above the earth, and surrounded by artificial EMFs. He called the pattern *magnetic field deficiency syndrome.*

Electromagnetic sensitivity syndrome

A contrasting syndrome, labeled *electromagnetic sensitivity syndrome,* appears to be an allergic response associated with electromagnetic fields. Practitioners have noted this syndrome in a number of workers with high EMF exposures, including operating room personnel, computer operators, and airline employees. Sufferers report symptoms common to other environmental illnesses: rashes, flulike complaints, nausea, dizziness, headache, low-grade fever, swollen glands, sound and light sensitivity, difficulty concentrating, vision disturbances, general malaise, and debilitating fatigue. In addition, people with this syndrome report increasing sensitivity to a diverse range of electronic devices. To prevent symptom exacerbation, they find themselves avoiding areas with a multitude of electronic devices, such as television and appliance stores or radio and TV stations.

EMF exposure and cancer

Some studies, including a 1991 Environmental Protection Agency (EPA) study, have linked certain cancers with exposure to high-

Looking at electromagnetic pollution hazards *(continued)*

level EMFs. Among electrical workers and telephone cable workers, for example, the risk of brain tumors is reportedly 70% higher than in the general population. Some research indicates that children living near high-tension lines may have a double risk of brain tumors.

There may also be a genetic effect; children of fathers employed in EMF-related occupations reportedly exhibited a 50% higher incidence of central nervous system and brain stem cancers. Also, some studies have pointed to a statistically significant rise in leukemia following EMF exposure.

Electropollution and disease

Bioelectromagnetic theorists, such as Dr. Robert Becker, the orthopedic surgeon who promoted the use of electrical current to heal fractures, blame electropollution for causing a wide range of chromosomal and viral diseases — from chronic fatigue syndrome, autism, and sudden infant death syndrome to fragile X syndrome and acquired immunodeficiency syndrome. They also continue to argue for a causative relationship between EMF pollution and cancer, which hasn't yet been proven.

In addition, Dr. Becker and others suggest that changes in pre-existing diseases — such as Alzheimer's disease, Parkinson's disease, and cancer as well as mental disorders—may be due to effects of electropollution just as electromagnetic energy has produced global environmental changes. Exposure to EMFs that previously never existed has occurred to all living organisms, from viruses to humans. These human-made EMFs don't mimic anything in the natural environment; indeed, they operate in a contrary manner. The alternating current flowing through wires continually switches direction (polarity), and with each switch comes a corresponding switch in the surrounding magnetic fields, fields that penetrate whatever they come in contact with.

The subject of electropollution merits continued research to prove or refute the link to human disease. In addition, society may need to create safer means of transmitting power, microwave, and radio frequencies and dealing with the force fields that carry energy through space. In the meantime, agencies such as the EPA help to monitor health risks.

Electromagnetic fields in the body

The electrical and magnetic phenomena discussed so far are part of our external environment. The resulting external electromagnetic fields interact with the body's own subtle internal electromagnetic fields that are caused by the complex electrochemical reactions taking place inside every living cell.

Electromagnetic fields exert many of their effects at the level of the cell membrane. The flow of positively charged sodium and potassium ions and negatively charged chloride ions across cell membranes forms the basis of bioelectricity. Nearly all cells develop a voltage difference across their membranes, due to the separation of these positive and negative ionic charges. The cell membranes of muscle and nerve cells, in particular, are capable of initiating and conducting electrochemical impulses generated by momentary and reversible changes in the transmembrane voltage. These impulses are detectable in brain, heart, and muscle tissues.

Diagnostic tests — such as electroencephalograpy, electrocardiography, and electromyography — can measure and analyze these electrical impulses. The impulses generate corresponding magnetic fields that can be measured by magnetoencephalography, magnetocardiography, and magnetomyography. Both principles merge in MRI, which uses a steady state magnetic field and an oscillating electric field to excite hydrogen nuclei in body tissues. The returned signals are stored and processed by a computer to yield a detailed three-dimensional picture of internal structures.

Beyond the obvious merits of these diagnostic modalities, some researchers believe that electromagnetic changes at the cell membrane level may affect the action of hormones, growth factors, and other biologically important molecules to influence health and disease.

Magnetic substances in the body

Most substances found in the body are considered relatively nonmagnetic. Such materials as water and fatty substances, which are weakly repelled by a magnetic field, are called *diamagnetic*. Other substances, such as deoxyhemoglobin in blood cells, are weakly attracted to a magnetic field and are called *paramagnetic*.

The only known metallic compound produced by living organisms is a ferromagnetic material called magnetite. Mag-

> *Magnetite's presence in the pineal gland and its susceptibility to external EMFs may affect the function of this master gland that's believed to be the seat of the body's biological clock.*

netite has the strongest magnetic properties and highest electrical conductivity of any cellular material, is known to interact with the earth's magnetic field, and is distributed throughout human brain tissue. Its presence in the pineal gland and its susceptibility to external EMFs may affect the function of this master gland that's believed to be the seat of the body's biological clock. The pineal gland produces melatonin, a neurohormone that controls other hormones and is a factor in the regulation of enzymes, immune function, oxidation, carbohydrate metabolism, pigmentation, and the sleep-wakefulness cycle. Overexposure of the pineal gland and other body tissues to external EMFs may produce systemic effects.

Body substances also possess another characteristic called *piezoelectricity,* the ability to generate electrical fields when deformed by compression or bending forces. Connective tissue, which is continuous throughout the body, is considered piezoelectric because of the crystalline structure of collagen tissue. Collagen acts as a semiconductor, forming an integrated electrical structural communication network. Through this network, patterns of strain caused by physical or emotional trauma are communicated to adjacent structures in the body.

Bone is also piezoelectric. It's capable of transforming mechanical stress into electrical energy, as demonstrated by studies of bone healing.

Electromagnetic therapy — then and now

The first documented bioelectromedical therapy was in 46 AD, when a physician named Scribonius Largus recommended applying an electric torpedo fish (which can generate powerful shocks) to the body to treat headaches and gouty arthritis.

The systematic application of electromedical equipment for therapeutic treatment was initiated in the 1700s. In 1745,

Pieter van Musschenbroek from the University of Leyden in the Netherlands invented the Leyden jar. This glass container lined with metal foil can store a charge of static electricity. The jar was used to stimulate the muscles in a patient's paralyzed hand. After 3 months of treatment with static electrical charges, the paralysis disappeared.

> 66 *Electrical stimulation of acupuncture needles was first demonstrated in Japan in 1764.* 99

Electrical stimulation of acupuncture needles was first demonstrated in Japan in 1764. In France in 1825, practitioners treated rheumatic conditions by applying static electrical current from Leyden jars to inserted acupuncture needles. In the 1950s, practitioners of traditional Chinese medicine used bioelectrical acupuncture for anesthesia.

In 1950, a French physician and student of Chinese acupuncture, Paul Nogier, developed *auriculotherapy*, or ear acupuncture. He formulated the original map of ear points used in contemporary acupuncture and created an electric device for stimulating those points.

In the 1940s, Reinhold Voll developed an instrument called a Dermatron for measuring the electrical resistance of acupuncture points as an overall measure of a person's health. His assessment technique became known as *electroacupuncture according to Voll*.

Electromagnetic devices, such as MRI devices, have long been used in conventional medicine to diagnose human illness. Contemporary examples of electrical therapy include electroconversion of the heart muscle during an arrhythmia or asystole, implanted cardiac pacemakers, electroconvulsive therapy for continuous severe depression, and extremely low-frequency devices such as transcutaneous electrical nerve stimulation (TENS) units for pain control.

Clinicians are also using bioelectromagnetic therapies for various indications, such as healing bone fractures and wounds that fail to heal spontaneously (pulsed EMF, extremely low frequency, and radiofrequency therapies), reducing anxiety (transcranial electrostimulation), and substituting for electroshock treatments for major depression (neuromagnetic stimulation). Now alternative practitioners are using some of the same EMF therapies to enhance traditional acupuncture, stimulate the immune system, and combat cancers.

With the exception of the historical therapeutic application of lodestone (naturally occurring mineral magnets) or magnetite, bioelectromagnetic literature seems to ignore magnet therapy or brush it off as too trivial to mention. Yet magnets are being used therapeutically in Japan, Russia, and Europe. Also, the scientific community still strongly resists the converse idea—that electrical, radio, and microwave systems may be biohazards. Because research in these areas isn't funded, a plethora of unsubstantiated "scientific claims" use the language and theory of bioelectromagnetism.

> ❝ *Bioelectromagnetic interventions are used to assess and restore a person's electromagnetic balance, the flow of electromagnetic energy in the body.* ❞

Bioelectromagnetic (BEM) interventions are used to assess and restore a person's electromagnetic balance—that is, the flow of electromagnetic energy in the body. BEM devices provide a tool for preventive screening to detect potential electromagnetic imbalances that may lead to disease, and they may be used to enhance healing (as with electric current applied to fractures to stimulate bone regrowth) or to rebalance endogenous electromagnetic fields before further structural or chemical disturbances occur.

Magnets work to balance the person by applying a static magnetic field at the site of the person's physical complaint. Electrical devices use pulsed DC microcurrents (from a rechargeable battery) to assess resistance at acupuncture or trigger points and stimulate the sites. BEM devices are noninvasive and appear to provide results more economically than comparable standard medical treatments. They're based on the holistic principle that restoring the balance of a patient's bioelectromagnetic fields assists the patient in self-healing.

Most BEM devices aren't regulated by the Food and Drug Administration (FDA), so no direct medical claims can be made about their effectiveness. However, based on current health standards, alternative therapy bioelectromagnetic devices fall within the FDA's acceptable safety range for BEM exposure.

Today, little concrete knowledge exists of the bioelectromagnetic nature of the human organism, and we know even less about the biological effects of EMFs and electropollution. Further research is needed on the efficacy of BEM therapies, the safety of BEM devices, the potential effects of electropollution, and the role of BEM therapies in counteracting these effects.

Specific BEM therapies used include radiofrequency (RF) hyperthermia, RF diathermy, microwave resonance therapy, and the use of TENS units.

Magnetic field therapy

Magnetic field therapy (also called biomagnetic therapy, magnet therapy, electromagnetic therapy, or magnetotherapy) involves the use of magnetic fields in the prevention and treatment of disease and first-aid treatment for injuries. Its goal is to restore a person's internal bioelectromagnetic balance. With successful therapy, the patient should learn to maintain this internal balance without the need for continued external intervention. (See *Understanding magnetic field therapy.*)

Therapeutic magnetism isn't a new idea. Natural mineral magnets, called lodestones, were used for thousands of years in Chinese, Egyptian, and Greek medicine to treat various ailments. Today's magnets consist of iron, iron-containing ceramics, neodymium, or other materials that can be permanently magnetized.

Practitioners of magnetic field therapy range from the self-healing layperson to licensed health care professionals, including massage therapists, nurses, physician assistants, acupuncturists, chiropractors, physical therapists, medical physicians, and dentists. The nurse's role is to be knowledgeable about magnetic field therapy as a possible health-enhancing therapy. The Bio-Electro-Magnetics Institute in Reno, Nevada, offers BEM education as well as technical assistance, research, and information about this field.

HOW IT WORKS

⟷ Understanding magnetic field therapy

One theory of magnetic field therapy suggests that diseased cells have lost their magnetic equilibrium and that topically applied magnets work on a molecular level to restore this equilibrium within the cells. This, in turn, benefits surrounding cells and the entire organism.

Another theory, based on the magnetic nature of red blood cells, supposes a magnetically induced increase in blood and oxygen supply to diseased tissues. This increased blood and oxygen supply yields accompanying pH adjustment and increased nutrient availability and relieves congestion and pain through improved circulation.

Reported effects

A survey of magnetic field therapy research identifies the following specific physiologic effects of treatment with magnets:
▶ increased blood and oxygen circulation along with the nutrient-carrying potential of blood
▶ changes in pH balance, often imbalanced in diseased tissues (Bionorth [–] fields promote beneficial alkalinity and biosouth [+] fields promote harmful acidity.)
▶ enhanced migration of calcium ions, which facilitates the healing of nervous tissue and bones and helps reduce the pathologic buildup of calcium in arthritic joints
▶ changes in the production of certain endocrine hormones
▶ enhanced enzyme activity and other related physiologic processes.

Therapeutic uses

Practitioners claim that therapeutic magnets benefit a wide range of conditions, from acute and chronic pain, strains, and swelling to systemic illness. In addition, magnets and electromagnetic therapy devices are now being used to help heal broken bones and counter the effects of stress. A negative magnetic field applied to the top of the head stimulates melatonin, producing a calming and sleep-inducing effect on the brain and body.

Magnetic field therapy has been recognized in sports medicine for its effectiveness in relieving sprains and strains. Magnetic field therapy has also been used in conjunction with other therapies, such as nutrition, herbs, and acupuncture. For example, practitioners believe that having a patient lie on a magnetic mattress enhances the effectiveness of craniosacral therapy.

Although the scientific basis of magnetic field therapy has yet to be established, thousands of patients have reported relief of pain or discomfort from such conditions as arthritis, back pain, pressure ulcers, carpal tunnel syndrome, diabetic neuropathy, gout, rheumatism, shoulder pain, trigeminal neuralgia, toothache, and ulcers. People who have been treated with magnetic field therapy say that it relieves their pain, helps heal injuries, relieves headaches, and has an overall beneficial effect on the body. Magnetic field therapy has been used to treat various orthopedic problems, musculoskeletal disorders, arthritis, and temporomandibular joint pain. Additionally, practitioners claim that it can be used to treat hepatitis, ulcers, epileptic seizures, optic nerve atrophy, migraine headaches, hypertension, and postsurgical swelling. Furthermore, magnetic field therapy has been used to restore electromagnetic field balance in patients with such diseases as multiple sclerosis, breast cancer, Parkinson's disease, osteoporosis, joint disease, heart disease, and diabetes.

> *Researchers at Baylor College of Medicine concluded that delivering static magnetic fields of 300 to 500 gauss over a pain trigger point brought significant and prompt relief.*

RESEARCH SUMMARY Most benefits attributed to magnetic field therapy in the United States are based on anecdotal evidence, rather than clinical studies. Empirical research has been conducted extensively in Japan, Russia, and India but is only now picking up in the United States. For example, in 1997, investigators at Baylor College of Medicine in Houston, Texas, performed a double-blind, randomized, clinical trial of pain response to static magnetic fields, using 50 volunteer patients who were suffering from postpolio syndrome. They found statistically significant evidence of pain relief for the patients who received treatment from an active magnetic device as opposed to those treated with a placebo. The researchers concluded that delivering static magnetic fields of 300 to 500 gauss over a pain trigger point brought significant and prompt relief. This study used bionorth (−) magnets. ■

The Bio-Electro-Magnetics Institute in conjunction with the Veterans Administration Hospital in Prescott, Arizona, plans to conduct another double-blind study that will examine the effectiveness of magnets in treating lower back pain. Clinical research is under way at other centers to investigate the use of magnets to treat such conditions as fibromyalgia and phantom limb pain.

Low-gauss strength exposure to alternating magnetic poles for short periods of time has been shown empirically to relieve symptoms quickly, perhaps more so than a unipolar application. Because of the vasodilation believed to occur with this bipolar treatment, it isn't recommended for acute injuries associated with bleeding until after 24 hours, to avoid potential clotting delays.

Practitioners agree that biomagnetic therapy effectively relieves pain, swelling, and discomfort, but they disagree over whether therapeutic effects are best obtained using the bionorth (−) pole, the biosouth (+) pole, or both together. Practitioners also disagree about which gauss strengths are most appropriate. Russian researchers have found beneficial effects from magnetic field therapy, regardless of polarity. Unfortunately, no scientific studies have yet been done to evaluate competing claims.

Equipment

Magnets used for magnetic field therapy should be high-quality medical magnets. Therapeutic magnets come in all sizes, shapes, and strengths. Because they aren't regulated as medical devices, quality and consistency may vary from one manufacturer to another. True bionorth (−) and biosouth (+) poles can be determined by using a simple compass: Bionorth (−) is south-seeking (attracted to the south or positive pole), and biosouth (+) is north-seeking (attracted to the north or negative pole). Gauss meters are also available for measuring the external field strength of the magnet. A magnet view device, which is filled with iron particles that respond when placed on a magnet, shows the pattern of plastic strip magnets.

Buying plastic magnet sheets at the craft store may be adequate in the short run, but they lack the consistency and quality of medical magnets. Craft magnets may stick to the refrigerator, but their field strength isn't rated and their therapeutic value is unknown. If no better magnet is available, a refrigerator magnet might work for treating a minor injury.

Biomagnetic appliances range from small adhesive pads to belts and mattresses. The typical magnet pad or mattress for a queen-sized bed contains anywhere from 200 to 550 small magnets, spaced from 1½ to 4″ (4 to 10 cm) apart, with surface field strength ranging from 75 to 1,075 gauss. The magnets are typically oriented with the bionorth (−) side closest to the person but may also be oriented with the biosouth (+) side closest to the person. Mattresses are said to be beneficial for promoting restorative sleep, increasing melatonin production, stimulating the body's natural healing ability, and facilitating the rebalancing of the body's electromagnetic flow from the adverse effects of electropollution.

Magnetic car seats and cushions offer comfort for driving or sitting in office chairs. They come in varying gauss strengths, and most are oriented with bionorth (−) facing the person — but some products are reversible.

Magnetic insoles are thin, flexible, magnetoform plastic inserts that may be bipolar or unipolar with bionorth (−) on one side and biosouth (+) on the other. They're said to improve circulation and reduce foot discomfort for people who must stand for long periods of time, such as hairdressers, bartenders, food service workers, and nurses.

Bipolar magnets, in the form of small magnetic pads, come in varying sizes and shapes for easier application over specific areas of discomfort. The bipolar pads usually have a metallic foil on the side worn away from the body, which directs the magnetic field more effectively toward the source of discomfort.

Magnetic pads come in various shapes and sizes and can be applied to the back, knees, elbows, wrists, ankles, face, neck, and shoulders. These wraps conveniently hold the magnets in place, directing the magnetic field toward the area of discomfort.

Acuband magnets are tiny (1 to 2 mm in diameter), disk-shaped magnets that are easily attached to the body with round adhesive bandages. Despite their small size, they have impressive internal field strengths ranging from 3,000 to 9,000 gauss. Some discs have marked bionorth (−) poles for easier identification. These magnets can be applied to acupuncture points that relate to the person's symptoms. They may also be applied at the site of a bone fracture to promote healing.

At the other end of the scale are large block magnets — industrial magnets made of iron ferrite. These magnets come in various sizes and shapes and usually have high-gauss field strength. Some people use these large block magnets to polarize and purify their drinking water.

Biomagnets are also available to be worn as jewelry. Necklaces deliver magnetic field therapy to areas of the neck, throat, thymus, shoulders, and heart, whereas bracelets can be worn for wrist, hand, and arm pain. Some designs position magnets at pulse points, which theoretically can regulate blood pressure. Rings and earrings are also available. The field strength of jewelry items ranges from 700 to 1,300 gauss.

Magnetic pet beds and collars are also available, which may be beneficial in treating a pet's joint pain or other ailments.

Procedure

Handbooks of magnetic field therapy describe the best placement and magnet strength for self-treatment of various illnesses. (See *Using magnets for basic first aid,* pages 216 and 217.) High-gauss treatments and those involving prolonged exposure to the biosouth (+) pole should be supervised by a qualified practitioner.

The simplest home remedy for pain involves applying a low- to medium-gauss (800-gauss or less) magnet to the area of discomfort and leaving it in place until well after the discomfort disappears. The longer the treatment, the more quickly the healing and the greater the symptom relief. If the pain decreases with treatment, the magnet is correctly oriented; if the pain increases, even if the magnet's bionorth side is facing the patient, the magnet needs to be turned over.

Therapy may be of short duration (1 to 2 hours) if high-gauss magnets are used; magnets may also be used overnight or for 24 hours or more for maximum effect. Nutrition and diet therapy may be used in addition to magnetic field therapy for optimal healing.

Using magnets for basic first aid

According to magnetic field therapy proponents, magnets can be used to treat minor complaints. If your patient uses magnetic field therapy, tell him to seek medical treatment for serious or nonresponsive burns or injuries. If he's allergic to insect bites, urge him to keep an anaphylactic kit handy and to seek immediate medical attention for an insect bite.

Insect bites
Because bites and stings are acid, practitioners recommend negative magnetic energy to reduce acidity, inflammation, and pain. Magnets are usually applied soon after occurrence.

Burns
Practitioners recommend applying negative magnetic energy to burns before tissue deterioration occurs. They prefer a 2" × 5" (5 × 12.5 cm) or 4" × 6" (10 × 15 cm) ceramic magnet.

Headache
Practitioners suggest applying ceramic magnets or stacked plastiform magnets directly over the painful area. If this brings no relief, they suggest placing magnets on opposite sides of the head to pull fluid away from the painful area. Alternatively, they suggest applying two ceramic cube magnets or 4" × 6" ceramic magnets bitemporally. Finally, they recommend placing one plastiform strip and one neodymium round magnet on the back of the head at the base of the skull along with ceramic or plastiform magnets on the forehead at the hairline.

Insomnia
Practitioners recommend the magnetic bed to reduce the stress, muscle tension, and musculoskeletal pain that disrupt sleep.

Muscle spasms
Practitioners suggest treating muscle spasms by placing ceramic magnets or three or four stacked plastiform magnets directly over the painful area. They recommend relieving leg cramps by placing ceramic magnets under the soles of the feet.

Using magnets for basic first aid *(continued)*

Sprain or strain
Practitioners suggest applying ceramic magnets or three or four stacked magnetic strips directly to the injured area to reduce inflammation and swelling.

Adapted with permission from Philpott, W.H., and Taplin, W.S.L. *Biomagnetic Handbook: Today's Introduction to the Energy Medicine of Tomorrow.* Choctaw, Okla.: Enviro-Tech Products, 1990.

Complications

Positive (biosouth) magnetic energy should be used only under medical supervision because some investigators believe that overstimulation of the brain may occur, producing seizures, hallucinations, insomnia, hyperactivity, and magnetic addiction. It has also been claimed that positive magnetic energy may stimulate growth of tumors and microorganisms.

A bedridden patient who uses a magnetic bed 24 hours a day risks suppressed adrenal function and slowed energy recovery. A magnetic bed should be used only 8 to 10 hours at a time.

Nursing perspective

▶ Practitioners report that older people respond especially well to overall energizing effects of magnetic field therapy as well as to specific treatment for chronic pain or illness. However, because of the complex range of symptoms that many older patients experience, you should encourage these patients to continue to seek conventional treatment and to report any alternative therapies they're undergoing.

▶ Because of the experimental nature of magnetic field therapy, it isn't recommended for children younger than age 5 or for pregnant women.

▶ Patients with pacemakers or defibrillators shouldn't use magnetic beds, and no magnets should be placed closer than 6″ (15 cm) to such devices to avoid interfering with their function.

Care and handling of therapeutic magnets

Observe the following care measures when handling magnets, and teach patients to do the same:

▶ Recognize that magnets may alter magnetic instruments, such as pacemakers, battery-powered wristwatches, hearing aids, and other equipment in use around a patient. Keep magnets away from magnetic resonance imaging machines. Also keep them away from patients who have metallic parts in their body. Post signs above a patient's bed to warn other staff and visitors.

▶ Avoid dropping or banging magnets. Don't heat a magnet above 500° F (260° C) because this can dissipate its strength.

▶ When not using a U-shaped magnet, connect the ends with a magnet keeper to prolong magnet strength.

▶ Don't keep different-sized magnets together; it alters their strength.

▶ Keep magnets away from computer hard drives and magnetic media — such as diskettes, recording tapes, credit or bank cards, videos, and compact disks — to prevent damage or erasure of contents. Any item with a magnetic strip on it, such as an identification card, can be ruined by exposure to a magnet.

▶ Because magnet polarity is important in treatment and industrial magnets typically have different pole labels than medical or therapeutic magnets, caution your patients to use a magnetometer or a compass to check the poles on a magnet they plan to use. With a compass, the tip of the arrow marked *N* or *north* will point toward the magnet's negative pole.

▶ Inform patients to avoid using magnets on the abdomen for 60 to 90 minutes after meals so that peristalsis can take place.

▶ Application of therapeutic magnets is considered relatively safe. However, some experts claim that using the positive pole of a medium- to high-gauss magnet for a protracted time may exacerbate symptoms rather than eliminate them.

▶ Monitor a patient who is undergoing magnetic field therapy for adverse reactions and the subsequent need to decrease or discontinue use. The danger exists that people will turn to magnetic field therapy as a cure-all rather than seek medical attention for significant health problems.

▶ Inform patients seeking magnetic field therapy that more and stronger magnets aren't necessarily better. No research documents the possible long-term adverse effects of static magnet fields.

▶ Warn patients to remove all magnets before undergoing surgery because magnets may cause life-threatening instrument malfunction.

▶ If your patient is treating himself with magnets, inform him about safe magnet use. (See *Care and handling of therapeutic magnets.*)

Bioelectrical acupuncture

Bioelectrical acupuncture, or electroacupuncture, involves application of electrostimulation to acupuncture needles during traditional acupuncture treatment. Another form of bioelectrical acupuncture is a needleless technique applying direct electrostimulation to acupuncture points.

Licensed acupuncturists can apply electrostimulation to acupuncture needles during acupuncture. Direct electrostimulation of acupuncture points can be performed by licensed acupuncturists or trained health care workers or self-administered by a layperson under the supervision of a practitioner.

Nurses who work in massage or pain clinics, those trained in acupressure and the acupuncture energy channels (meridians), or those who do body work with their patients may also practice this therapy. If not, the nurse's role is to be well informed about the process of bioelectrical acupuncture, its effectiveness and limitations, the potential adverse effects of such treatment, and the appropriate timing of referrals for other methods of care.

Electroacupuncture according to Voll (EAV) is the basis of subsequently developed bioelectrical acupuncture biofeedback devices, also called electrodermal screening devices. In the United States, these devices are approved only for use as experimental screening devices, not yet for treatment. Using low frequencies, these devices provide information that can be used to treat conditions that are identified by bioelectrical acupuncture assessment.

Therapeutic uses

As with traditional acupuncture, therapeutic application of bioelectrical acupuncture would appear limitless, depending on the ability and experience of the practitioner. Reportedly,

> 66 *Controlled studies have demonstrated the benefits of bioelectrical acupuncture to treat postoperative pain, chemotherapy-induced illness, and renal colic and to induce contractions in postterm pregnancy.* 99

it's particularly effective for treating physical injury and acute and chronic pain.

RESEARCH SUMMARY Controlled studies have demonstrated the benefits of bioelectrical acupuncture to treat postoperative pain, chemotherapy-induced illness, and renal colic and to induce contractions in postterm pregnancy. In research using rats, bioelectrical stimulation of acupuncture points has enhanced peripheral motor nerve regeneration and sensory nerve growth. ■

Equipment

Bioelectrical acupuncture devices can be used to assess a patient's condition and provide treatment as well, following the concepts of traditional Chinese acupuncture. These meters measure the flow of energy along the meridians at specific acupoints (points along a meridian where energy flow can best be measured and manipulated). A steady flow indicates health, whereas an impaired flow suggests disease, with different organs associated with specific meridians. Some acupoints, called control measurement points (CMP), give an overall indication of health in an organ or tissue. Other acupoints relate to specific parts of the organ and can show the specific site of the imbalance in that organ. Over 2,000 CMPs have been identified with this type of meter. Each acupoint has a standard measure that represents health. With deteriorating health, the measurement changes.

Various bioelectrical acupuncture devices are available. They range in sophistication from simple handheld, battery-operated, point-locator treatment devices to multifaceted, computerized units. Some of the devices are assessment tools, others deliver treatments, and still others do both.

Dermatron

Assessment devices such as the Dermatron, developed by Reinhold Voll, use sensors to measure the electrical resistance at acupoints. Higher-than-normal resistance at a specific acupoint indicates irritation or inflammation in the corresponding organ, whereas lower-than-normal resistance at the acupoint indicates degeneration or fatigue.

Thus, the Dermatron provides a way of screening for the existence of disease. It can also test the energetic effects of certain remedies. For example, when a patient takes a homeopathic dilution prescribed for his disease, the EAV reading returns to normal. In this way, EAV screening resembles an electronic version of kinesiology, the muscle-testing method that assists the therapist to similarly identify what weakens or strengthens the muscular system.

Computerized bioelectrical acupuncture devices can be used to perform multiple screenings quickly, and they support research with a detailed patient database. Most of these bioelectrical acupuncture devices are battery-operated, using direct current to avoid introducing the possible adverse effects of a pulsating or fluctuating alternating current into the system.

Locator-stimulator

The locator-stimulator (shown below) is another example of a bioelectrical acupuncture assessment tool. This simple, battery-operated device is used to locate and treat acupoints and trigger points (any point responding with pain upon palpation).

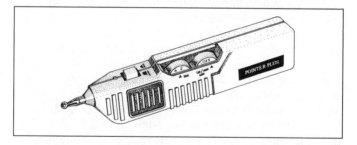

One dial adjusts to location, emitting a flashing light and sound when a point is located. The stimulation control delivers a fixed frequency signal (10 Hz) for treating the point. For self-treatment, a metal plate on the side of the device can be used to complete the necessary grounding circuit. A separate grounding pole is used to complete this circuit when being used by a practitioner.

SOLITENS device

A treatment unit, the SOLITENS is categorized as a transcutaneous electrical nerve stimulation (TENS) device. TENS units were originally developed to block pain by directing a stimulating current into local nerves, using a relatively high-frequency signal. This sometimes created muscle spasm instead of the intended pain relief. Used at low frequencies, TENS devices have been found effective for reducing pain by stimulating acupuncture and trigger points without the use of needles.

The SOLITENS has point location abilities, a timer, a ground, and the capability of delivering a stimulation pulse rate of 15 Hz for treating acupoints and trigger points. Therapeutic applications include symptomatic relief of chronic intractable pain, posttraumatic acute pain (in athletic injuries, for example), and postsurgical pain.

MORA

A combination assessment and treatment device developed by Franz Morrel, MD, the MORA works under the assumption that all biological processes are bioelectromagnetic and can be recognized by a distinctive, complex waveform. A smooth wave indicates health, and higher or lower wave deviations indicate disease. The MORA collects electromagnetic signals directly from the acupoints, manipulates and adjusts any aberrant wave forms to create normal waves, and then feeds these corrected waves back into the patient through the same acupoints. Proponents of this device describe it as a truly natural therapy because it uses specific wave information from the patient without introducing any artificial electrical signal.

Therapeutic applications of the MORA include treatment of skin disease and circulation problems; relief of headaches, migraines, and muscular aches and pains; and treatment in conjunction with homeopathy. The MORA doubles as an EAV diagnostic instrument. It can also be used in color therapy to transmit individual color frequencies of the electromagnetic field (EMF) spectrum, which are believed to impart beneficial effects.

Electro-Acuscope

The Electro-Acuscope (shown on next page) is a treatment device that uses extremely low-frequency current — microamperage rather than the milliamperage used by standard TENS devices.

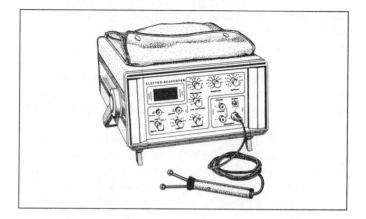

Microamperage is used to stimulate tissue repair. Rather than delivering a premeasured current, the device matches current delivery to the resistance sensed in the damaged tissue; such self-regulation facilitates the repair process.

This treatment works at the cellular level. Microcurrent stimulation is believed to induce extracellular calcium ions to enter the cell through pores in the cell membrane (called voltage-sensitive calcium ion channels). Higher levels of calcium, in turn, encourage increased synthesis of adenosine triphosphate, which activates mechanisms that control deoxyribonucleic acid and protein synthesis. The result is an increase in the rate of cellular repair and replication.

Treatment with this device is highly interactive between the patient and a well-trained practitioner. Popular as a treatment instrument in sports medicine, the Electro-Acuscope is used to treat musculoskeletal injuries, such as lumbosacral sprains, shoulder strains, whiplash, trauma, temporomandibular joint pain, bursitis, carpal tunnel syndrome, and muscle spasms. It's also used for arthritis, bruises, herpes zoster infections, local skin infections and skin ulcerations, chronic fatigue syndrome, migraines, neuralgia, surgical incisions, and palliative care of a ruptured disk in patients unwilling or unable to undergo surgery.

Nogier auriculotherapy device
The Nogier auriculotherapy treatment device uses direct current (DC) electricity or laser energy to treat acupoints on the ear. Similar to reflexology, which uses the foot, auriculotherapy operates on the concept that the entire body and all its or-

gans can be identified at different points on the ear. Auriculotherapy can also be practiced with acupuncture needles, therapeutic magnets, and a glass rod technique for point massage.

While using the Nogier device to treat the patient, the practitioner takes a radial pulse. The increase or decrease in radial pulse amplitude, called the vascular autonomic signal, is used as an indicator for the progression of treatment.

Considerable training is required before using this device. Therapeutic applications include addictions, dyslexia, pain control (acute or chronic pain, back pain, and pain from trauma), tinnitus, and parkinsonian tremors. Its use is contraindicated for severe conditions, such as renal insufficiency and heart disease.

Other devices

Similar to the MORA, many bioelectrical acupuncture devices apply other frequencies from the low range of the electromagnetic spectrum. For example, a light beam generator has been used to direct photons of light to assist in restoration of the cells' normal energy state, thus promoting healing. Able to attain deep body penetration, it's described as effective for treating organ as well as skin problems.

Sound probes are reported to destroy parasites and anything not in resonance with the body, by emitting a tone of three alternating frequencies. Radiofrequency diathermy devices use radio waves to send penetrating heat deep into the tissues for improved blood flow, pain reduction, and healing.

Procedure

Most bioelectrical acupuncture devices are used in similar ways. First, the practitioner uses the device to locate either traditional acupoints or a patient's trigger points of complaint. The practitioner is searching for tissue impedance, which generates a pitched signal from the device. Then the practitioner uses the device to provide treatment consisting of low-level DC directed back into the identified points. Treatment lasts 30 minutes to 1 hour, and the patient may need to return for additional visits. Some patients can use the devices at home.

Complications

Headache, nausea, and unpleasant sensations can occur with invasive or noninvasive bioelectrical acupuncture, requiring adjustment in the frequency and amperage of the device. Skin irritation and rash are also possible. If alterations in skin integrity occur, treatment may need to be postponed or treatment frequency reduced.

Nursing perspective

▶ Bioelectrical acupuncture devices are contraindicated for pain of unknown cause and for severe conditions, such as renal insufficiency and heart disease. Also, they shouldn't be used for patients with demand-type cardiac pacemakers, transcerebral electrode placement (because of the remote risk of seizures), or electrode placement over the carotid sinus region (which regulates blood pressure).

▶ Whether these devices may be used safely during pregnancy hasn't been established. However, in Europe, TENS units have been used during labor and delivery to facilitate contractions.

▶ Bioelectrical acupuncture devices have been incorporated into the modern biofeedback approach. Although bioelectrical acupuncture is "alternative," its reliance on technology makes it subject to the same concerns nurses face in conventional treatments — that the human patient is in danger of being reduced to a treatable electric potential.

Cell-specific cancer therapy

The Center for Cell-Specific Cancer Therapy, located in Santo Domingo, Dominican Republic, and staffed by a nuclear engineer and a medical doctor, uses pulsed electromagnetic field therapy against various cancers. According to the center, cancer cells emit an excessive amount of positively charged ions, making them a logical target for the center's bioelectromagnetic therapy called cell-specific cancer therapy (CSCT). No other cells in the body produce such an energy signature, and different cancers have distinctively different ionic signatures.

The goal of the Center's therapy is to detect cancer cells by their signatures and destroy them, using a pulsed electromagnetic field. This field reportedly alters the cancer cells' metabolism without harming surrounding healthy cells. Since opening in August 1996, this outpatient clinic has treated 150 clients and claims a success rate of 50%. Its claims haven't been verified independently.

Therapeutic uses

The Center claims that CSCT best detects actively growing cancers. It purports to have successfully treated even stage IV cancers.

RESEARCH SUMMARY CSCT bases its efficacy claims on operating principles that are grounded in scientific knowledge of cancer. Although CSCT is considered noninvasive and nondestructive of healthy tissue, precise and objective research is needed to verify its effectiveness.

The use of pulsed magnetic fields for cancer therapy has been questioned on the grounds that such fields may stimulate cancer growth while simultaneously stimulating the immune system through a stress response. At the onset of treatment, it appears that the immune system wins out and the cancer subsides. However, when the stress response declines, the cancer may again rapidly replicate. ■

Equipment

The Center uses a proprietary electromagnetic device, the CSCT-200, which is described as producing a pulsed electromagnetic field.

Procedure

According to the Center, CSCT treatment consists of scanning the body and then marking the cancerous sites on a body map and on the person. The CSCT device reportedly identifies the sound frequency of the cancer cells, matches it, and then sends the signal back into the cells, causing them to vibrate, rupture, and die.

Treatment sessions generally last for 30 minutes and are given twice a day for up to 3 weeks. The center considers the treatment successful when the CSCT-200 can no longer detect the cancer signals and when conventional laboratory tests no longer detect cancer markers.

The Center for Cell-Specific Cancer Therapy focuses only on the scanner treatment without attention to other factors related to achieving long-term remission, such as nutrition, diet therapy, detoxification, dental work, and counseling.

Complications
The Center doesn't accept patients who have received conventional chemotherapy and radiation therapy because it maintains that such therapies can hinder the effectiveness of the CSCT treatment. The scanner reportedly can't perceive previously treated cancer cells that have received high doses of chemotherapy or radiation and yet survived, presumably because their metabolism has slowed and their ionic pattern is undetectable. These undetectable cells could recover to multiply again. By delaying conventional treatment, the patient also risks cancer progression if CSCT fails.

CSCT scanning also carries the potential risk of cumulative radiologic exposure.

Nursing perspective
Because the Center maintains that conventional treatment can inhibit CSCT, the danger is that a patient may reject or postpone conventional treatment in favor of this alternative treatment, potentially risking his life.

Static electromagnetic field therapy
Static electromagnetic field therapy is another bioelectromagnetic treatment that's being applied to cancer. This therapy uses magnets, which create a static electromagnetic field (EMF), as opposed to electromagnets, which create a pulsed EMF.

Although many substances are known carcinogens, biomagnetic researcher William Philpott, MD, has postulated that cancer is a single disease with a single root cause: acid-hypoxia — that is, an acidic, hypoxic environment makes tissues more susceptible to carcinogens. This theory holds that corrective treatment requires the creation of an alkaline-hyperoxic environment.

Therapy with a static bionorth (−) magnetic field is believed to produce such a state. As with cell-specific cancer therapy (CSCT), in static EMF therapy, targeted cancer cells don't revert to a normal state; instead, they die. According to this theory, tumors may still be present after treatment, but they're no longer cancerous.

Therapeutic uses

Practitioners apply static EMF therapy to various cancers. As with conventional cancer treatments, they report that single, nonmetastatic lesions are more successfully treated than obstructive or metastatic lesions.

RESEARCH SUMMARY   Similar to CSCT, practitioners justify static EMF therapy as being in line with current knowledge of cancer. It's considered noninvasive and nondestructive of healthy tissue but requires further and independent research. ■

Equipment

Static EMF therapy uses high-gauss magnets. The higher the gauss, the better; practitioners prefer high-strength neodymium magnets. Equipment also includes magnetic chair pads, a 5″ × 6″ (12.5 × 15 cm) flexible magnet, and a magnetic mattress.

Procedure

According to its practitioners, treatment with static EMF therapy consists of continuous, intense therapy with high-gauss magnets for at least 3 months. The bionorth (−) pole of the magnet is placed directly over the lesion and kept there 24 hours a day for 3 months and is removed only for bathing. In addition, the patient sits on a magnetic chair pad placed atop still another 5″ × 6″ magnet. When walking around, the patient wears a 5″ × 6″ flexible magnet over the heart. At bedtime, this flexible magnet is placed across the face, and the patient sleeps on a magnetic mattress, adding several other strong magnets as directed.

During the course of intense magnetic exposure, the patient is instructed to avoid toxic substances, such as tobacco, alcohol, pesticides, and other known carcinogens. The patient is

> 66 The goal of static electromagnetic field therapy is to create a more alkaline internal environment and subsequently more oxygenation of tissues, the opposite required by cancer cells, which are anaerobic. 99

also placed on a 4-day rotation diet that reduces exposure to individual foods and eliminates possible allergens, thereby supporting the immune system.

The goal of treatment is to create a more alkaline internal environment and subsequently more oxygenation of tissues, the opposite required by cancer cells, which are anaerobic. Practitioners believe that placing magnets over the forehead, eyes, and large intestine also helps increase production of melatonin, which is known to have antineoplastic values.

Complications
Some practitioners believe that prolonged therapy with the biosouth (+) pole of the magnet—especially a high-gauss magnet—can overstimulate tissues and worsen the pain and symptoms of infection.

Nursing perspective
▶ Be aware that patients with pacemakers or defibrillators shouldn't use magnetic beds; furthermore, no magnets should be placed closer than 6″ (15 cm) to such devices, to avoid interfering with their function.

▶ As with most proven and unproven therapies, caution is urged with young children and pregnant women. Also, older patients may warrant special consideration; as with many treatments, these patients may be more sensitive and may require shorter and milder treatment.

▶ Pregnant patients should never use magnets on the abdominal area.

▶ Patients should avoid using magnets on the abdomen for 60 to 90 minutes after meals.

▶ To ensure patient safety, caution your patients to seek practitioners who are affiliated with a medically supervised magnetic therapy research project.

Selected references

Becker, R.O. *Cross Currents: The Promise of Electromedicine, the Perils of Electropollution.* Los Angeles: J.P. Tarcher; New York: Distributed by St. Martin's Press, 1990.

Becker, R.O., and Selden, G. *The Body Electric: Electromagnetism and the Foundation of Life.* New York: William Morrow, 1985.

Bronzino, J.D., ed. *The Biomedical Engineering Handbook.* Hartford, Conn.: CRC Press, 2nd ed. Boca Raton: CRC Press: IEEE Press, 2000.

Burton Goldberg Group. *Alternative Medicine: The Definitive Guide.* Puyallup, Wash.: Future Medicine Pub., 1993.

Cassileth, B.R. *The Alternative Medicine Handbook: The Complete Reference Guide to Alternative and Complementary Therapies.* New York: W.W. Norton & Co., 1998.

Fetrow, C.W., and Avila, J.R. *Professional's Handbook of Complementary and Alternative Medicines,* 2nd ed. Springhouse, Pa.: Springhouse Corp., 2001.

Kirschvink, J.L., et al. "Magnetite Biomineralization in the Human Brain," *Proceedings of the National Academy of Sciences USA* 89(16):7683-687, August 1992.

Kirschvink, J.L., et al. "Magnetite in Human Tissues: A Mechanism for the Biological Effects of Weak ELF Magnetic Fields," *Bioelectromagnetics Supplement* 1:101-13, 1992.

Levitt, B.B. *Electromagnetic Fields: A Consumer's Guide to the Issues and How To Protect Ourselves.* San Diego: Harcourt Brace, 1995.

Malmivuo, J., and Plonsey, R. *Bioelectromagnetism: Principles and Applications of Bioelectric and Biomagnetic Fields.* New York: Oxford University Press, 1995.

National Institutes of Health. *Alternative Medicine: Expanding Medical Horizons. A Report to the National Institutes of Health on Alternative Medical Systems and Practices in the United States prepared under the auspices of the Workshop on Alternative Medicine, Chantilly, Virginia, September 14-16, 1992.* NIH pub. 94-066. Washington, D.C.: U.S. Government Printing Office, 1994.

Novey, D. *Clinician's Complete Reference to Complementary Alternative Medicine.* St. Louis: Mosby–Year Book, Inc., 2000.

Philpott, W.H. "Cancer Prevention and Reversal: The Magnetic Answer," *Magnetic Health Quarterly* 2(4):1-26, 1996.

Philpott, W.H. *Critical Reviews of Currently Practiced Magnetic Therapy.* Choctaw, Okla.: Enviro-Tech, 1997.

Philpott, W.H. "Magnetic Resonance Bio-Oxicative Therapy for Major Mental Disorders," *Magnetic Health Quarterly* 3(3):1-44, 1997.

Philpott, W.H., and Taplin, S. *Biomagnetic Handbook: Today's Introduction to the Energy Medicine of Tomorrow.* Choctaw, Okla.: Enviro-Tech, 1990.

Rosenfeld, I. *Dr. Rosenfeld's Guide to Alternative Medicine: What Works, What Doesn't, and What's Right for You.* New York: Random House, 1996.

Rubik, B. "Can Western Science Provide a Foundation for Acupuncture?" *Alternative Therapies in Health and Medicine* 1(4):41-47, September 1995.

Rubik, B., et al. "Bioelectromagnetics Applications in Medicine," in National Institutes of Health. *Alternative Medicine: Expanding Medical Horizons. A Report to the National Institutes of Health on Alternative Medical Systems and Practices in the United States prepared under the auspices of the Workshop on Alternative Medi-*

cine, Chantilly, Virginia, September 14-16, 1992. NIH pub. 94-066. Washington, D.C.: U.S. Government Printing Office, 1994.

Spencer, J., and Jacobs, J. *Complementary Alternative Medicine: An Evidence-Based Approach.* St. Louis: Mosby–Year Book, Inc., 1999.

Tierra, M. *Biomagnetic and Herbal Therapy.* Twin Lakes, Wisc.: Lotus Press, 1997.

Ulett, G.A. "Conditioned Healing with Electroacupuncture," *Alternative Therapies in Health and Medicine* 2(5):56-60, September 1996.

Vallbona, C. et al. "Response of Pain to Static Magnetic Fields in Post-polio Patients: A Double-Blind Pilot Study," Archives of *Physical Medicine and Rehabilitation* 78(11):1200-203, November 1997.

Zimmerman, J.T. "An explanation about the Assignment of North and South Magnetic Polarities," *BEMI Currents: Journal of the Bio-Electro-Magnetics Institute* 2(3):5, 1990.

Zimmerman, J.T. "Comparisons between Different Brands of Magnetic Bed Products," *BEMI Currents: Journal of the Bio-Electro-Magnetics Institute* 4(1):11, 1995.

Zimmerman, J.T., and Hinrichs, D. "Magnetotherapy: An Introduction," *BEMI Currents: Journal of the Bio-Electro-Magnetics Institute* 4(1):3-7, 1995.

Internet resources

www.bioelectromagnetics.com
www.healthweb.org
www.holistic-online.com
www.nccam.nih.gov

7

Manual healing therapies

I n all of the therapies discussed in this chapter, the practitioner uses his hands to treat the patient and, in some cases, diagnose him. Most of the therapies — such as chiropractic, Rolfing, massage, and the Feldenkrais, Alexander, and Trager techniques — involve physical manipulation or pressure of some sort. Some, such as Therapeutic Touch, involve not physical touch but moving energy fields within and around the patient. Others, such as acupuncture, *qigong,* and reflexology, combine physical actions and energy-based principles.

Like the mind-body therapies discussed in chapter 5, all of the therapies reviewed here look at the patient as an integrated whole, consisting of body, mind, and spirit. However, whereas mind-body therapies aim to improve physical health by training the mind, manual healing therapies — also known as "bodywork" therapies — attempt to improve or maintain individual functioning by restoring the physiologic integrity of the body at some level. (See *Types of manual healing therapies.*)

Most of these techniques are aimed at enhancing well-being — for example, by reducing pain and stress, soothing injured muscles, promoting relaxation, and stimulating circulation — rather than at curing specific diseases.

Classification
The four main categories of manual healing are energetic healing, movement repatterning, adjustment-based techniques, and

Types of manual healing therapies

The diagram below shows the different types of manual healing therapies and how they can overlap.

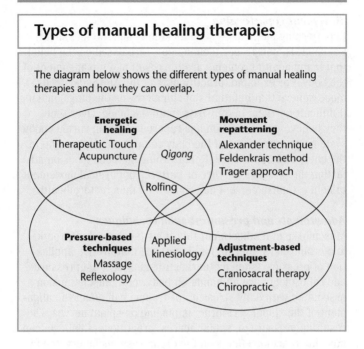

pressure-based techniques. Many manual healing practitioners use a combination of these techniques to achieve the desired results.

Energetic healing

Energetic healing therapies, such as Therapeutic Touch, are based on a belief in the existence of a universal life force, or energy, that can be used for healing purposes. Practitioners claim that these therapies balance or unblock the flow of energy in the body, thereby restoring health. In many cases, the practitioner and the patient believe that they can actually feel this energy. This method of healing is closely associated with the practice of "laying on of hands." Practitioners of energetic healing achieve their effects primarily by redirecting energy rather than by physically manipulating the patient. Acupuncture, qigong, and reflexology are also based on a belief in human energy fields, but these therapies redirect the energy through physical means—insertion of needles, exercise, and application of pressure, respectively.

Movement repatterning

Repatterning methods — such as Rolfing and the Alexander, Feldenkrais, and Trager techniques — are based on the belief that many health problems are the result of a misalignment of the body. For example, practitioners of the Alexander technique believe that habitual slouching crowds the lungs, making it difficult for them to fully oxygenate the blood. Over time, they believe, this condition has repercussions on various body systems as other parts of the body compensate for tension in the chest and upper back. Repatterning methods focus on adjusting the patient's posture or patterns of physical movement to help establish correct movement and thus restore health.

Adjustment- and pressure-based techniques

Musculoskeletal adjustment therapies (such as chiropractic and craniosacral therapy) and methods that involve application of pressure (such as therapeutic massage, acupressure, and reflexology) are all hands-on bodywork. Muscle tension associated with daily stressors or trauma can affect the alignment of the spinal vertebrae, impinging on spinal nerves. The resulting pressure on spinal nerves, practitioners believe, can have far-reaching effects on the organ systems innervated by those nerves. Manual adjustment of the vertebrae removes this pathologic pressure on the nerves and thereby relieves apparently unrelated symptoms.

Similarly, applying pressure to tense muscles, as in therapeutic massage, can help relieve that tension. Acupressure and reflexology practitioners apply pressure to specific points based on traditional Chinese medicine's concepts of energy traveling along channels within the body. Thus, these two techniques are a combination of pressure-based and energetic healing methods.

Patients can be taught to perform some of these techniques themselves — for example, massaging their own tense muscles. However, most manual healing therapies are performed by trained professionals.

Nursing's role

Many nurses are trained in the use of certain manual healing techniques, particularly Therapeutic Touch and therapeutic massage, and integrate them into a holistic nursing approach. These techniques can be easily implemented in standard hospital nursing care and are already practiced in numerous hospitals.

Even if you don't practice these therapies, you should be knowledgeable about them. As more and more patients seek alternative methods of healing, they'll rely on your knowledge and experience to help them in that search. You'll need to be able to review with them the appropriateness of different therapies and make sure they have realistic expectations.

Acupuncture

A key component of traditional Chinese medicine, acupuncture dates back nearly 5,000 years to the legendary Yellow Emperor, believed to have lived around 2700 B.C. The Yellow Emperor is actually a composite of numerous ancient Chinese physicians, whose medical knowledge was passed down through the centuries and collected in *The Yellow Emperor's Classic of Internal Medicine,* a classic treatise on traditional Chinese medicine. Written in the 2nd or 3rd century B.C., this book provides the earliest known record of acupuncture.

In the West, acupuncture began to attract widespread attention after President Richard Nixon's visit to China in 1972. During that trip, *New York Times* reporter James Reston underwent an emergency appendectomy and wrote an article on the acupuncture anesthesia that was used during the procedure. His article piqued the interest of American physicians, who began traveling to China to observe this procedure firsthand. They discovered a medical practice that was used not only as a substitute for surgical anesthesia but also as a treatment for pain and numerous disorders.

Basic principles

Acupuncture is based on the same principle that underlies traditional Chinese medicine: the existence of a vital life force — *qi* — that circulates in the body through channels known as meridians. The 12 major meridians are believed to be connected to specific organ systems. (There's also a network of collateral and minor meridians.) The meridians, used in diagnosis and treatment, act as a road map that allows the practitioner to locate specific acupuncture points.

According to the Chinese theory, an organ that's experiencing an energy imbalance or diseased state may manifest signs or symptoms at its corresponding meridian. Such signs and symptoms may include pain, aching, a change in skin temperature, sensitivity to touch, and alterations in skin texture or color along a portion of the channel. These signs and symptoms help the practitioner determine which organ systems are affected and, thus, which acupoints should be used in the treatment. The stimulation of these points by acupuncture needles is believed to balance, release, or enhance the flow of *qi* and thus relieve pain or restore health. (See *Understanding acupuncture.*)

Acupuncture involves the insertion of very thin metal needles — usually no more than 12 — just under the skin at specific points determined by the practitioner. The needles are typically kept in place for 20 to 30 minutes and may be set in motion or connected to low-voltage electric generators to enhance their intended effects.

Acupuncturists also commonly use other treatments involving the acupoints, including moxibustion and cupping. In *moxibustion,* a small piece of an herb called moxa (*Artemisia vulgaris,* commonly known as mugwort) is burned either directly on the skin on the needle tip or on another substance (such as salt or a slice of gingerroot) that's then placed over the designated acupoint. Alternatively, it may be rolled into a large cigarlike wrapper and used to warm the acupoints. This supplementary technique is intended to stimulate or increase the flow of *qi* in the body. In *cupping,* glass or bamboo cups are placed on the skin to create a vacuum suction, which is believed to draw out pathogenic substances.

❝ *Americans spend about $500 million and make 9 to 12 million office visits per year for acupuncture treatments.* ❞

Some acupuncturists don't use needles at all; instead, they substitute electrostimulation, ultrasonic waves, or laser beams for the steel needles. In Chinese massage, or acupressure, the practitioner applies deep finger pressure to the acupoints. (See *Relieving a headache with acupressure,* page 238.)

A more recent form of acupuncture, auriculotherapy, was developed in France after World War II and involves inserting needles at specific points on the outer ear that are believed to

HOW IT WORKS

⤴ Understanding acupuncture

Although acupuncture is one of the most thoroughly researched of the alternative therapies, Western scientists aren't really sure how it works. The following theories provide a possible explanation:

▶ *Stimulation of endorphins* — According to this theory, acupuncture needles stimulate peripheral nerves, which in turn stimulate the release of endorphins and enkephalins, the body's inherent pain-killing chemicals. Researchers have found that endorphin levels rise in blood and cerebrospinal fluid and fall in specific brain regions during acupuncture analgesia.

▶ *Neurotransmitter effect* — This theory proposes that acupuncture affects levels of certain neurotransmitters, such as serotonin and norepinephrine, the substances that transmit nerve impulses across the synapses.

▶ *Gate control* — This popular theory is based on the belief that pain perception is controlled by a part of the nervous system that regulates the pain impulse. Known as the "gate," this part of the nervous system becomes overwhelmed and closes if it's bombarded by too many impulses, as occurs with acupuncture needles. Thus, the insertion of the needles is believed to "close the gates" on the nerve fibers that carry pain impulses to the brain.

▶ *Electrical conductance* — Based on researchers' findings that the acupuncture points have a higher level of electrical conductance than other areas, some scientists theorize that these acupoints act to amplify the minute electrical signals as they travel through the body and that the acupuncture needles interrupt that flow, thus blocking the transmission of pain impulses.

▶ *Enhanced immunity* — According to this theory, acupuncture raises the white blood cell count as well as prostaglandin, gamma globulin, and overall antibody levels.

▶ *Circulation control* — This theory maintains that acupuncture works by constricting or dilating blood vessels, possibly through control of vasodilators.

affect other regions of the body. This method is being used in the United States to treat alcohol, cigarette, and drug addiction.

Growing mainstream acceptance

Today, acupuncture is practiced in numerous mainstream medical settings and is a widely accepted treatment for pain and

Relieving a headache with acupressure

Also known as Chinese massage, acupressure is simply acupuncture without the needles. It involves placing firm finger pressure on designated points of the body—known as acupoints—to relieve symptoms such as pain. Each acupoint is believed to be connected to a particular organ system. The particular acupoint used may be far away from the site of the patient's symptoms.

Locating the acupressure points

You can practice acupressure on yourself or your patient with a minimum of training. The diagrams below show useful points to use for releasing a muscle tension headache. The points known as GB 20 are located at the base of the skull (shown at left); the point known as LI 4 (Hoku point) is located at the base of the thumb and index finger (shown at right).

Breathe in; then slowly exhale as you press the designated point. (Use both thumbs to press on each GB 20 point simultaneously.) Press until you feel resistance or pain; then maintain pressure until you finish the exhalation, releasing the pressure as you inhale. Press each point three to five times. Repeat, if needed, after 10 minutes.

Acupressure shouldn't be applied directly over cuts, wounds, sores, scar tissue, or infected areas.

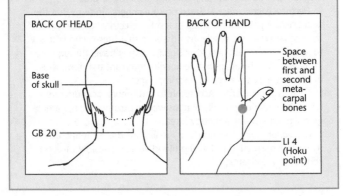

BACK OF HEAD

Base of skull

GB 20

BACK OF HAND

Space between first and second meta-carpal bones

LI 4 (Hoku point)

certain addictions. According to the World Health Organization, there are about 10,000 acupuncture practitioners in the United States, of whom about 3,000 are medical doctors. Americans are estimated to spend $500 million and make 9 to 12 million office visits per year for acupuncture treatments.

In November 1997, a National Institutes of Health (NIH) consensus panel found "clear evidence" that needle acupuncture is effective in treating postoperative dental pain as well as nausea and vomiting due to surgery, chemotherapy, and pregnancy. The 12-member panel also listed a number of conditions for which acupuncture might be used as an adjunctive therapy or an "acceptable alternative" therapy. Those conditions include addiction, stroke rehabilitation, low back pain, menstrual cramps, headache, tennis elbow, fibromyalgia, carpal tunnel syndrome, and asthma.

To promote greater public access to acupuncture, the panel also urged insurance companies and governmental insurance programs, including Medicare and Medicaid, to reimburse patients for appropriate acupuncture treatments.

In another sign of acupuncture's growing acceptance, the U.S. Food and Drug Administration (FDA) recently removed acupuncture needles from its list of "experimental medical devices" and now regulates them just as it does scalpels, syringes, and other common medical instruments.

Licensing

The licensing of acupuncturists varies widely from state to state. Most states have laws specifically licensing or registering acupuncture professionals, but the scope of practice varies widely. New Mexico recognizes the Doctor of Oriental Medicine (DOM) as a primary care provider, but a number of states allow only MDs or DOs to practice acupuncture or allow an acupuncturist to practice only under the supervision of an MD.

Acupuncture schools are accredited by the Accreditation Commission for Acupuncture and Oriental Medicine. The National Commission for the Certification of Acupuncturists (NCCA) provides a national certification examination (similar to the NCLEX examination of the National Council of State Boards of Nursing) that's used by a number of states as their certifying examination. The American Academy of Medical Acupuncture is the professional organization that represents practitioners who are also physicians.

The NIH consensus panel urged national standardization of training and licensing requirements for acupuncture practitioners to increase public confidence in them.

Therapeutic uses

The World Health Organization has listed more than 100 conditions that may benefit from treatment with acupuncture, including neurologic disorders (migraines, Ménière's disease, trigeminal neuralgia, and peripheral neuropathy), GI disorders (colitis, gastritis, ulcers, diarrhea, constipation, and hiccups), pulmonary and respiratory conditions (bronchitis, asthma, sinusitis, and rhinitis), eye disorders (myopia, conjunctivitis, and central retinitis), sciatica, and various rheumatoid and arthritic conditions. In China, acupuncture is commonly used as a surgical anesthetic. (See *A portrait of brain surgery using acupuncture.*)

In the United States, millions of people use acupuncture, primarily to relieve or prevent pain, to relieve nausea and vomiting, and to help overcome drug and alcohol addictions. (More than 300 substance abuse programs in the United States use acupuncture.) Some practitioners claim acupuncture can improve immune system function and reduce symptoms in patients with acquired immunodeficiency syndrome (AIDS).

RESEARCH SUMMARY Although acupuncture is one of the most widely researched of all the alternative and complementary therapies, most of the published reports have been case studies that don't meet modern scientific standards for assessing efficacy. Double-blind randomized studies are difficult to perform for acupuncture because the treatments are so individualized; two people with the same disease label would probably be treated differently.

Despite these problems, the 1997 NIH consensus panel concluded that "the data in support of acupuncture are as strong as those for many accepted Western medical therapies." The panel also encouraged practitioners to make acupuncture part of a comprehensive management program for asthma, addiction, and smoking cessation. ■

Equipment

Acupuncturists use very fine, solid filiform needles made of metal. Most needles are made of stainless steel but other metals, such as gold and silver, are used occasionally. Single-use, disposable needles are now a standard for most acupuncturists in the United States.

If moxibustion is used, the acupuncturist needs the herb moxa; if cupping is used, glass or bamboo cups; if nonneedle methods of stimulation are used, the appropriate devices, such as laser, ultrasound, or electrostimulation equipment.

PERSONAL ACCOUNT
A portrait of brain surgery using acupuncture

From 1979 to 1980, David Eisenberg, a Harvard medical student, spent a year in China as the first American medical exchange student with the People's Republic. During this year, he studied and practiced traditional Chinese medicine and witnessed many amazing applications, which he later described in a memoir called *Encounters with Qi: Exploring Chinese Medicine.*

One such experience was the use of acupuncture anesthesia in a patient undergoing brain surgery. The 58-year-old male patient was diagnosed with a chestnut-size brain tumor in the center of his brain. The tumor was too large to be accessed through his nose—the usual access point for such tumors; his skull had to be cut open. The neurosurgeon convinced the patient to undergo the surgery using acupuncture anesthesia because it produced fewer adverse effects than conventional anesthesia. He said that more than 90% of the head and neck operations performed at the Beijing Neurosurgical Institute were done using this form of anesthesia. Conventional anesthesia would be available in the operating room in case the acupuncture didn't work.

"Do you have the *qi?*"

The patient received a mild preoperative sedative I.V. Then the anesthesiologist, who was trained in both Chinese and Western medicine, inserted six needles to achieve anesthesia: two in the eyebrow area, two near the right temple, and two in the area of the left shin and ankle. The needles were wired to a device that delivered a low-voltage electric current at regular intervals.

"Do you have the *qi?* " the anesthesiologist asked the patient after each point was stimulated. "Obtaining the *qi*" meant experiencing a sensation of fullness and a mild electric shock, indicating that the needles had reached the *qi.* "I have it," the patient replied. While the surgeons waited 20 minutes for the analgesia to take effect, Eisenberg checked the patient's vital signs.

The doctors encouraged Eisenberg (who had learned Chinese) to chat with the patient during the procedure and asked him to continue to monitor the vital signs. As the surgeons made the incision in his scalp, the patient didn't wince or show any sign of pain. He was calm and responsive. He said he was aware of pressure being applied on his skin but didn't feel any discomfort. His pulse and blood pressure remained the same.

(continued)

A portrait of brain surgery using acupuncture
(continued)

During the entire 4-hour procedure, the patient remained conscious and his vital signs remained stable. "We conversed the whole time he was on the operating table," Eisenberg wrote. When the surgery was completed, the patient rose from the operating table, thanked the doctors, shook hands with everyone, and left the room unassisted. The tumor turned out to be benign.

Impressive results
Soon after this procedure, Eisenberg witnessed two thyroidectomies using acupuncture anesthesia that were "even more impressive" than the brain surgery. In these procedures, usually performed under general anesthesia, the patients received no drugs at all. The anesthesia consisted only of two needles in the hand. As in the earlier brain operation, "the patient remained alert and comfortable, the vital signs remained stable, and the clinical results were most impressive," Eisenberg wrote.

Eisenberg has continued his explorations into Chinese medicine and other alternative therapies. Today, he's director of the Center for Alternative Medicine at Harvard Medical School's Beth Israel–Deaconess Medical Center.

Procedure

A visit to an acupuncturist is usually similar to a visit to a traditional Chinese medicine practitioner, except that herbs may not be prescribed and the treatment is done at the time of the visit. Before treatment begins, the practitioner determines the patient's overall condition by the traditional Chinese methods of diagnosis: inspecting, listening, smelling, questioning, and palpating. The assessment includes intensive pulse measurements and questions about eating and sleeping habits, digestive complaints, urine color, and stress.

Treatment is based on the results of the assessment, which indicate the balance of *qi* flow in the network of channels. However, the particular channels and points chosen for treatment may also be influenced by the practitioner's style and experience as well as the specific school of acupuncture in which he was trained.

Acupuncture as practiced in the United States today isn't a monolithic body of knowledge similar to Western biomedicine; rather, it's based on a number of medical traditions from China, Viet Nam, Korea, Japan, England, and France. A practitioner trained in a school following the mainland Chinese model will practice differently from one trained in the Japanese model. The underlying theory of all the schools is identical, but the vast tradition of Chinese medicine allows for quite divergent emphases in practice. Thus, a practitioner may emphasize the five phases theory, the eight principles theory, or the three yin–three yang theory in making a diagnosis. (For an explanation of these theories, see "Traditional Chinese medicine" in chapter 4, page 84.) These different diagnostic frameworks result in very different approaches to therapy in each model.

The basic technique is similar in all schools of acupuncture. Very fine filiform needles made of solid metal — usually stainless steel — are inserted into the skin. The needles (usually no more than 10 to 12) are placed in designated acupuncture points on the body, depending on the patient's diagnosis. Although most acupuncture points are located on meridians, several points located away from any channel have been discovered to have therapeutic effects; these are called miscellaneous points.

Because the needles are so fine and aren't hollow, the patient feels relatively little pain compared to the insertion of tunneling needles used in Western injections. Although single-use, disposable needles have become customary, strict standards of sterilization are required for nondisposable needles and implements. Treatments can last anywhere from a few seconds to 45 minutes or more. A typical treatment session lasts from 20 to 30 minutes.

Complications
The 1997 NIH consensus panel reported that the incidence of adverse effects from acupuncture treatment is lower than that for many accepted medical procedures used for the same conditions. For example, it said the steroids and nonsteroidal anti-inflammatory drugs (NSAIDs) commonly used to treat painful musculoskeletal conditions, such as fibromyalgia and epicondylitis, could cause serious adverse effects, yet they have no more compelling evidence supporting their usefulness than acupuncture.

Because of the slight risk of life-threatening reactions (such as pneumothorax) from some types of acupuncture, the panel urged practitioners to take appropriate safeguards, such as carefully explaining the procedure to their patients and following FDA guidelines on needle sterility.

Nursing perspective

▶ Be aware that some third-party payers provide coverage for acupuncture treatments by qualified practitioners. However, inability to pay continues to be a problem for many patients seeking alternative therapies.

▶ If your patient is considering acupuncture, inform him that he can obtain a referral from the NCCA.

Alexander technique

The Alexander technique is a form of bodywork that focuses on the dynamic interaction of the head, neck, and trunk based on the belief that various physical ailments can be linked to faulty posture. The goal of this therapy is to learn proper use of the body to prevent injury and maximize pleasure in work and leisure.

Frederick M. Alexander, an Australian actor in the late 1800s, developed his theory while trying to determine why he frequently lost his voice during performances. Medical doctors were unable to cure his problem with medication and rest, nor could they explain what might be causing this condition that threatened his livelihood.

Alexander was convinced that something he did while using his voice caused the problem and that if he could uncover that habit, he could work to alter it. By observing himself in mirrors, he saw that he unconsciously moved his head a certain way and sucked in his breath whenever he began to speak. When he made this unconscious movement, the muscles at the back of his neck contracted in such a way as to pull his head down and back. He concluded that this movement also strained his vocal cords and affected his voice.

Experimenting with his body over several years, Alexander practiced postures that were the opposite of the unconscious ones he had observed. In time his voice problem disappeared. He began helping others with posture and movement problems and eventually abandoned the stage to teach his posture technique around the world.

> 66 *Alexander taught that the stresses and strains we place on our bodies by incorrect sitting and standing are at the root of many of our ailments.* 99

The core of Alexander's teaching was that people use their bodies incorrectly for such routine activities as sitting and standing and that the stresses and strains we place on our bodies through these faulty postures are at the root of many medical problems. By learning to consciously change the way our bodies move when we sit, stand, walk, and talk—specifically, by properly aligning the head, neck, and trunk—Alexander believed that people could treat various ills and improve overall health.

Today, the Alexander technique is especially popular with people in the performing arts. The North American Society of Teachers of the Alexander Technique has approved 17 teacher-training programs in the United States. To become certified, each teacher must complete 1,600 hours of training over 3 years. There are about 600 certified teachers in the United States.

Therapeutic uses

The Alexander technique has been used for nearly a century for a broad range of physical complaints, from asthma to paralysis, but few scientific studies in mainstream medical literature have evaluated its efficacy for such disorders. The technique is taught primarily as a preventive method to promote relaxation and enhance movement and posture; actors, musicians, and athletes use it to improve their performances.

Proponents claim the technique is useful in treating chronic conditions—such as neck and back pain, postural disorders, myalgia, breathing problems, hypertension, and anxiety—and in preventing repetitive stress injuries.

RESEARCH SUMMARY Although many articles have been written about the Alexander technique, most of them don't meet the scientific community's standards for proving a treatment's efficacy. Despite this lack of mainstream research, Barrie Cassileth, a member of the Advisory Council to the NIH's Office of Alternative Medicine, says those who are curious may want to try the technique because it's gentle and unlikely to cause harm. "It may indeed work for you, bringing pain relief, relaxation, and the more efficient body function it claims to bestow," he says. ◼

Equipment
The Alexander technique requires no specific equipment other than comfortable clothing and a room large enough to practice in.

Procedure
It's possible to learn the basic elements of the Alexander technique from books. However, ideally one should learn from a teacher because the technique must be specifically tailored to the individual based on his movement patterns. A teacher can assess precisely how the person moves and then tailor a program to his needs.

The teacher usually begins by simply observing the student as he sits and gets up from a chair and walks around the room. The teacher will offer suggestions on making proper use of the body, guiding the student's movements with his hands. The focus is on slow, steady development of habits of tension-free movement, which the student continues in everyday life. The result is improved balance, posture, and coordination.

Complications
The Alexander technique should cause no complications if taught and performed correctly.

Nursing perspective
▶ If the patient has a chronic muscle or joint condition, advise him to consult his physician to make sure this technique won't exacerbate the condition or interfere with medical treatment.
▶ Make sure the patient closely follows the practitioner's recommendations—as in other areas, a misapplied technique can be worse than none at all.

Applied kinesiology
Kinesiology is the scientific study of the movement of body parts—how the body moves through space as a unit and how each body part "relates" to the others. Applied kinesiology, also known as muscle testing, is a method of assessment and evaluation. It focuses on the relationship of muscle strength

and energy flow; as muscles become strong, circulation and other vital functions become strong. George Goodheart, Jr., an American chiropractor, developed this system in the 1960s based on the theory that particular muscles correlate to specific body systems or organs and can therefore be used to diagnose a wide range of disorders.

Practitioners of applied kinesiology believe that health is a balance between three major factors. The first, the chemical factor, includes nutrition and the effects of drugs and other chemicals such as environmental toxins. The second, the structural factor, includes anatomy and physiology—the structural relationships of bones, muscles, and organs. The third, the mental factor, includes attitudes, moods, and emotions.

These practitioners also believe that the three factors are interdependent—for example, an alteration in body chemistry from poor diet or environmental pollution can affect a person's mood and body organs. This effect is apparent in the decreased functioning of the whole person, either in the form of a frank disease state or a chronic condition of low energy and malaise, with no apparent cause.

The type of therapy chosen depends on the cause of the condition, as determined by the practitioner. After muscle testing, two persons with what appear to be the same symptom—for example, neck pain resistant to standard therapies—might receive two different treatments. One might be treated with spinal adjustment, based on the structural factor, but the other might be treated primarily with dietary supplements, based on the chemical factor. Most treatments are aimed at restoring neuromuscular function. They include joint manipulation and mobilization, spinal and cranial adjustments, myofascial therapies, stimulation of acupuncture points, and reflex procedures. Dietary and nutritional measures may also be used.

The International College of Applied Kinesiology in Shawnee Mission, Kansas, offers information, publishes a newsletter, and provides referrals to practitioners of applied kinesiology.

Therapeutic uses

Applied kinesiology is commonly used to assess and treat such chronic problems as musculoskeletal imbalances, joint problems, and structural imbalances. It's especially popular for assessing athletic injuries. People with vague symptoms, such as malaise and tiredness, or illnesses that seem to have no identifiable cause or that are unresponsive to standard treatments may be good candidates for this diagnostic method.

Equipment
Applied kinesiology requires no particular equipment.

Procedure
After taking the patient's history, including diet and lifestyle, the practitioner examines the patient's posture, gait, and any obvious physical problems, such as a limp or drooping shoulder. Then he methodically assesses the strength of various muscles and muscle groups. He does this by placing the patient's limbs in various positions and asking the patient to resist as the practitioner attempts to push against the resistance. By comparing the left and right sides as well as the relative strength of muscles, the practitioner identifies muscles that are weak. (See *Assessing muscle strength.*)

Because applied kinesiology holds that each muscle is associated with specific diseases or organ conditions, once the practitioner identifies the weak muscles, he knows where the patient's problem originates — for example, a weak psoas muscle indicates kidney disease. Depending on the cause, he then prescribes a treatment, such as spinal manipulation, a change in diet, or dietary supplements.

Complications
When performed by a properly trained practitioner, applied kinesiology shouldn't result in any complications.

Nursing perspective
▶ If your patient expresses an interest in applied kinesiology, inform him that this technique isn't intended to replace conventional physical examinations and diagnostic measures.
▶ Be aware that applied kinesiology is a highly specialized technique that should be performed only by a licensed professional trained in differential diagnosis. Despite the existence of several self-help systems for muscle testing, most patients lack the knowledge to interpret the tests properly and reach appropriate diagnostic conclusions.

Assessing muscle strength

In this illustration, an applied kinesiology practitioner tests the strength of the patient's deltoid muscles by holding the arm firmly and asking the patient to resist the practitioner's pulling action.

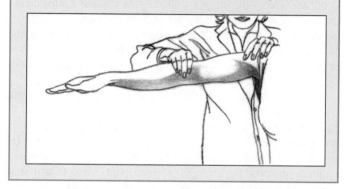

▶ Advise your patient to consult his physician before undergoing applied kinesiology, to make sure the technique won't exacerbate his condition or interfere with treatment.

Aston-Patterning

Aston-Patterning is an integrated system of movement education, bodywork, ergonomics, and fitness training. It helps patients use their bodies more efficiently, to release tension and pain and to improve posture and movement.

The premise is that an injury or dysfunction in one part of the body causes the rest of the body to compensate in ways that reinforce the original symptoms. All movement is considered a three-dimensional, ascending or descending, asymmetrical spiral, due to the body's asymmetries and the play of gravity and ground reaction force. For any activity, an optimal base of support comes from the legs while standing and the pelvis while sitting. The width, depth, and length of this base of support vary according to the task, ensuring an adequate foundation for the body segments above to prevent strain or injury.

Aston-Patterning teaches that the basic components of all movements are weight transfer, rocking across the hinge joints of the legs and pelvis, and matching flexion and extension of the spine, arms, and legs. Understanding what these movements are and how and when they should be combined for a given activity results in added support for the whole body, better use of momentum, better shock absorption, and more stability and mobility.

In 1963, with a B.A. and M.F.A. in dance from the University of California, Los Angeles, Judith Aston started a movement education program for athletes, dancers, and actors at Long Beach City College in California. Exploring the way movement communicates emotion, she worked with psychotherapists to develop a format of body consciousness to assist in the therapy process.

Needing rehabilitation after two car accidents, Aston sought treatment with Ida Rolf in 1968. Rolf's myofascial treatment, called Rolfing, facilitated Aston's recovery and expanded her understanding of how the body can change. Rolf asked Aston to develop a movement education counterpart to Rolfing to help patients preserve the changes they achieved. Aston taught students how to make patients aware of and change the ways they move their bodies in work and play and how to help them use their bodies with minimum effort and maximum precision. These contributions to Rolfing became known as Rolf-Aston Structural Patterning.

By the mid-1970s, Aston had added environmental modification to her work. She maximized patient comfort by adjusting their chairs at work, using pillows in sleep postures, and modifying their use of sports equipment. This work developed into a line of products designed to help maintain alignment while sitting or exercising.

Aston abandoned her linear viewpoint of bodywork in favor of three-dimensional spiral patterns, in which she perceived retained tension. She taught patients to release this tension by incorporating their asymmetries into their movements, rather than resisting their nature by moving in straight lines. Increasingly aware that her paradigm differed from Rolfing, she dissolved the Patterning Institute associated with Rolfing in 1977 and continued to develop her work as Aston-Patterning.

Basic principles
The three basic principles of Aston-Patterning are neurokinetics, bodywork, and ergonomics. Neurokinetics, the movement education aspect, begins with learning more efficient and less stressful ways of performing the simple movements of every-

day life and progresses to more complex activities. All aspects of the movement work aim to evoke easy and efficient activity.

The bodywork aspect consists of Aston massage, myokinetics, and arthrokinetics. The massage uses noncompressive touch to help release functional holding patterns (patterns of tension that are maintained by the nervous system and haven't yet created physiologic change in connective tissue) from both superficial and deep layers. Myokinetics uses precise strokes to release structural (more strongly held) holding patterns in the fascial network. Arthrokinetics addresses structural holding patterns at bone and joint surfaces.

The ergonomics aspect of Aston-Patterning identifies environmental factors (such as seating conditions and shoe type) that may be compromising body structure. The practitioner then suggests ways of changing body usage or modifying objects to make them more "body friendly."

Another aspect of Aston-Patterning is Aston fitness training, which includes vertical and horizontal loosening (self-massage techniques), toning, stretching, and cardiovascular fitness.

Aston-Patterning draws on all of these tools as needed. Patients are taught to be more self-aware so they can understand the source of their tension and movement. The diversity of techniques available helps them neutralize the negative effects of their past on their body and move into more knowledgeable and comfortable patterns.

The Aston-Patterning Practitioner Program, a continuing education program for health professionals, includes training in neurokinetics, myokinetics, and ergonomic evaluation, plus advanced massage techniques and fitness. The 84-day program is scheduled in five 3-week segments over a period of 1½ to 2 years. Blocks of time between the levels allow the student to apply and practice the skills in work situations. The training is intended to prepare the practitioner to address a wide range of situations from athletic endeavors to rehabilitation.

Therapeutic uses

Aston-Patterning is a noninvasive technique used in people with injuries involving the spinal axis, peripheral joints, and multiple pain sites. It can be an adjunct to physical therapy and medication, or it can be used in place of other treatment for an active rehabilitation approach. When the body's segments — legs, pelvis, spine, shoulder girdle, head, and neck — are optimally aligned, movement becomes easier and more natural.

This treatment is considered useful in clients, such as dancers or runners, who encounter chronic overuse problems. It's considered particularly helpful in individuals who have anterior knee pain (chondromalacia), chronic piriformis syndrome, chronic adductor strains, and various lumbar and sacroiliac joint problems. Aston work may also be useful in preventing pain, joint wear and tear, and so forth, caused by stressful body use.

RESEARCH SUMMARY The concepts behind the use of Aston-Patterning and the claims made regarding its effects haven't been scientifically proved. ■

Equipment

Aston-Patterning requires a quiet room to make the assessment. This room may be in the patient's home or work area, in order to better assess his movements during the problem activity. If massage is being used, a massage table is required.

Procedure

An Aston-Patterning session begins with a patient history (physical, psychological, and emotional), a review of everyday activities (work, home, sports, and leisure activities), and a discussion of when or where the patient feels fatigue or pain.

A baseline pretest follows — usually involving a basic activity, such as walking, sitting, standing, reaching, bending, or lifting, or a particular problem activity such as using a keyboard. This enables the practitioner to evaluate the client's movement and potential for improvement. To make the patient aware of his movements during the activity, the practitioner may call attention to details, such as how the hand is held when keyboarding, what position the shoulders take as they move, or how the foot is planted on the ground. Movement education, or bodywork, is included in virtually every session, to release unnecessary tension and make the new movement easier and more efficient. Continual emphasis on self-awareness gives the patient the knowledge to keep the changes as part of future patterns of movement. During pretesting, the practitioner makes a chart of the patient's postural alignment and tension-holding patterns. A new chart is made at each session to document the patient's progress.

Posttesting essentially repeats the pretesting movements, allowing the patient to see and feel the changes that have taken place and to integrate them into daily life. If the session focused on arm and shoulder movements, the patient may apply the new movements to a golf swing or to computer keyboarding.

Complications

Aston-Patterning drills and exercises can be extremely demanding. A patient with a heart condition or respiratory problems should check with his physician before undertaking this form of therapy. The program can be adjusted to meet the needs of older adults, those in poor health, and those with special rehabilitation requirements.

The deep massage used in Aston-Patterning could be an issue if the patient has osteoporosis or tends to bruise easily. If he has a bleeding disorder, takes anticoagulants, or is undergoing long-term steroid therapy, which can make the tissues fragile, Aston-Patterning may not be an appropriate therapy.

For people in good physical condition, most complications are the result of overly intensive training. Exhaustion and pain are the principal problems.

Nursing perspective

▶ Ask the patient if he has a heart or respiratory condition before he begins this form of therapy.

▶ Advise the patient to voice any pain or discomfort during the sessions. The experienced practitioner will know how hard to push and when it's best to stop.

▶ If the patient has circulation problems, such as those resulting from diabetes or varicose veins, advise him not to receive deep massage in the legs and feet.

▶ The Aston Fitness Program may be a useful approach to physical fitness training for the elderly.

Chiropractic

With more than 50,000 practitioners, chiropractic is the fourth largest health profession (after physicians, dentists, and nurses) in the United States and may be the most commonly used alternative therapy today. Stemming from the Greek words for "done by hand," chiropractic is a therapeutic system based on the belief that most medical problems are caused by misalignments of the vertebrae and can be corrected by manipulating the spine.

Like osteopathy, chiropractic originated in the Midwest in the late 19th century as a reaction to medical orthodoxy. Daniel Palmer, its founder, was a grocer and self-educated healer from Iowa. His theory that the spine plays a major role in health was sparked by an encounter with a janitor who had been stooped and deaf for 17 years after suffering a spinal injury. Palmer noticed a misaligned vertebra in the man's spine and manipulated it back into place. Surprisingly, the man was able to stand up straight without pain and his hearing was restored.

The story of the janitor illustrates the two primary benefits that practitioners ascribe to chiropractic: the relief of musculoskeletal pain and disability (the janitor was able to stand upright without pain) and the re-establishment of internal organ function (his hearing returned).

The body's innate healing power

Palmer, who later opened the first school of chiropractic, taught that the human body seeks to maintain a state of homeostasis and has an innate ability to heal itself. This "innate intelligence" regulates all body functions through the nervous system. Because the nerves originate in the spine, Palmer reasoned that displaced vertebrae could disrupt nerve transmissions, a condition he called *subluxation*. He taught that the chiropractor's job was to eliminate the subluxations so the body could carry out its job of maintaining equilibrium unimpeded.

Palmer believed that almost every disease was ultimately caused by subluxation and that spinal manipulation could treat them all — an idea that became known as "one cause–one cure." Although few chiropractors today still adhere to this theory, the core of the chiropractic profession remains the detection and correction of vertebral misalignment.

Growing mainstream acceptance

Conventional medical doctors repudiated chiropractic for many years because of its emphasis on the one cause–one cure principle. This belief, combined with the lack of a clearly demonstrated physiologic explanation of how spinal adjustment could affect organ function, prevented rational communication between medical doctors and chiropractors for decades.

However, recent advances in the understanding of neurophysiology may provide a theoretical basis for visceral organ responses to chiropractic adjustment. (See *Understanding spinal manipulation,* page 256.)

> 66 *Even the American medical establishment has recently ceased to condemn the practice of chiropractic as harmful or at best useless.* 99

Today, more than 15 million people a year use chiropractic to relieve pain, injuries, and some internal ailments, and its efficacy in treating musculoskeletal complaints is widely accepted. Chiropractors are licensed in all 50 states (after completing a 5-year course of study) and regulated by state chiropractic boards. Their services are covered by Medicare and many other insurance providers. The American Chiropractic Association in Arlington, Virginia, provides information and referrals.

Even the American medical establishment has recently ceased to condemn the practice of chiropractic as harmful or at best useless. This transformation occurred as the result of a 1991 Supreme Court ruling against the American Medical Association (AMA). The Court affirmed a lower court decision that found the AMA guilty of conspiring to contain and eliminate the competitive profession of chiropractic — an antitrust violation. As a result of this judgment, the AMA was required to reverse its ban on professional cooperation between chiropractors and medical doctors and to pay a substantial settlement, much of which is being used for chiropractic research. Today, interprofessional cooperation between chiropractors and other health care practitioners is growing; some physicians are even referring patients to chiropractors for specific problems.

Therapeutic uses

Although back pain is the most common reason that people see a chiropractor, any musculoskeletal condition clearly related to spinal or vertebral malfunction is a likely candidate for a chiropractic consultation. Other common problems treated by chiropractors are neck and shoulder pain, headaches, sports injuries, and work-related injuries such as carpal tunnel syndrome.

HOW IT WORKS
⤳ Understanding spinal manipulation

Early theories of how spinal adjustment worked were based on the anatomic understanding of the time. Misaligned vertebrae were thought to put pressure on spinal nerves, blocking the flow of impulses along the nerves. Spinal manipulation restored the free flow of neural impulses, relieving symptoms. Because patients commonly reported significant relief of their complaints as well as an increase in function after an adjustment, this explanation was deemed satisfactory for many years. However, an increased understanding of anatomy and physiology over the years has made this explanation less acceptable.

Another difficulty with the original explanation is that positive changes in health status aren't always reflected in vertebral alignment—that is, an adjustment may result in immediate and dramatic relief from pain, but an X-ray may show no detectable alteration in spinal alignment. In addition, there is no clearly demonstrated physiologic connection between spinal manipulation and the organ responses ascribed to them. Because of these problems with the original explanation, alternative theories of how chiropractic achieves its results have been put forward.

Current theories
The most widely accepted theory is that of intervertebral motion and segmental dysfunction, which states that the key concept is loss of correct spinal joint mobility rather than vertebral misalignment. Neighboring pairs of vertebrae and their surrounding tissues consist of a motion segment; loss of mobility within a segment is called a fixation. These fixations are most amenable to spinal manipulative therapy.

Recent advances in neurophysiology may provide the explanation for how spinal manipulation can lead to visceral organ responses. These studies indicate that spinal adjustment initiates nerve signals that are transmitted by autonomic nervous system pathways to internal organs, thus providing a physiologic connection between spinal manipulation and the visceral organs.

RESEARCH SUMMARY In 1994, the Agency for Health Care Policy and Research of the U.S. Department of Health and Human Services released "Acute Low Back Problems in Adults: Clinical Practice Guideline Number 14," a report developed by a panel of medical doctors, chiropractors, and other health professionals based on extensive research. This report endorsed spinal manipulation — either alone or in combination with nonsteroidal anti-inflammatory drugs — as an effective therapy for acute lower back pain, adding that it brought relief as well as functional improvement. The report rejected many standard medical treatments for this condition, such as bed rest, traction, and the use of "disorienting painkillers." It also cautioned against lumbar surgery, except in extreme cases.

Similar research is being conducted to determine whether headaches — particularly the muscle tension type — respond better to chiropractic than to conventional medications.

Some chiropractors still claim they can cure any disease — from allergies and impotence to heart disease and cancer — with spinal manipulation. However, such claims haven't been scientifically proved. ■

Equipment

Spinal manipulative therapy is typically delivered with little more equipment than a practitioner's hands. Some chiropractors use a special treatment table that can be adjusted to numerous positions. Others use various devices to help them control more precisely the force and direction of adjustments and administer higher-force adjustments if necessary.

Some practitioners also combine chiropractic with other adjunctive therapies, such as massage, nutrition, heat or cold application, and ultrasound; some of these methods require special equipment.

Procedure

Chiropractic emphasizes the importance of taking a holistic approach to the diagnosis and treatment of a specific problem. The chiropractor looks not merely at the patient's specific complaint but at the whole person, seeking to understand how, for example, pain in the knee might actually stem from a lower back dysfunction that isn't causing pain in the back.

The chiropractor begins by taking the patient's history — including family history, diet, and work and lifestyle factors — paying special attention to the history of his chief symptom. Next, the chiropractor performs a physical examination — focusing on possible subluxations, muscle strength, and postural and structural problems — to determine whether spinal manipulative therapy is appropriate. He may order X-rays as well.

Performing a spinal adjustment

In this illustration, the chiropractor is manipulating the patient's right superior sacroiliac joint fixation. With one hand stabilizing the patient's shoulder, he thrusts his other hand against the affected ilium. Bracing his thigh against the patient's leg, the chiropractor institutes a quick thrust using his body weight.

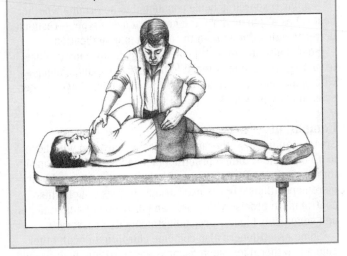

If the chiropractor concludes that manipulation is needed, he'll perform a specific type of adjustment, depending on the patient's condition. The most common technique is the *high-velocity, low-amplitude thrust* (also known as osseous adjustment). It's performed by moving a joint to the end point of its current normal range of motion and then imparting a swift, low-amplitude, specifically directed thrust. This generally painless maneuver moves the joint beyond its normal range of motion, while keeping within the anatomic limits of its range. (See *Performing a spinal adjustment.*)

Other low-velocity adjustments are used when this standard adjustment isn't appropriate. In addition, many chiropractors perform other manual therapies, such as massage and joint mobilization. As a practitioner who embraces a holistic perspective, the chiropractor may also integrate other treatments into his plan of care, such as stress reduction, exercise, and nutritional interventions.

Complications

Chiropractors claim that if performed by a trained profession-al, spinal manipulation should produce few if any complica-tions. However, those who don't support chiropractic say ma-nipulation of the lower spine can lead to such complications as leg weakness, bladder disturbance, and rectal and genital mal-function. They also note reports of life-threatening dissection of an artery during an adjustment.

Nursing perspective

▸ Chiropractic manipulation is contraindicated in patients with a condition that might worsen as the result of a spinal ad-justment, such as osteoporosis or advanced degenerative joint disease.

▸ Inform your patient that chiropractic hasn't been proved ef-fective in treating serious illnesses such as cancer.

Craniosacral therapy

An offshoot of chiropractic and osteopathy, craniosacral thera-py is based on the theory that an unimpeded flow of cerebro-spinal fluid (CSF) is the key to good health. CSF normally cir-culates from the cranium to the base of the spine — the cran-iosacral system. Practitioners believe that anything that impedes this flow or affects its rhythm can cause physical and mental problems.

Craniosacral therapy was developed in the early 1900s by William G. Sutherland, an American osteopathic physician who believed that the bones of the skull move rhythmically through-out the day in response to the production of CSF in the ventri-cles. Craniosacral therapists claim that they can actually pal-pate the flow of CSF by running their fingers over the skull or along the spine. According to their theory, any bumps or blows to the head can knock the skull bones out of alignment or cause them to become stationary or move improperly. By gen-tly manipulating these bones through massage or light pres-sure at the suture lines, they believe they can realign the bones, restore the free circulation of CSF, and remove strains and stresses built up in the meninges, allowing the entire body to function optimally.

Craniosacral therapy is most commonly practiced by osteo-pathic and chiropractic doctors who have been trained in the technique. The Upledger Institute in Palm Beach Gardens, Florida, provides information and referrals.

Conventional medical practitioners say craniosacral therapy is based on theories that are inconsistent with the basic principles of anatomy taught in the West today. The current understanding of skeletal anatomy holds that the skull bones fuse together by age 2 and therefore can't be moved by hand pressure. And no one except craniosacral therapists has been able to detect the rhythmic skull motion that lies at the heart of this technique.

Therapeutic uses

Proponents say craniosacral therapy can be used to treat chronic headaches, back or neck pain, sciatica, temporomandibular joint syndrome, depression, anxiety, and chronic fatigue in adults. However, they claim the most success in treating disorders in infants and children, including earaches, hyperactivity, and irritability, which they believe result from cranial injuries during birth At least one practitioner has claimed success in treating cerebral palsy.

RESEARCH SUMMARY The mainstream scientific community has been unable to find evidence that the bones of the skull expand and contract in a rhythmic pattern that's palpable, as Sutherland claimed. As a result, even many osteopathic physicians have failed to embrace this therapy. However, the massage aspect may at least decrease stress and muscle tension and promote relaxation. ■

Equipment

Craniosacral therapy requires no special equipment except a table on which the patient can lie.

Procedure

Craniosacral therapy is usually performed with the patient lying in a prone position and the therapist sitting behind the patient's head. The therapist begins by holding the patient's head and examining the placement and movement of the skull bones. He then gently pulls, lifts, and stretches the bones into alignment. Patients report a feeling of deep relaxation during this process, which usually lasts from 30 to 60 minutes. Results of the therapy sometimes include relief of symptoms in distant parts of the body such as leg pain. (See *Craniosacral therapy techniques.*)

Craniosacral therapy techniques

The following illustrations show some techniques used in craniosacral therapy.

In the illustration below, the therapist attempts to relieve eyestrain and sinus pressure by decompressing the frontal bone and stretching the membrane beneath it.

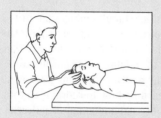

To help alleviate tinnitus, the therapist places his hands on the temporal bones and attempts to bring them back into alignment (as shown below).

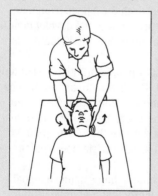

To relieve maxillary sinus conditions, the therapist applies pressure to the bones in the roof of the mouth, which balances the upper jaw (as shown below).

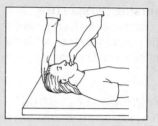

The jawbone is stretched to its limit to relieve temporomandibular joint syndrome (as shown below).

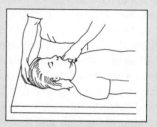

To relieve headache and stress, the therapist balances the large parietal bones on either side of the skull and stretches the membrane beneath them (as shown below).

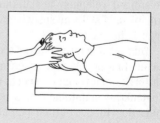

Complications
Some conventional medical doctors warn that craniosacral therapy shouldn't be performed on infants or toddlers because their skull bones haven't become fused and manipulation of the delicate bone plates might be harmful.

Nursing perspective
▶ Craniosacral therapy may be an appropriate intervention for the patient who is uncomfortable with the physical intimacy of other manual healing techniques, such as Rolfing or massage.

Feldenkrais method
The Feldenkrais method is a form of somatic education. Students become aware of their habitual neuromuscular patterns and rigidities and expand options for new ways of moving. This method works with one's ability to regulate and coordinate movement by working through the nervous system. It's considered a functional approach of learning how to reorganize your body and behavior in new and more expanded motor patterns.

Moshe Feldenkrais, a Russian-born Israeli physicist, mechanical engineer, and judo expert, developed his gentle method of bodywork in an attempt to rehabilitate his own knee, which he injured in an athletic accident. He studied anatomy, physiology, and psychology in the hope that he might avoid surgery. The result of this search for a deeper understanding of the body and its functioning was the development of an entire philosophy of life that underlies the Feldenkrais method.

Feldenkrais came to believe that people practice a skill only until they achieve a desired goal. For instance, an infant sees adults and children moving around and doing things for themselves, and strives to do the same. Once he achieves that goal, he stops developing the skill that got him there. The same is true of such skills as speech and social interaction, Feldenkrais believed.

This settling for whatever technique helps achieve a goal means that people tend to learn inefficient and unhealthful patterns of movement, speech, and emotional and social skills, Feldenkrais maintained. As a result, most people learn to make do with 5% of their potential without realizing that their development has been stunted. In terms of movement, this means that people learn unconscious patterns of musculo-skeletal behavior that limit their ability to function optimally.

> *Feldenkrais believed that his exercises could not only increase flexibility, coordination, and range of motion but also lead to enhanced functioning in other aspects of life.*

Feldenkrais argued that habitual patterns of muscle movement underlie human self-awareness as well as emotional actions and reactions. "We know what is happening within us as soon as the muscles of our face, heart, or breathing apparatus organize themselves into patterns, known to us as fear, anxiety, laughter, or any other feeling," he wrote. Because of the key role of the muscular system in the development and ordering of mental, emotional, social, and physiologic systems, Feldenkrais believed that his exercises could not only increase flexibility, coordination, and range of motion (ROM) but also lead to enhanced functioning in other aspects of life.

Classes in the Feldenkrais method are taught in either group sessions or private one-on-one sessions. Practitioners must complete 800 to 1,000 hours of training over a 3- to 4-year period. The Feldenkrais Guild of North America in Oregon sponsors training programs, provides information to the public, makes referrals, and maintains the Web site *www. feldenkrais.com.*

Therapeutic uses

Feldenkrais never considered his technique a medical therapy, but rather a training method to improve coordination, flexibility, ROM, and function. Practitioners say the method can benefit anyone — young or old, physically fit or physically challenged — but is especially useful for people experiencing chronic or acute pain of the back, neck, shoulder, hips, legs, or knees. They also claim success in dealing with central nervous system disorders (such as multiple sclerosis, cerebrovascular accident, and cerebral palsy).

The program is popular with many athletes (including Julius Erving, according to the Feldenkrais Guild) and musicians (such as Yehudi Menuhin and Yo-Yo Ma), who claim it improves their performance.

Equipment
The group classes require no special equipment. The private sessions require a table or chair on which the student can lie down or sit; pillows, blankets, and other props may be used to facilitate certain movements.

Procedure
The Feldenkrais method uses two trademarked approaches: Awareness Through Movement, which consists of group lessons, and Functional Integration, which offers private lessons tailored to the individual student. In the group classes (which last 30 to 60 minutes), the teacher verbally leads the students through a series of exercises designed to help them become more aware of their bodies and develop new patterns of movement. The exercises are performed in a slow, relaxed way, progressing from easy movements to movements of greater range and complexity. The emphasis is on enjoyment and avoiding pain. Numerous different lessons may be used, depending on the student's needs.

Functional Integration consists of gentle bodywork attuned to the individual student's needs. The student is fully clothed and may lie on a table or be in a sitting or standing position. Through touch, the teacher senses the student's patterns of neuromuscular "organization" and suggests new, more comfortable and more functional patterns. The result ideally is more fluid movements and a decrease in "restrictive" patterns that create pain, tension, and stiffness. A typical session lasts 45 to 60 minutes.

Complications
Because of its gentle technique, the Feldenkrais method is unlikely to cause complications.

Nursing perspective
▶ The Feldenkrais method may be appropriate for patients with limitations caused by accidents. It can be incorporated into a rehabilitation program.

▶ Tell the patient that it may take time to retrain himself to properly align his body.

▶ The patient must be able to follow verbal commands for the awareness-through-movement part of the method.

 RESEARCH SUMMARY The concepts behind the Feldenkrais method and the claims made haven't been scientifically proved. ■

Hydrotherapy

Hydrotherapy, which is the use of water to treat disease and maintain health, has been practiced in one form or another by most cultures throughout history, from the ancient Babylonians, Greeks, and Israelites to the Hindus, Chinese, and Native Americans. The best-known American medical doctor who used hydrotherapy and performed many experiments on its effects was J.N. Kellogg. In 1900, he published a hydrotherapy textbook that's still considered an important publication. Today, water-based treatments are used primarily to treat wounds, burns, and injuries; to aid physical rehabilitation; and to relieve tension. The water can be hot or cold; liquid, solid (ice), or steam; and applied externally or internally.

The three types of external hydrotherapy are hot, cold, and contrast. *Hot water therapies,* including saunas and application of heat, work by dilating the blood vessels and increasing circulation in the area being treated. Increasing the supply of blood to muscles can relieve pain as well as soothe and relax the body. Proponents believe these therapies also stimulate immune system functioning, encouraging white blood cells to leave the blood vessels and migrate into the surrounding tissues, where they scavenge for toxins and help eliminate them from the body. The copious sweat stimulated by these heat treatments is also believed to help release toxins from the body.

Cold water therapies, such as application of ice and cold packs, cause vasoconstriction, which decreases circulation to the body part being treated. These treatments are used to reduce swelling and inflammation. Cold water may also tone muscle weakness by stimulating muscle contractions. If cold application continues long enough, a secondary effect is achieved as the body gets used to the cold and returns to normal function. Many hydrotherapy techniques are directed at producing this secondary reaction. More blood is pumped to the area, and the body reacts with greater activity. Alternating between hot and cold application in the same treatment, known as *contrast therapy,* is believed to stimulate endocrine function, reduce inflammation, decrease congestion, and improve organ function.

Therapeutic uses

Hyperthermia, or fever induction therapy, is used to stimulate the immune system by inducing fever in a patient too debilitated by a disease to mount a defense. Many alternative practitioners see fever as the body's natural response to a pathogen. Fever has been shown to stimulate immune system production of antibodies and may also enhance the body's excretion of toxins, such as pesticides and drug residues (especially when combined with cold treatments). Steam baths and hot packs are used in this way. Hyperthermia can also be effective in relieving muscle aches, combating tiredness, and improving blood circulation.

Whirlpool baths (heated baths with jets that force water to circulate) are used to assist in the rehabilitation of injured muscles and joints. The water temperature can be either hot or cold, depending on the desired effect; the jets of water act as a massage on soothing muscles. These baths are also used to treat burn patients and to aid healing of skin sores and infected wounds. Patients suffering from paraplegia and polio receive whirlpool baths to increase circulation in atrophied muscles.

A *neutral bath* is the full immersion of the body up to the neck in water that's near body temperature. This soothing bath calms the nervous system and is used to treat emotional disturbances and insomnia. In a *sitz bath,* the pelvic area is immersed in a tub of warm water; this treatment is used to relieve perianal pain, swelling, or discomfort; to increase circulation; and to reduce inflammation.

Ice, usually applied locally, is another common therapy used to relieve sprains, strains, and inflammation. Contrast hydrotherapy can be used for trauma relief.

Equipment

The equipment needed depends on the type of hydrotherapy used. It may include tub, steam, sauna (a sealed, steam-filled room), pool, hose, hot or cold pack, or Jacuzzi or whirlpool bath.

Procedure

Depending on the type of therapy used, the patient enters the water (hot, cold, or warm) or the sauna and remains in it for the prescribed amount of time. The desired temperature is maintained to prolong the therapy's benefits. If hot or cold packs are used, they're applied to the target body area for the specified length of time and changed as needed to maintain the desired temperature.

Complications

Hydrotherapy treatments can be used for people in relatively good health or with debilitating disease. The effects are complex and need to be prescribed with care and understanding. Keep in mind that any therapy involving heat can produce harmful effects, such as burns, if applied improperly. In addition, very hot treatments can cause elderly people and children to become exhausted or faint. Cold may aggravate painful spasms or acute lung congestion and some traditional hydrotherapy practitioners consider ice therapies inappropriate and thus don't use them.

Nursing perspective

▶ Hot baths, saunas, and immersion baths aren't recommended for pregnant women, children, elderly patients, or patients with diabetes, multiple sclerosis, hypertension, or hypotension. Tell patients using these therapies to stop the treatment if they feel light-headed, dizzy, or faint (which are possible symptoms of decreased blood pressure).

▶ Cold applications are contraindicated for patients with conditions that would be exacerbated by vasoconstriction, such as Raynaud's disease and sickle cell anemia.

▶ Use caution when administering a hot bath or steam bath to prevent burns, light-headedness, and falls.

▶ Patients shouldn't remain in a sauna for more than 20 minutes and should wipe their faces frequently with cool cloths to avoid becoming overheated.

▶ Many hydrotherapy treatments, such as whirlpool and steam baths, can be performed at home, but more intensive forms are best performed in a clinical setting, where response to the therapy can be monitored by experienced therapists.

Hyperthermia

Hyperthermia (also referred to as heat therapy, thermotherapy or fever therapy) is used to stimulate the immune system by inducing fever in a patient whose body is too debilitated by a disease to mount a defense on its own. Many alternative practitioners see fever as the body's natural response to a pathogen. Fever has been shown to stimulate immune system production of antibodies and may also enhance the body's excretion of toxins, such as pesticides and drug residues (especially when combined with cold treatments). Hyperthermia can also be effective in relieving muscle aches, combating tiredness, and improving blood circulation.

Exogenous heat sources can be applied to the entire body or a single body part. Whole body application of exogenous heat — commonly referred to as heat therapy — is done with heating sources, such as hot baths (see "Hydrotherapy," page 265), diathermy, or hot air (wet and dry saunas). Local application of exogenous heat, called thermotherapy, uses radiant heating devices that give off infrared rays, and conductive heating devices, such as hot water bottles, paraffin baths, moist hot packs, or computerized application of microwaves.

Licensed naturopathic physicians who graduated from a 4-year training program are instructed in general and local hyperthermia techniques. However, there are no certification programs for focused microwave hyperthermia. The best option here is a licensed conventional physician with at least 1 year of special training in hyperthermia treatments.

Therapeutic uses

Hyperthermia is used to treat various conditions, ranging from viral and bacterial infections to cancer and acquired immunodeficiency syndrome (AIDS). Therapeutic effects of hyperthermia vary based on the degree of body involved and the modalities used to increase the tissue temperatures. Body involvement may range from the entire body to the extremities to focused tissues such as specific tumor tissues. Alternative practitioners have successfully treated acute and chronic infections with simple, whole-body methods of inducing general hyperthermia. The same methods are used to precipitate detoxification — a complementary therapy useful in treatment of chronic illnesses and cancer. High-tech local hyperthermia has gained acceptance as a promising new complementary procedure in cancer therapy.

RESEARCH SUMMARY Multiple studies have shown that whole-body hyperthermia plays a positive role in several aspects of the healing process — destruction of the invading organism, stimulation of the immune system, and general detoxification of the body — all of which are needed to regain and maintain optimum health. Studies have also shown that focused hyperthermia of specifically targeted tissues can modify cell membranes in a manner that actually protects the healthy cells and makes the cancer cells more susceptible to chemotherapy and radiation treatments. Used as adjunctive therapy, focused microwave diathermy may thus permit lower doses of these potent and toxic forms of therapy. ■

Bacterial and viral infections

Whole-body hyperthermia is successful in treating both acute and chronic infections, such as upper and lower respiratory tract infections (colds and flu), urinary tract infections, and Lyme disease. Its effects range from potentiation of white cell antimicrobial activity to direct viricidal and bactericidal activity. Hyperthermia alone may not destroy all the invading organisms, but it can significantly reduce their numbers and thus the overall load on the immune system.

HIV infection

Studies have shown the human immunodeficiency virus (HIV) is very sensitive to temperatures above the normal body temperature of 98.6° F (37° C). Treatment of 107.6° F (42° C) for 30 minutes showed a 40% decrease the HIV activity. Patients with HIV infections experienced a decrease in night sweats, decreased frequency of secondary infections, and a greater sense of well-being after hyperthermia treatments.

Cancer therapy

The concept of treating cancerous cells with heat began with serendipitous findings of spontaneous tumor regression in patients with smallpox, influenza, tuberculosis, and malaria, who had experienced fevers of 104° F (40° C). This lead to a period of experimentation with fever therapy (hyperpyrexia), which is done by injecting blood products, vaccines, pollens, and benign forms of malaria. This method proved to be unreliable and dangerous, and was rejected by the medical community. Heat therapy wasn't considered a reliable modality until medical scientist Haim I. Bicher began experimenting with focused microwave diathermy.

Equipment

Treatment can be given on an outpatient basis in the office or clinic, and typically nothing more than a bathtub, heat lamps, sauna, or steam room and dry sheets and blankets are needed. Additionally, an ultrasound machine is needed if ultrasound is used, a microwave apparatus if microwave diathermy is used, and an external blood heating device if extracorporeal heating of the blood is used.

Procedure

Low-tech methods of hyperthermia include immersion hot water baths, wet and dry saunas, and radiant heat. High-tech methods of hyperthermia include ultrasound therapy for deep heating of body parts, microwave diathermy for heat directed to specific cells or tissues, and extracorporal heating of the blood, which is invasive and affects the entire body.

Heating and diaphoretic herbs, such as *Achillea millefoliu* (yarrow) tea, are helpful in promoting hyperthermia and are particularly useful during whole-body hyperthermia therapies.

Extracorporeal heating of the blood

With extracorporeal heating of the blood, blood is removed from the body, delivered to an external heating device, heated, and returned to the body at the higher temperature. The procedure is used in patients with HIV.

Immersion hot water baths

Immersion hot water baths are usually done in a deep, stainless steel tub. The water is typically heated to between 101° and 108° F (38.3° and 42.2° C), although temperatures as high as 115° (46.1° C) may be used if the patient can tolerate them. The goal is to keep the body temperature at between 102° and 104° F (38.8° and 40° C) for about 20 minutes. The typical treatment requires about 30 minutes — 10 minutes for the body temperature to rise and 20 minutes of maintained high temperature. The individual is removed from the water and wrapped in a dry sheet and several blankets for 30 more minutes to continue the internal heating.

Treatment frequency and duration depends on the patient's chief symptom. For upper and lower respiratory tract infections, patients typically undergo only 1 or 2 treatments before improving in a few days. For more serious conditions, however, therapy can take much longer. Cancer patients typically begin with 15 treatments over a 3-week period followed by a 3-week rest. The cycle is then repeated four more times and, in some cases, may continue for as long as a year.

Microwave diathermy

Microwave radiation is a high-frequency oscillatory current used to heat specific, target cells. All metal must be removed from the general area of treatment to prevent current arcing. The microwave apparatus is placed 1″ to 5″ (2.5 to 12.5 cm) from the target area. Placement and duration of treatment vary, depending on the desired effect. Microwave radiation shouldn't be used over pacemakers or metal implants.

Radiant heat

Radiant heat can be applied with heat lamps and ultraviolet (UV) lamps. The body should be kept 30″ (76 cm) from the ultraviolet lamp source. Treatment duration begins at 15 seconds and increases to 3 minutes as the sessions proceed. When the 3-minute time frame is reached, the UV lamp can be drawn closer by 2″ (5 cm) per treatment session until a distance of 18″ (46 cm) is achieved.

Saunas

General external application of dry or moist heat causes vasodilation (swelling of the arteries) and diaphoresis (sweating), which is the body's attempt to prevent the internal increase in temperature. Superficial vessels in the skin initially contract, increasing the blood pressure. This can make the patient feel as if his head is full and bursting, an uncomfortable effect that dissipates in a short time and can be avoided by applying a cold compress or ice bag to the head. Patients must be monitored carefully; apparent discomfort and the state of pulse, respiration, and skin coloring are observed to be certain the patient doesn't become dehydrated or suffer heat exhaustion.

Ultrasound

In ultrasound, special equipment emits inaudible sound in the frequency range of 20,000 to 10 billion (109) cycles/second. The sound directs its thermal effects deep into the targeted tissues. Ultrasound waves can be transmitted through a coupling agent applied directly onto the skin or through water with the transmitting head held 1″ (2.5 cm) from the skin.

Treatment duration varies, depending on the condition; treatment for acute conditions lasts 4 minutes and for chronic conditions 10 minutes. Care should be taken when placing the transmitting ultrasound head because these sound waves can fracture bones, melt myelin sheaths, and burn the periosteum if used incorrectly.

Complications

Safe and appropriate use of hyperthermia requires an understanding of the safe limits of induced temperature and the contraindications to heat therapy. The lower limit of body temperature for human survival is 74° F (23.3° C); the upper limit, 113° F (45° C). Normal cells die at a temperature of 110° F (43.3° C).

Hyperthermia therapists find that adults in good health can tolerate temperatures of 107.6° F (42° C) for periods of 8 to 10 hours. However, the therapist must take into account the patient as a whole, including age, health status, and medical history. For example, hyperthermia should be strictly avoided in pregnant patients, due to potential danger to the unborn child, and in individuals with temperature regulation problems, especially the very old and very young.

Heat therapy should also be restricted in patients with a cardiovascular disease, such as arrhythmias or tachycardia, and in those with severe hypertension or hypotension. People with arrhythmias and tachycardia risk an increased chance of myocardial infarction from altered blood blow dynamics caused by systemic or local application of heat. Severely hypertensive patients risk hemorrhagic stroke and severely hypotensive patients risk syncope and tissue ischemic damage.

Heat shouldn't be applied to extremities of patients with peripheral vascular disease such as arteriosclerosis, advanced diabetes, Raynaud's syndrome, or Berger's disease due to their compromised sensation of heat and increased risk of burns. Sensitivity to extreme temperatures is seen in other chronic conditions, such as anemia, heart disease, diabetes, thyroid disease, seizure disorders, and tuberculosis; patients with these conditions may require a reduction in the number of treatments, a reduction in the intensity of heat applied, or another method of treatment.

Patients with acute illness may initially have difficulty tolerating the extreme temperatures, but this usually subsides after hyperthermia is initiated. Use heat therapy with caution in these individuals. Other reported risks in weakened individuals are herpes outbreaks and liver toxicity.

Patients should avoid induced hyperthermia, also called hyperpyrexia or fever therapy, which is a state of artificially induced fever. Hyperpyrexia is induced by injecting a pyrogen, such as a blood product, vaccine, pollen, or benign form of malaria. This experimental method of inducing general hyperthermia is dangerous and unreliable and isn't recommended.

Nursing perspective

▶ Factors to consider before using hyperthermia include the patient's age and overall health status and current drug therapy. High temperatures can increase the efficacy of certain drugs to the point of toxicity.

▶ Heat therapy can cause or exacerbate internal bleeding, so use extreme caution if the patient has anemia, heart disease, or diabetes because of the increased risk of hemorrhage. Periodically check vital signs to catch early signs of increased blood loss and hypovolemic shock.

▶ Hyperthermia shouldn't be used in patients with a history of seizure disorders because of the increased risk of seizure activity and possible nervous system damage.

▶ Hyperthermia shouldn't be used in patients with tuberculosis because the increased heat stress on the body may reactivate the latent bacteria.

▶ Electrical devices shouldn't be used to heat moist dressings because of the high risk of electrical shock. Microwave diathermy can burn periocular tissues and is contraindicated in people with pacemakers. Radiant heat lamps are safely used to promote local hyperthermia; however, misuse, overexposure, or direct skin contact with the heat lamp can cause blistering, dermal burns, and even heatstroke.

▶ Local hyperthermia can be used with constant monitoring.

▶ Heatstroke is characterized by hyperthermia (107.6° F [42° C]), delirium, coma, and anhidrosis, a breakdown of the hypothalamic heat regulatory mechanisms, which has a mortality rate as high as 80% if untreated. Survivors can develop neurologic deficits, including cerebellar ataxia and severe dysarthria. Therapists must be alert to changes in the patient and be prepared to rapidly dissipate the heat. Continuous sponging with tepid water and continuous gentle massage promotes cutaneous vasodilation and dissipation of heat.

▶ Promoting hyperthermia via hyperpyrexia is unreliable and dangerous and isn't recommended.

▶ If the patient experiences any adverse effects, the hyperthermia treatment should be stopped immediately. Improvements should be noted after the first few treatments for conditions other than cancer and AIDS. If no improvement is apparent, other forms of therapy should be considered.

▶ Instruct your patient to check with his insurance company about reimbursement for hyperthermia treatments. Hyperthermia was given legal status as an approved medical procedure in 1984. Hyperthermic oncology, for which Medicare and most insurance companies provide reimbursement, has now joined surgery, radiation, and chemotherapy in the expanding arsenal of proven, effective treatments for both primary cancer and locally recurrent tumors.

Myotherapy

Myotherapy (also referred to as deep tissue therapy, manual ischemic compression, or trigger-point therapy) is a noninvasive, therapeutic approach developed in 1976 for relief of symptoms associated with muscular pain and dysfunction. Trigger points — localized areas of hyperirritable tissue in muscle, fascia, ligaments, and periosteal tissue — are tender when compressed. If sufficiently hypersensitive, trigger points give rise to referred pain and tenderness, and sometimes to referred autonomic phenomena and distortion of proprioceptions. In addition, trigger points may cause muscle spasm, limited range of motion (ROM), numbness, weakness, and fatigue. Therapeutic goals of myotherapy include relaxation of muscle spasms, improved circulation, and pain relief. Myotherapy enhances the function of muscles and joints, improving ROM and general body tone. Pain relief minimizes the need for muscle relaxants and analgesics.

Bonnie Prudden developed myotherapy in 1976 while working with Desmond Tivy, a trigger-point practitioner who treated chronic pain with injection therapy. While preparing patients for treatment, Prudden discovered that compression of trigger points decreased their sensitivity. After testing this theory on a number of patients, she found that ischemic compressions for 5 to 20 seconds allowed passive muscle stretching without procaine injections. Prudden also found she could usually return the patient to a normal state of painless activity in fewer than 10 sessions.

Basic principles

Trigger points (also called trigger zones, trigger spots, or trigger areas) occur when tissue is damaged as a result of an accident, a sports activity, occupational stress, a disease, or a nutritional deficiency. Objective and subjective findings identify trigger points in the absence of laboratory and radiologic findings. Objective findings include a palpable, firm, tense band of muscle, production of a local twitch response of the muscle during palpation, restricted stretch ROM, weakness without atrophy, and the absence of neurologic deficits. Subjective findings include stiffness and easy fatigability, spontaneous pain in a referred pain pattern predictable for the trigger point, and an exquisite, deep tenderness, specifically at the trigger point. Some muscles may produce autonomic concomitants in the pain reference zone, such as localized vasoconstriction, sweating, lacrimation, coryza, salivation, and pilomotor activity (gooseflesh).

Acute or chronic overload of the muscle or undue physical or emotional stress can activate these trigger points. When activated, the points cause the muscle to increase tonus until it induces a painful spasm or cramp — a sharp, disabling pain or deep muscle ache. The pain causes more spasms, and the spasm-pain-spasm cycle is set in place. Active trigger points can entrap nerves (sciatica), limit circulation, and pull muscles into a shortened state, which can cause weakness and interfere with coordination. Myotherapy interrupts this spasm-pain-spasm cycle.

Certified Bonnie Prudden myotherapists train for 1,300 hours. After completing the program, students must then pass board examinations to be certified. Myotherapists must undergo 45 hours of continuing training every 2 years in order to maintain certification. Many myotherapists are also licensed massage therapists.

Therapeutic uses

Myotherapy is useful in relieving any chronic myofascial pain, such as chronic back pain, headache, temporomandibular disorder, carpal tunnel syndrome, tendinitis, or bursitis. It's also effective in cases of imbalanced muscle training, acute or repetitive sprain or strain injuries, and occupational injuries or overuse syndromes. This treatment relieves the swelling and discomfort associated with such diseases as lupus, multiple sclerosis, rheumatoid arthritis, osteoarthritis, and fibromyalgia.

RESEARCH SUMMARY The concepts behind the use of myotherapy and the claims made regarding its effects haven't been scientifically proved. ■

Equipment

This therapy requires no special equipment. Only a treatment table and a quiet room in which to perform the assessment and treatment are necessary.

Procedure

A myotherapy patient should be cleared by a physician, nurse practitioner, or physical therapist, or, in the case of temporomandibular joint disease, a dentist, to rule out a pathologic condition requiring medical treatment.

The treatment protocol to interrupt the pain-spasm-pain cycle and deactivate trigger points consists of three parts: First, a pretreatment assessment is done; second, the trigger point is deactivated, the spasm is released, and the involved muscles are stretched; third, a posttreatment prescription of exercise, nutrition, and stress management is issued.

In the pretreatment assessment, a thorough patient history is taken to develop a customized plan of care, based on the individual's specific medical condition and lifestyle. Locations of the trigger points are identified by palpation of the involved muscles. In trigger-point deactivation, various methods may be used to release trigger-point spasms. Biofeedback has been successfully used to assist relaxation of the spasmed musculature. Passive stretching and myomassage is performed immediately after the trigger point is released, to help lengthen the shortened muscles and increase movement and flexibility. Deep-stroking myomassage can then be used to advance healing by increasing local blood circulation and lymph drainage.

In *ischemic compression,* direct, firm pressure is applied to the trigger point using knuckles, hands, elbows, or *bodos* (small, wooden dowels with handles). Manual pressure usually releases the muscle spasm, diminishing the patient's experience of pain, allowing for myomassage and passive stretching, which lengthen the involved musculature. Imagery exercises designed to increase skin temperature have been used to help promote warmth and muscle relaxation at trigger-point sites, decreasing their pressure-pain sensitivity.

Patients are given a home therapeutic plan, with corrective exercises to re-educate the involved musculature and suggestions for balanced nutrition and stress management. Patients may also be taught self-care methods using ischemic pressure maneuvers to increase the effectiveness of long-term maintenance. A well-designed exercise program incorporates full ROM for injured muscles, thus preventing the shortening of newly lengthened muscles; recovers normal muscle activity levels; and maintains an effective level of fitness and function. Stress management is taught to diminish the effects of stress on trigger-point activation. And, finally, nutritional deficiencies are addressed so the body can achieve the biochemical balance necessary for proper muscle function. Special nutritional concerns with myofascial pain syndromes include vitamins B_1, B_6, B_{12}, and C, folic acid, calcium, iron, and potassium.

Complications

Adverse effects may include sensation of pain during trigger-point desensitization. Minor bruising may occur at the site of compression. Bruising is more common in women, in patients undergoing anticoagulant therapy, and in patients with vitamin C deficiency. Patients should be advised to increase their activity level gradually, otherwise they may risk injury.

Nursing perspective

▶ Advise your patient that bruising may occur after myotherapy.
▶ Assess your patient's pain status before, during, and after treatment.
▶ Advise your patient to alert his therapist of any health conditions he has or medications he's taking.
▶ Instruct your patient to check with his insurance company about coverage for this therapy. Many private insurance companies, personal injury protection plans, and workers' compensation insurance carriers cover myotherapy when it's prescribed by a physician.

Qigong

Qigong (pronounced "chee goong") is a system of gentle exercise, meditation, and controlled breathing that's used by millions of Chinese people daily to increase strength and relax the mind. Practitioners believe that when practiced daily over time, *qigong* can improve strength and flexibility, reverse damage due to injury or disease, relieve pain, restore energy, and induce relaxation and healing.

This ancient practice, like acupuncture and tai chi chuan, is based on the principles that underlie all traditional Chinese medicine. The cornerstone belief is the existence of a vital life force, known as *qi*, which flows through the body and is responsible for maintaining health. (See chapter 4, Alternative systems of medical practice, for more information on *qi*.) *Qigong*, which means "energy work," is believed to enhance or balance the flow of *qi* through a system of repetitive motions, intense concentration, and breathing exercises.

Qigong is even less physically demanding than tai chi chuan (discussed in chapter 5, Mind-body therapies) and is suitable for people of all ages and physical conditions. Those who are disabled can even practice it while sitting or lying in bed. In the United States today, *qigong* is taught by qualified instructors in adult education centers, fitness centers, YMCAs, and even some hospitals. It can also be self-taught through videos and books.

> 66 Qigong *masters have learned through years of practice to transmit the force of their* qi *outside their bodies to heal others or move inanimate objects.* 99

Internal vs. external

There are two forms of *qigong*: internal and external. Internal *qigong* focuses on manipulating the *qi* within one's own body to maintain health and self-healing. This type can consist primarily of meditation and breathing exercises (quiescent *qigong*), or it can include active, dancelike movements (dynamic *qigong*). In the quiet form, the body is relaxed while the mind aims to control the *qi* through breathing and concentration. In the dynamic form, the body is active while the mind is quiet and relaxed.

External *qigong* is the domain of *qigong* masters, who have learned through years of practice to transmit the force of their *qi* to others for healing purposes. Many can even move inanimate objects and display their skills in exhibitions. (See *Encounter with a* qigong *master.*)

Encounter with a *qigong* master

Qigong masters are revered in China for their ability to perform superhuman feats. During the Cultural Revolution, they were dismissed as superstitious and backward. By 1979, however, they were again on television, in magazines, and performing in public.

David Eisenberg, a Harvard medical student, witnessed some of these performances during the year he spent in China in 1979–80 studying traditional Chinese medicine as a medical exchange student. He later wrote about his experiences in his book, *Encounters with Qi: Exploring Chinese Medicine.* He saw *qigong* masters splitting thick marble blocks with their foreheads, bending thick iron bars with their hands, and even being run over by a jeep without injury. These were all examples of internal *qigong,* manipulating the *qi* within one's own body.

Exploring external *qi*

Eisenberg was more intrigued by the stories of external *qigong,* the apparent ability of some masters to emit *qi* outside their bodies and move inanimate objects or even heal people. One day a friend arranged a private demonstration.

The *qigong* master began with a warm-up exercise aimed at helping him gain control of his *qi.* He swallowed two iron balls about 2″ (5 cm) in diameter and weighing 1½ lb (0.7 kg), then regurgitated them, spitting them at Eisenberg's feet. He next took a fist-size stone and cracked it against his forehead.

Eisenberg asked him if he could move a 4′ (1.2 m)–high Chinese lantern hanging from the ceiling without touching it. The master said he had never done this before but would try. He began to breathe deeply, performing some short martial arts steps and tracing circles in the air with his hands. Then from 3′ (0.9 m) away, he pointed his left foot and right arm directly at the lantern. Slowly, the lantern began to swing back and forth.

The master's perspective

Afterward, the exhausted master shared his thoughts with the young American. He believed in the existence of *qi* unequivocally. He said some *qi*-related feats were easy, whereas others required years of practice and dedication.

The master said he could actually "feel" the *qi* flowing in his body but didn't really understand its power. "It's a part of me, like an arm or a breath. Emitting *qi* is like exhaling for me. Can anyone fully understand a breath?"

Therapeutic uses

Chinese researchers say that regular practice of *qigong* lowers heart rate, blood pressure, metabolic rate, and oxygen demand—the effects known as the relaxation response. Proponents claim a wide range of therapeutic uses, from treatment of nearsightedness and hemorrhoids to coronary artery disease and arthritis. Chinese practitioners often combine *qigong* with conventional therapies to treat cancer, bone marrow disease, heart disease, acquired immunodeficiency syndrome, and diseases associated with old age.

RESEARCH SUMMARY Chinese researchers in the past 15 years have done extensive research on the healing effects of *qigong*. They've reported success in treating (or improving) numerous conditions, including asthma, insomnia, depression, anxiety, pain, diabetes, and hypertension. Several studies have reported significant improvement in patients with terminal cancer who practiced *qigong* in addition to receiving chemotherapy.

Because the Chinese studies generally aren't the rigorous, controlled studies that Western science demands, the medical establishment for the most part doesn't accept the claims of *qigong's* effectiveness in treating specific diseases. However, an increasing number of mainstream physicians believe that *qigong*, like meditation and other therapies that induce the relaxation response, may be effective in reducing stress and anxiety, relieving pain from arthritis, improving sleep, and enhancing overall well-being. ■

Equipment

No special equipment is required for *qigong*, other than loose, comfortable clothing and an open, flat area in which to practice.

Procedure

Quiescent *qigong* is a meditative state that can be achieved sitting, standing, or lying down. The body is relaxed and quiet while the mind controls the *qi* with breathing, visualization, and mental concentration. The person begins by inhaling as he visualizes a concentration of *qi* in the abdominal area (believed to be the source of this vital force). As he exhales, he visualizes the *qi* leaving the abdomen and entering the organs, glands, extremities, and other parts of the body. These thoughts are augmented by deep breathing and relaxation to circulate the healing energy of *qi*.

A simple *qigong* exercise

Begin by rubbing your hands together to build up heat, which is thought to increase the flow of *qi*. Your hands will become warmer if you're relaxed. Stroke your warmed palms across your face, eye, and forehead as if you were washing your face.

Follow the diagram below to continue to trace your hands over the top and sides of your head, down the back of the neck, and forward along the shoulder to the joint, down the rib cage, around the back, down to the back and sides of the legs, and then out to the sides of the feet. Then, with the same continuous motion, continue the path inside the feet and inner surface of the legs up the front of the torso and back onto the face.

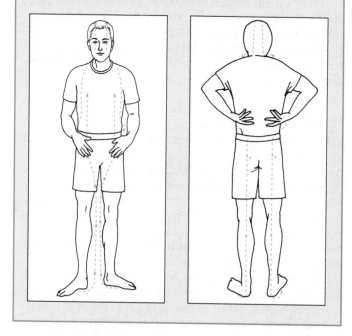

In dynamic *qigong*, the body moves from one posture to another, almost as in a dance. While the body is in motion and active, the mind is quiet and relaxed. Practitioners believe that both forms of *qigong* are important, just as in life there must be a balance of activity and relaxation.

Basic *qigong* exercises can be learned from books or videos. (See *A simple* qigong *exercise*.) After learning the basics, the patient can design his own daily practice regimen. To receive the full benefits of these exercises, the patient should practice for at least 20 to 30 minutes each morning and add an afternoon or evening practice if possible.

Complications
When properly performed, *qigong* is a gentle and invigorating exercise with no adverse effects.

Nursing perspective
▶ Be aware that patients with respiratory problems may not be able to integrate the breathing aspect of *qigong* into their therapy.

▶ If your patient has a serious illness, inform him that *qigong* may be beneficial as a complementary therapy, but not as a substitute for conventional treatment.

▶ Tell your patient that it's best to learn *qigong* from a qualified teacher than from books or videos to ensure that he's doing the movements properly.

Reflexology
Reflexology is a widely practiced form of manual therapy that involves the application of pressure to specific parts of the body, usually the soles of the feet (but sometimes the palms of the hands). It's based on the theory that these parts of the body correspond to and can therapeutically affect various organs and glands. For example, the top of the big toe is said to connect to the brain, and the arch area to the solar plexus. Some practitioners believe that these points follow the same meridians used in acupuncture.

The roots of reflexology can be traced back 3,000 years to folk medicine traditions in China, India, and Egypt. The current revival of interest in this technique began in the early 1900s with an American ear, nose, and throat specialist, William Fitzgerald, who discovered that his patients felt less pain when he applied pressure to specific points on their soles or palms before surgery. In the 1930s, Eunice Ingham, a physical therapist, expanded upon Fitzgerald's work. Ingham believed that applying varying levels of pressure to certain areas could not only decrease pain but also provide other health benefits.

Right foot reflex zones

The illustration below, showing the organs and body parts associated with specific regions of the right foot, serves as a map that guides reflexologists in performing therapy.

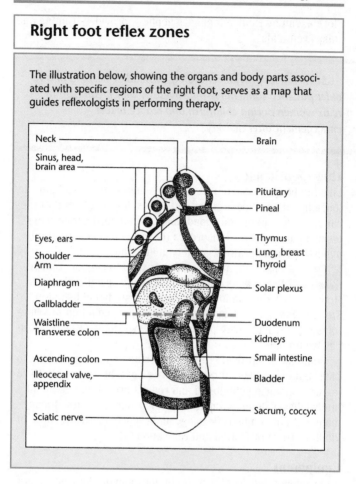

Neck — Brain
Sinus, head, brain area —
— Pituitary
— Pineal
Eyes, ears — — Thymus
Shoulder — — Lung, breast
Arm — — Thyroid
Diaphragm — — Solar plexus
Gallbladder —
Waistline — — Duodenum
Transverse colon — — Kidneys
Ascending colon — — Small intestine
Ileocecal valve, appendix — — Bladder
Sciatic nerve — — Sacrum, coccyx

She mapped the specific reflex zones on the feet that reflexologists use today. (See *Right foot reflex zones*.)

Reflexologists, most of whom are masseurs or physical therapists with special training, say that their technique works by reducing the amount of lactic acid in the feet and breaking up calcium crystals that accumulate in the nerve endings, blocking the flow of energy.

Many health clubs and spas offer reflexology treatments. No specific license or certification is needed to practice reflexology. The International Institute of Reflexology in St. Petersburg,

Florida, run by Eunice Ingham's nephew, provides training and makes referrals.

> *66 Some nurses provide reflexology instead of sleeping pills to older patients; some nurse-midwives say that it can help to relax women during childbirth and reduce breast engorgement after delivery. 99*

Therapeutic uses

Like full body massage, reflexology relieves stress and muscle tension and produces relaxation. Reflexologists claim that they can also treat numerous conditions, including skin disorders (eczema and acne), GI disorders (diarrhea and constipation), hypertension, migraines, anxiety, and asthma.

RESEARCH SUMMARY Little scientific evidence exists to support that reflexology is effective in treating specific illnesses. However, a 1993 randomized controlled study published in *Obstetrics and Gynecology* found a significant reduction in symptoms in 35 women with premenstrual syndrome after reflexology treatment.

Some nurses provide reflexology instead of sleeping pills to older patients; some nurse-midwives say that it can help to relax women during childbirth and reduce breast engorgement after delivery. Even without scientific evidence of its efficacy, many patients enjoy reflexology and report positive results, including stress reduction and relaxation. ■

Equipment

Reflexology requires only a treatment table or chair or a stool to elevate the feet. A quiet environment is preferred.

Procedure

The patient is either seated comfortably in a reclining chair or placed in a supine position on a treatment table, with feet raised and supported. The therapist is seated facing the patient's soles. After an initial assessment of the patient's feet for alterations in skin thickness and abnormalities in foot structure, the therapist feels for tender areas and signs of tension or thickening on the sole.

A treatment session typically begins with relaxation techniques designed to release tension and make the patient comfortable with the manipulation of his feet. The therapist uses thumbs and fingers to apply gentle but firm pressure to the reflex zones of the foot, paying more attention to zones that are tender to the touch. Working systematically, the therapist begins with the toes and proceeds in small, creeping movements proximally toward the heel. (For therapy using the hand, the therapist starts with the fingers and moves proximally toward the wrist.) A typical session lasts 20 to 60 minutes.

Complications

Treatments may produce what practitioners call a "healing crisis," consisting of a fever, rash, diaphoresis, or urinary changes or a worsening of symptoms related to the patient's chief symptom — for example, worsening diarrhea or nausea in a patient with a GI disorder. These crises are said to result from the release of toxins — proof that the treatment is working and the body is healing itself.

Nursing perspective

▶ Advise your patient to postpone reflexology treatments if he has cuts, boils, bruises, or other injuries on his feet.

▶ If the patient has diabetes, peripheral vascular disease, or another vascular problem in his legs, such as thrombosis or phlebitis, instruct him to check with his physician before trying reflexology.

▶ If the patient is pregnant, advise her to get her physician's consent before trying this therapy.

▶ Many people who claim to perform reflexology are actually providing a simple foot massage. If your patient wants treatment for a specific symptom, he should make sure the practitioner has been trained in reflexology.

Rolfing

Formally known as Structural Integration, Rolfing is a system of bodywork developed in the 1940s by Ida Rolf, a biochemist. Rolf, who was greatly influenced by the principles of yoga and osteopathy, believed that body structure affects all physiologic processes and that maintaining the proper balance of head, torso, and pelvis is the key to improving function and health.

Rolf's work began almost by accident in about 1940, when she met a music teacher who had been injured in a fall and could no longer teach or play the piano. Rolf made a deal with her: If she could help the teacher recover from her injuries, the teacher would give Rolf's children piano lessons. The teacher accepted, and Rolf began to work with her. They started working with yoga exercises, and by the fourth session the woman was able to resume teaching piano. Word spread, and soon Rolf was treating all sorts of people with the new system she was developing. Rolf's system of bodywork was influenced by three key principles: osteopathy's belief that structure determines function; homeopathy's emphasis on the integration of physical, mental, and emotional aspects of the human being; and yoga's focus on body-lengthening positions to achieve a balanced body.

Rolf combined these three principles but took them a step further: She maintained that repositioning bones wasn't enough to alter body structure; one also needed to focus on the fascia — the fibrous tissue that covers all muscles and organs. She believed that chronic stress, bad posture, and injury cause the fascia to thicken (the feeling of a "knot" in a muscle), leading to restricted movement in the muscles and joints and interfering with proper body alignment. By manipulating the thickened fascial tissues, Rolf believed one could stretch and "unwind" them, restoring the proper alignment of bones and muscles and improving overall body functioning.

66 *Rolf's aim in advancing Structural Integration, was not just to relieve symptoms but to develop new, better human beings.* 99

The Rolf Institute in Boulder, Colorado, teaches Structural Integration and certifies instructors. Once certified, instructors become members of the Rolf Institute and are entitled to use the trademarked term *Rolfing*. Members are required to abide by the Institute's code of ethics and standards of practice. The Institute also provides referrals to certified Rolfers.

Therapeutic uses

Rolf's aim in advancing Structural Integration was the development of "new, better human beings." Bringing the physical body back into balance and alignment, she believed, would cause symptoms to disappear and ultimately make the person integrated and healthy.

Rolfing practitioners don't claim to cure disease. They *do* claim that they can reduce pain and muscle spasms; increase range of motion, flexibility, and energy; and release tension. Rolfing may be most helpful for chronic pain and muscle stiffness related to structural imbalances.

RESEARCH SUMMARY A study done at UCLA found that patients who underwent Rolfing had smoother, more energetic movements and improved posture. Another study at the University of Maryland found that Rolfing reduced chronic stress, improved neurologic function, and reduced curvature of the spine in patients with lordosis. ■

Equipment

A treatment table may be used for some Rolfing techniques. Also, a mirror may be provided to help the patient understand how his body moves and to observe changes as they occur.

Procedure

Rolfing is usually administered in a series of 10 weekly sessions each lasting 60 to 90 minutes. The sessions are designed to work systematically on the whole body, beginning at the surface and progressing deeper into the tissues. Practitioners use their thumbs, fingers, knuckles, and sometimes their elbows and knees to apply pressure to the fascia in all areas of the body. This gradually releases tension in overstressed muscles, lengthens muscles, and allows the skeletal structure to assume its natural position.

As the muscles and fascia move more smoothly together and bones move into a more normal relationship, joints move with greater ease and the body becomes more relaxed and open. According to Rolfing proponents, as the physical body becomes more fluid, blood and lymph circulation improves and the patient generally experiences a sense of greater well-being.

Complications

Rolfing may be painful at times, but shouldn't result in any complications when performed by a properly trained practitioner.

Nursing perspective

▶ Patients suffering from coagulopathy shouldn't undergo Rolfing because of the risk of bruising.

▶ If your patient expresses an interest in Rolfing, help him locate a certified practitioner.

▶ Inform the patient that some aspects of Rolfing may be painful.

Therapeutic massage

Throughout history, human beings have used touch to help ease pain and further healing. Touching, stroking, and kneading movements are almost automatic when people feel pain or are injured. Massage has played an important role in traditional medical systems, such as the Chinese system, through the centuries. Today, it has emerged as a therapeutic discipline in the West, embraced by millions who use it to relieve pain and tension and generally to feel better.

The beginnings of modern massage in the West are often traced to Pehr Henrik Ling, a Swedish physician who developed his own style of massage and exercises in the early 1800s that came to be called Swedish Remedial Massage and Exercise. By 1900, modern therapeutic massage techniques were being used throughout the developed world, primarily for rehabilitation. Gertrude Beard, an American nurse who served in the army in World War I, is credited with establishing therapeutic massage as a vital intervention for the stimulation of self-healing in patients.

Most massage therapists in the United States practice some variation of Swedish massage, applying several basic strokes to the body's soft tissue. Beyond this, many individual therapists have their own style and techniques. (See *Understanding therapeutic massage*.)

Massage therapists are licensed in 25 states and the District of Columbia. Licensing requirements vary from state to state; most states require that the therapist undergo at least 500 hours of training from a recognized program and pass an

ff *Elderly patients may benefit from improved circulation and muscle tone as well as the personal attention and social interaction that a good massage provides.* ™

HOW IT WORKS

⤳ Understanding therapeutic massage

The primary physiologic effect of therapeutic massage is improved blood circulation. As the muscles are kneaded and stretched, blood return to the heart increases and toxins, such as lactic acid, are carried out of the muscle tissue to be excreted from the body.

Improved circulation also results in increased perfusion and oxygenation of tissues. Improved oxygenation of the brain helps us think more clearly and feel more alive; improved perfusion and oxygenation of other organ systems leads to improved digestion and elimination as well as quicker wound healing. Massage also appears to trigger the release of endorphins, the body's natural pain relievers.

examination. The American Massage Therapy Association in Evanston, Illinois, and the National Certification Board for Therapeutic Massage and Bodywork in McLean, Virginia, provide information and referrals.

Therapeutic uses

Therapeutic massage is used primarily for stress reduction and relaxation, but it can serve as a complementary therapy for a broad range of conditions. By improving circulation, massage can help relieve the pain and stiffness of arthritic joints and speed the healing of broken bones. Through its muscle-toning effects, massage stimulates peristalsis, helping relieve constipation and indigestion from a sedentary lifestyle.

The stress-reducing effects of massage may help people with hypertension or anxiety. Elderly patients may benefit from improved circulation and muscle tone as well as the personal attention and social interaction that a good massage provides. Massage has even been used to reduce irritability in infants. (See *Indications for therapeutic massage*, page 290.)

RESEARCH SUMMARY   In her classic reference *Beard's Massage*, Gertrude Beard, former Associate Professor of Physical Therapy at Northwestern University Medical School, summarizes the research findings on this form of therapy. According to the studies, massage:

Indications for therapeutic massage

The following conditions may benefit from therapeutic massage:
- chronic pain
- circulatory disorders
- digestive disorders
- inflammation
- intestinal disorders
- joint mobility disorders
- muscle tension
- overstimulated or under-stimulated nervous system
- skin conditions
- swelling.

- increases blood flow through the muscles, promoting muscle relaxation and relieving some types of pain
- has a sedative effect on the nervous system
- increases peristalsis
- loosens mucus and induces drainage of sinus fluids from the lungs
- increases lymphatic circulation
- reduces swelling from fractures
- decreases scar tissue, adhesions, and fibrosis due to injury or immobilization. ■

Equipment
Massage therapy requires a sturdy massage table (or a chair with a head rest for chair massages), lubricating oil, and a quiet room with relaxing music.

Procedure
The patient undresses in private and covers himself with the sheet or towel provided. With the patient on the massage table, the therapist may begin playing a tape of quiet, soothing music to induce relaxation. To respect the patient's modesty, the therapist keeps the body fully draped, exposing only the area being worked on at the moment.

The therapist usually uses a scented oil to prevent friction between her hands and the patient's skin while she kneads various muscle groups in a systematic way from head to toe. (See *Basic massage techniques*.)

Basic massage techniques

Theraputic massage uses five basic techniques: effleurage, pétrissage, friction, tapotement, and vibration.

Effleurage

In *effleurage,* the therapist performs a long, gliding stroke using the whole hand or the thumb. This motion is a warm-up technique that lets the patient get used to the therapist's hands. The gliding stroke, which should always move toward the heart, improves circulation.

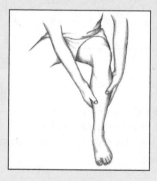

Pétrissage

Pétrissage is a kneading and compressing motion in which

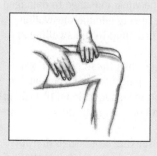

the muscles are grabbed and lifted. This motion relieves sore muscles by clearing away lactic acid and increasing circulation to the muscle tissue.

Friction

In *friction,* the therapist uses the thumbs and fingertips to work around the joints and the thickest part of the muscles. Circular motions break down adhesions and may also help make soft tissue and joints more flexible. For larger muscles, the therapist may use the palm or heel of the hand.

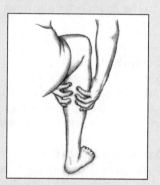

Tapotement

In *tapotement,* the therapist uses the sides of the hands, fingertips, cupped palms, or slightly closed make chopping, tapping, and beating motions. These motions invigorate and stimulate the muscles, resulting in a burst of energy. However, when muscles are cramped, strained, or spastic,

(continued)

Basic massage techniques (continued)

tapotement performed for a longer period has the opposite effect of relaxing the muscles.

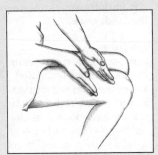

Vibration
In *vibration,* the therapist presses her fingers or flattened hands firmly into the muscle and then "vibrates" (transmits a trembling motion to) the area rapidly for a few seconds. She repeats this motion until the entire muscle has been vibrated. This helps to stimulate the nervous system and may increase circulation and improve gland function.

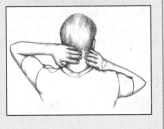

Complications

A trained massage therapist will pay close attention to body language as well as the patient's comments to avoid causing pain or discomfort. Other than this, there are no complications from properly performed massage.

Nursing perspective

▶ Be aware that massage is contraindicated in those with any of the following conditions: diabetes, varicose veins, phlebitis, or other blood vessel problems (because massage to damaged tissue can dislodge a blood clot); pitting edema; or swollen limbs (use only gentle massage, proximal to the swelling and in the direction of the heart).

▶ If you'll be performing massage, take these precautions: Avoid massaging the abdomen of a patient with hypertension or gastric or duodenal ulcers, and massage at least 6″ (15 cm) away from bruises, cysts, broken bones, and breaks in skin integrity.

▶ Advise your patients who are seeking a massage therapist to get recommendations from people who have been satisfied with their treatment. They should also make sure the therapist is properly trained and licensed and belongs to a professional organization such as the American Massage Therapy Association.

Therapeutic Touch

Developed in the 1970s, Therapeutic Touch is a widely used complementary therapy developed *by* nurses *for* nurses in an attempt to bring a more humane and holistic approach to their practice. Rooted in the ancient art of "laying on of hands," this technique focuses on "healing" rather than "curing" and is built on the belief that all healing is basically self-healing.

> 66 *By using their hands to manipulate the energy field above the patient's skin, practitioners say they can restore equilibrium, thereby reactivating the mind-body-spirit connection and empowering the patient to fully participate in his own healing.* 99

Central to Therapeutic Touch is the concept of a universal life force (similar to the Ayurvedic concept of *prana* and the Chinese concept of *qi*) that practitioners believe permeates space and sustains all living organisms. Practitioners believe that in healthy people, this vital energy flows freely in and through the body in a balanced way that nourishes all body organs and that when people get sick it's because their energy field is out of equilibrium.

By using their hands to manipulate the energy field above the patient's skin, practitioners say they can restore equilibrium, thereby reactivating the mind-body-spirit connection and empowering the patient to fully participate in his own healing. Although the existence of a human energy field hasn't been proved scientifically, nurses claim that they can actually feel something best described as energy when performing this technique. (See *Human energy field*, page 294.)

Despite its name, Therapeutic Touch doesn't require actual physical contact during a treatment. In most cases, the nurse's hands remain several inches above the patient's body.

Human energy field

Practitioners of Therapeutic Touch and other energy-based therapies believe that the human body emits several energy fields, as indicated in the illustration below. However, the layers aren't as separate as the illustration suggests; rather, each successive layer encompasses some of the preceding one.

Intuitive (or spiritual) layer

Mental layer

Emotional layer

Ether (or vital) layer

Background
Therapeutic Touch was developed in the early 1970s by Dolores Krieger, a nursing professor at New York University (NYU), and her mentor, Dora Kunz, a healer. The two women had been studying the work of well-known healers who practiced the laying on of hands. In 1971, Krieger did a study comparing 19 people who received treatment by a world-famous healer and 9 people who received routine nursing care. All those who were treated by the healer had an increased hemoglobin level; the 9 in the control group had no increase. When this study was replicated with a group of Krieger's nursing students, it yielded the same results.

Krieger developed a formal instruction method for this healing process, which she termed Therapeutic Touch, and began teaching it at NYU. The publication of Krieger's experiment in the *American Journal of Nursing* in 1975 marked the beginning of Therapeutic Touch's acceptance as a recognized clinical method. In the early 1980s, Martha Rogers, dean of NYU's nursing school, postulated her human energy field theory, which complemented Krieger and Kunz's theory that Therapeutic Touch could interact in a specific way within the human energy field to promote healing.

Current status

Today, Therapeutic Touch is widely used by practitioners of holistic nursing and other health professionals and is practiced in many hospitals, hospices, long-term care facilities, and other settings. It's taught in more than 100 colleges and universities worldwide, and it has been taught to more than 40,000 health care providers. The North American Nursing Diagnosis Association recognizes "energy field disturbance" as a nursing diagnosis, and professional organizations, such as the American Nurses Association and the National League for Nursing, have supported Therapeutic Touch as a nursing intervention.

The Nurse Healers–Professional Association is the official organization representing nurses who practice Therapeutic Touch. (The American Holistic Nurses Association endorses Healing Touch, an offshoot of Therapeutic Touch developed in the 1980s that also incorporates the practices of other energetic healers, including Rev. Roselyn Bruyere, Rev. Rudy Noel, Brugh Joy, MD, and Barbara Brennan, PhD.)

Although most practitioners are nurses, other health care professionals (massage therapists, physical therapists, dentists, and medical doctors) and nonprofessionals have incorporated this therapy in their practices. Practitioners say that anyone can study the technique and apply it to himself or others.

Therapeutic uses

Therapeutic Touch is used as a complementary therapy for virtually all medical and nursing diagnoses as well as surgical procedures. Practitioners say it's especially helpful for patients with wounds or infections because it eases discomfort and speeds up the healing process. However, the technique is best known for its ability to relieve pain and anxiety.

Because it helps reduce anxiety and promote relaxation, proponents say Therapeutic Touch is helpful in treating stress-related disorders, such as tension headaches, hypertension, ulcers, and emotional problems. It's also used in Lamaze classes and delivery rooms to induce relaxation and in neonatal intensive care units to help speed the growth of premature infants.

RESEARCH SUMMARY Since Krieger's 1971 experiment on patients treated by laying on of hands, numerous other studies have been done on this technique. Studies have shown that, like meditation and yoga, Therapeutic Touch produces signs of the relaxation response, including slower and deeper breathing, decreased muscle tension and heart rate, and altered brain wave activity.

Other studies have reported benefits in reducing headache pain, wound healing, easing breathing in asthmatic patients, decreasing fever and inflammation, and reducing postoperative pain.

In April 1998, a study by a fourth grade Colorado girl debunking Therapeutic Touch received widespread media attention when it was published in *JAMA*. To test proponents' claims that they can detect another person's energy field with their hands, the girl had 21 practitioners place their hands through holes cut in a cardboard partition and then placed her own hand over the subjects' right or left hand. The therapists were asked to say which hand could detect the girl's energy field. The average correct score was 44%, no more than would be expected by guessing.

Proponents of Therapeutic Touch criticized the study's premise and setup. They also condemned the study as biased because the girl's mother, a registered nurse, had been a vocal opponent of the practice for years. ■

Equipment
Therapeutic Touch treatments require no equipment beyond the nurse's hands and an environment conducive to relaxation in the patient and inward-focused concentration in the nurse. This may include a comfortable chair, bed, or massage table for the patient and possibly soothing music to help create a relaxing atmosphere.

Procedure

Therapeutic Touch incorporates the nursing process, beginning with assessment and continuing through diagnosis, treatment, and evaluation. In a typical session, the patient usually lies fully clothed on a massage table or a hospital bed. The nurse begins by "centering" herself — achieving a calm, meditative state that lets the practitioner be sensitive to whatever signs and symptoms the patient presents. This heightened sensitivity is also necessary in order to perceive subtle changes in the patient's energy field.

After becoming centered, the nurse begins the assessment. The Therapeutic Touch practitioner slowly moves her hands over the patient's body, 2″ to 4″ (5 to 10 cm) away from the skin surface, to detect any alterations in the energy field, such as feelings of cold or heat, vibration, or blockages. Depending on what this assessment reveals, the nurse then performs interventions aimed at balancing the energy field and removing any obstructions. These may include "unruffling" a chaotic and tangled field, eliminating "congestion," and acting as a conduit to direct the "life energy" from the environment into the patient. The nurse may alter her techniques based on the patient's response to the treatment or on changes in the patient's condition.

Throughout the treatment, the patient remains quiet and relaxed. He may actually feel the nurse's hands even though they aren't touching the body. Practitioners say that the patient doesn't have to consciously believe in the power of the procedure. However, in order to be effective in channeling energy into the patient, the nurse must have "conscious intent" — that is, the intent to become a calm, focused "instrument of healing," enabling the patient's body to ultimately heal itself.

Complications

Complications from Therapeutic Touch treatments are rare. Practitioners are careful to moderate the length and strength of the treatment for small children and the elderly because of their more fragile physiologies. A common sign of overtreatment in these age-groups is restlessness during or after the treatment.

Nursing perspective

▶ If you practice Therapeutic Touch, be careful to respect the personal preferences of those you treat. People have differing tolerances for touch, and some people regard energy work as an invasion of their personal space and boundaries.

▶ Certain patients warrant extra sensitivity and shorter treatment periods. These include infants, the elderly, pregnant women (especially during the last trimester), patients with head injuries or psychosis, emaciated patients, and patients in shock. Always ask for consent before proceeding with a Therapeutic Touch treatment.

Trager approach

Like the Alexander and Feldenkrais techniques, the Trager approach is a gentle method of movement reeducation that aims to help people recognize and "unlearn" mental and physical habits that limit their movements, cause muscle pain and tension, and prevent them from functioning optimally. This technique has two components: gentle, rhythmic bodywork designed to loosen stiff joints and muscles, increase range of motion (ROM), and enhance relaxation (known as Psychophysical Integration), and dancelike exercises (known as Mentastics, or mental gymnastics) designed to increase awareness of how the body moves and teach people how to move it more freely and pleasurably.

The method was developed by Milton Trager, an American physician who became a follower of Maharishi Mahesh Yogi, the founder of Transcendental Meditation. Trager believed that the subconscious mind transfers the stresses of daily life into musculoskeletal tension, which dictates the way we hold and move our bodies. To alleviate this physical tension, Trager focused on gentle movement as a way of repatterning the brain by loosening the body.

Rather than using set exercises, the Trager approach involves gently pushing, pulling, stretching, and rocking the body to loosen tense muscles and stiff joints. The emphasis isn't on moving particular muscles and joints, but on using movement to produce pleasant sensations of lightness, limberness, and deep relaxation. Eventually, Trager believed, the unconscious mind would mimic movements that produced these pleasurable sensations.

Founded in 1980, the Trager Institute in Mill Valley, California, provides training in this technique and certification. There are more than 1,000 certified Trager practitioners worldwide.

Therapeutic uses

Trager practitioners view this technique as a learning experience rather than a medical treatment and believe it can benefit anyone. Trager used it to improve the condition of people suffering from serious musculoskeletal disorders, such as multiple sclerosis, muscular dystrophy, and polio. Proponents say it has also benefited people with back problems, asthma, and emphysema. Athletes have also reported improved performance and increased stamina as a result of the Trager approach, which releases tension and allows athletes to function at full capacity.

Equipment

The Trager approach requires only a well-padded table and a room big enough to allow free movement.

Procedure

The practitioner begins by entering a relaxed, meditative state (which Trager called "hook-up") that allows him to connect with the patient and remain aware of the patient's slightest responses. In this state, the practitioner begins touching, rocking, pulling, and otherwise gently manipulating the patient's trunk and limbs, helping to induce a state of total relaxation. As the patient's body relaxes, the therapist continues performing the gentle, rhythmic movements to extend ROM, as if demonstrating to the patient's body that movements beyond its previous limits aren't only possible but also pleasurable.

A typical session lasts 60 to 90 minutes, and therapy continues as often as necessary. In addition to the table work, the patient receives instruction in the use of Mentastics; this system of effortless, dancelike movements is intended to enhance the sense of lightness, freedom, and flexibility produced by the table work.

Complications

The gentle movements used in the Trager approach are unlikely to cause complications.

Nursing perspective

▶ The Trager approach isn't recommended for those who are uncomfortable with physical contact.

Selected references

Acupuncture. NIH Consensus Statement Online 15(5):1-34, November 3-5, 1997. *www.odp.od.nih.gov/consensus/cons/107/107_statement.htm.*

Alpers, D., et al. *Manual of Nutritional Therapeutics*, 4th ed. Philadelphia: Lippincott Williams & Wilkins, 2002.

Alternative Medicine: Expanding Medical Horizons. A Report to the National Institutes of Health on Alternative Medical Systems and Practices in the United States. NIH pub. 94-066. Washington, D.C.: U.S. Government Printing Office, 1994.

Benford, M.S., et al. "Gamma Radiation Fluctuations during Alternative Healing Therapy," *Alternative Therapies in Health and Medicine* 5(4):51-56, July 1999.

Caplan, D. "The Alexander Technique and Its Application to Back Problems," from The Brighton Congress Papers. *DIRECTION* 1(4), 1988.

Chance, J. *Thorson Principles of Alexander Technique.* New York: HarperCollins, 1999.

Cibik, T. "An Introduction to Medical *Qigong,*" in *IDEA Health & Fitness Source* 19(2): February 2001.

Cross, J.R. *Acupressure: Clinical Applications in Musculoskeletal Conditions.* Boston: Butterworth, 2000.

Eisenberg, D., and Wright, T.L. *Encounters with Qi: Exploring Chinese Medicine.* New York: W.W. Norton & Co., 1995.

Freeman, L., and Lawlis, F. *Mosby's Complementary and Alternative Therapy: A Research Based Approach.* St. Louis: Mosby–Year Book, Inc., 2001.

Frost, R., and Goodheart, G. *Applied Kinesiology: A Training Manual and Reference Book of Basic Principles and Practices,* 2nd ed. Berkeley, Calif.: North Atlantic Books, 2001.

Gerber, R. *Vibrational Medicine for the 21st Century.* New York: Eagle Brook, an Imprint of HarperCollins Pub., 2000.

Haslam, R. "A Comparison of Acupuncture with Advice and Exercises on the Symptomatic Treatment of Osteoarthritis of the Hip – A Randomized Controlled Trial," *Acupuncture in Medicine* 19(1):19-26, June 2001.

Kuhn, M. *Complementary Therapies for Healthcare Providers.* Philadelphia: Lippincott Williams & Wilkins, 1999.

Levine, A.S., and Levine, V.J. *The Bodywork and Massage Sourcebook.* Lincolnwood, Ill.: Lowell House, 1999.

Micozzi, M. *Fundamentals of Complementary & Alternative Medicine,* 2nd ed. St. Louis: Mosby–Year Book, Inc., 2001.

Mitzel-Wilkinson, A. "Massage Therapy as a Nursing Practice," *Holistic Nursing Practice* 14(2):48-56, January 2000.

National Institutes of Health Consensus Development Statement: Acupuncture. Revised draft, Nov. 5, 1997. Electronic publication. URL: *www.healthy.net/LIBRARY/Articles/NIH/Report.htm.*

Nelson, C., et al. "Manual Healing Diversity and Other Challenges to Chiropractic Integration," *Journal of Manipulative and Physiological Therapeutics* 23(3):202-7, March-April 2000.

Novey, D.W. *Clinician's Complete Reference to Complementary and Alternative Medicine.* St. Louis: Mosby–Year Book, Inc., 2000.

Peters, D., and Woodlan, A. *Encyclopedia of Natural Healing,* 2nd ed. New York: Kindersey Press, 2000.

Reisser, P., et al. *Examining Alternative Medicine: An Inside Look at the Benefits and Risks.* Downers Grove, Ill.: InterVarsity Press, 2001.

Smith-Fassler, M.E., and Lopez-Bushnell, K. "Acupuncture as Complementary Therapy for Back Pain," *Holistic Nursing Practice* 15(3):35-44, April 2001.

Teschendorf, M., and Evans, C. "Hydrotherapy during Labor: An Example of Developing a Practice Policy," *MCN American Journal of Maternal Child Nursing* 25(4):198-203, July-August 2000.

Upledger, J.E., and Vredevoogd, M.F.A. *Craniosacral Therapy.* Chicago: Eastland Press, 1983.

Ren, Y.E. "Acupuncture in the Treatment of Hypertension and Stroke." *Acupuncture in Medicine* 18(1):54-60, June 2000.

8

Herbal
therapy

Most of us are familiar with herbs used as culinary accents—for example, dill and oregano used in sauces. However, numerous cultures around the world have used herbs and plants for thousands of years to treat illness. There's even archaeologic evidence that prehistoric man used plants for healing purposes.

Many drugs prescribed today are derived from plants that ancient cultures used for medicinal purposes. (The word *drug* comes from the Old Dutch word *drogge* meaning "to dry," because pharmacists, physicians, and ancient healers often dried plants for use as medicines.) In fact, about one-fourth of all conventional pharmaceuticals (including about 120 of the most commonly prescribed modern drugs) contain at least one active ingredient derived from plants. The rest are chemically synthesized. (See *Common drugs derived from plants.*)

Herbs and plants may be valuable not only for their active ingredients but also for their minerals, vitamins, volatile oils (used in aromatherapy), glycosides (sugar derivatives), alkaloids, and bioflavonoids. Herbalists may select leaves, flowers, stems, berries, seeds, fruit, bark, roots, or any other plant part for medicinal uses.

Modern usage

The World Health Organization estimates that 80% of the world's population uses some form of herbal medicine. Still,

Common drugs derived from plants

Many drugs commonly used today have botanical origins.

Drug	Use	Botanical origin
▶ aspirin, or salicylic acid	analgesic	white willow bark and meadowsweet plant
▶ atropine	antiarrhythmic	belladonna leaves
▶ colchicine	antigout drug	autumn crocus
▶ digoxin	inotropic	foxglove, a poisonous plant
▶ ephedrine	bronchodilator	ephedra plant
▶ morphine and codeine	narcotic analgesic	opium poppy
▶ paclitaxel	antineoplastic (for metastatic ovarian cancer)	yew tree
▶ quinine	antimalarial	cinchona bark
▶ vinblastine and vincristine	antineoplastics	periwinkle

traditional practitioners in the United States are largely unaware of successful herbal remedies, and patients are unaware of the significance of reporting herbal remedy use to their physicians and nurses.

Today, however, renewed interest in all forms of alternative medicine is encouraging patients, health care providers, and drug researchers to re-examine the value of herbal remedies. One of the most newsworthy of the plants being studied is St. John's wort. Recent studies have shown that this perennial herb, commonly used in Europe as a tonic for anxiety and depression, contains xanthones and flavonoids that act as monoamine oxidase inhibitors.

Because of the staggering number of stories touting herbal remedies in popular magazines, books, and television shows, you're likely to encounter patients who have read amazing claims about certain herbs and ask your opinion about them. This chapter will provide you with a general overview of the subject as well as a useful chart on specific herbs that will help you to answer some of your patients' questions.

However, in light of the almost mystical benefits ascribed to herbs in the popular literature, it may be wise to keep in mind (and to make sure your patients understand) that herbs are "nothing more than diluted drugs," according to Varro E. Tyler, author of *The Honest Herbal.* "They do not possess any magical or mystical properties, and like other drugs, they must be administered in proper doses for appropriate periods of time to produce their benefits.... Every herb is different from every other herb. Some are safe and effective. Some are neither. [Some] may produce undesirable side effects."

> 66 *In ancient times, medicinal plants were chosen because of their color or the shape of their leaves — for example, plants with heart-shaped leaves were used for heart disorders and plants with red flowers were used for bleeding disorders.* 99

History of herbal medicine

Also known as *phytotherapy* or *phytomedicine* (especially in Europe), herbal medicine has been practiced since the beginning of recorded history, and specific remedies have been handed down from generation to generation. In ancient times, medicinal plants were chosen because of their color or the shape of their leaves. For example, heart-shaped leaves were used for heart problems, and plants with red flowers were used to treat bleeding disorders. This primitive approach is known as the *Doctrine of Signatures.* The best use for each plant was determined by trial and error.

The formal study of herbs, known as *herbology,* goes back to the ancient cultures of the Middle East, Greece, China, and India. These cultures revered the power of nature and developed herbal remedies based on the plants that were found in their home environments. Written evidence of the medicinal use of herbs has been found on Mesopotamian clay tablets and ancient Egyptian papyrus.

The first known compilation of herbal remedies was ordered by the king of Sumeria around 2000 B.C. and included 250 medicinal substances, including garlic. Ancient Greece and Rome produced their own compilations, including the *De Materia Medica,* written in the 1st century A.D. Of the 950 medicinal products described in this work, 600 are derived from plants and the rest from animal or mineral sources. The Arab world added their own discoveries to the Greco-Roman texts, resulting in a compilation of more than 2,000 substances that was eventually reintroduced to Europe by Christian physicians traveling with the Crusaders.

Herbal therapy is also a major component of India's Ayurvedic medicine, traditional Chinese medicine, Native American medicine, homeopathy, and naturopathy. (See chapter 4, Alternative systems of medical practice.)

> ❝Interest in herbal preparations is reviving in the United States because of a general disillusionment with modern medicine, the high cost and adverse effects of prescription drugs, the widespread availability of herbal drugs, and the belief that natural remedies are superior to manmade drugs. ❞

In the United States, herbal remedies handed down from European settlers and learned from Native Americans were a mainstay of medical care until the early 1900s. The rise of technology and the biomedical approach to health care eventually led to the decline of herbal medicine. However, interest in herbal preparations is reviving in the United States for various reasons, including general disillusionment with modern medicine, the high cost and adverse effects of prescription drugs, the widespread availability of herbal drugs, and the belief that natural remedies are superior to manmade drugs.

Regulating herbal medicine

In the 19th century, many fake remedies were sold to gullible, desperate people in the United States. The federal government finally took action against disreputable purveyors of phony remedies with the 1906 Food and Drug Act. This law addressed problems of mislabeling and adulteration of plant remedies but failed to address issues of safety and efficacy.

Today, herbal remedies are still largely unregulated. The Food and Drug Administration (FDA) regulates these products only as dietary supplements, not drugs. This means that the FDA has the right to recall any herbal product shown to be harmful, but manufacturers aren't required to provide information about product contents or adverse effects or to prove their safety or efficacy. They need only provide "reasonable assurance" that the product contains no harmful ingredients.

In addition, although manufacturers aren't allowed to claim that a particular product cures or prevents a specific disease, they can make any other claim about its supposed benefits without providing supporting evidence. They need only add the following disclaimer: "This statement has not been evaluated by the Food and Drug Administration. This product isn't intended to diagnose, treat, cure or prevent any disease." In 2001, the FDA issued a letter to the food industry reminding manufacturers about the legal requirements regarding claims made on food products. This letter was the result of the significant growth in the marketing of foods containing botanicals and other ingredients.

> ❝ *In essence, herbal remedies in the United States are sold on a buyer-beware basis. Therefore, consumers should be well informed about the herbal products they plan to use.* ❞

In essence, herbal remedies in the United States are sold on a buyer-beware basis. Therefore, consumers should be well informed about the herbal products they plan to use and should seek the advice of a trained practitioner before trying a product, especially for a serious condition.

In Europe, where herbal and homeopathic remedies are used by millions of people, government bodies and the scientific community are much more open to natural remedies, especially those that have a long history of use. In Great Britain and France, traditional medicines that have been used for years with no serious adverse effects are approved for use under the "doctrine of reasonable certainty" when scientific evidence is lacking.

In addition, the European Economic Community has established guidelines that standardize the quality, dosage, and production of herbal remedies. These guidelines are based on the World Health Organization's 1991 publication *Guidelines for the Assessment of Herbal Medicines*, which addressed concerns about the safety and efficacy of herbal medicines and established guidelines for pharmacopoeia monographs. (See *World Health Organization guidelines*.)

World Health Organization guidelines

In 1991, the World Health Organization published Guidelines for the Assessment of Herbal Medicines, which established standards for determining the safety and efficacy of herbal preparations and the development of pharmacopoeia monographs. A summary of these guidelines appears below.

Guidelines regarding safety
▶ If the product traditionally has been used without demonstrated harm, no specific restrictive action should be taken unless new evidence demands a revised risk-benefit assessment.
▶ Prolonged and apparently uneventful use of a substance is considered testimony to its safety.

Guidelines regarding efficacy
▶ For treatment of minor disorders and for nonspecific indications, some relaxation is justified in the requirements for proof of efficacy, taking into account the extent of traditional use.
▶ The same considerations can apply to prophylactic use.

Guidelines regarding pharmacopoeia monographs
▶ If a pharmacopoeia monograph exists, it should be sufficient to make reference to this monograph.
▶ If a monograph doesn't exist, one must be supplied and should be set out in the same way as in an official pharmacopoeia.

Therapeutic uses

Herbal remedies are used primarily to treat minor health problems, such as nausea, colds and flu, coughs, headaches, aches and pains, GI disorders (such as constipation and diarrhea), menstrual cramps, insomnia, skin disorders, and dandruff. These therapeutic uses also serve as a method of categorizing herbal remedies. (See *Herbal classifications,* page 308.)

Some herbalists have also reported success in treating certain chronic conditions, such as peptic ulcers, colitis, rheumatoid arthritis, hypertension, and respiratory problems (such as bronchitis and asthma), as well as illnesses generally treated only with prescription drugs, such as heart failure, hepatitis, and cirrhosis. However, advise your patients with serious dis-

Herbal classifications

Herbs are commonly classified by their effects on patients, as follows:

▶ *Adaptogenic herbs* work on the adrenal gland to increase the body's resistance to illness.
▶ *Anthelmintic herbs* work to eliminate intestinal worms from the body.
▶ *Anti-inflammatory herbs* reduce the tissues' inflammatory response.
▶ *Antimicrobial herbs* boost the immune system by destroying disease-causing organisms or helping the body resist them.
▶ *Antispasmodic herbs* ease skeletal and smooth muscle cramps and tension.
▶ *Astringent herbs,* applied externally, work on the mucous membranes, skin, and other tissues to reduce inflammation, irritation, and the risk of infection.
▶ *Bitter herbs* work on the central nervous system, playing a major role in preventive medicine. Bitter herbs are recommended to increase the secretion of digestive juices, stimulate the appetite, and promote liver detoxification.
▶ *Carminative herbs (aromatic oils)* stimulate proper function of the digestive system, soothe the lining of the GI tract, and reduce gas, inflammation, and pain.
▶ *Delmucent herbs,* rich in mucilage, soothe and protect irritated or inflamed tissue.
▶ *Diuretic herbs* increase the production and elimination of urine.
▶ *Emmenagogic herbs* stimulate menstrual flow.
▶ *Expectorant herbs* work to eliminate mucus from the lungs.
▶ *Hepatic herbs* work to increase the strength and tone of the liver and to increase the flow of bile.
▶ *Hypotensive herbs* work to decrease abnormally high blood pressure.
▶ *Laxative herbs* relieve constipation.
▶ *Nervine herbs* are divided into three groups based on their role in helping the nervous system: those that strengthen and restore, those that ease anxiety and tension, and those that stimulate nerve activity.
▶ *Stimulating herbs* stimulate the body's physiologic and metabolic activities.
▶ *Tonic herbs,* the foundation of traditional Chinese medicine and Ayurvedic (Indian) medicine, enliven and invigorate.

orders who express an interest in herbal remedies not to discontinue any ongoing medical treatments and to consult their physicians about possible interactions between prescribed drugs and herbal remedies.

RESEARCH SUMMARY Numerous studies have been done on herbal remedies in Europe and Asia, where phytomedicine has a long history. European studies have shown benefits from such herbs as ginkgo, bilberry extract, and milk thistle in treating various chronic disorders. Chinese researchers have done extensive studies on many herbs, such as ginseng, fresh ginger rhizome, foxglove, licorice root, and wild chrysanthemum. And Indian researchers using modern scientific methods have recently studied various Ayurvedic herbs, including Indian gooseberry and turmeric.

The United States lags behind other countries in herbal medicine research for a number of reasons:

▶ Until the establishment of the Office of Alternative Medicine (OAM) in 1992, there was no federal support for research on natural remedies.

▶ Pharmaceutical companies have no financial incentive to develop herb-based drugs because botanical products can't be patented; therefore, the companies could never recoup their research investment.

▶ There's an inherent difficulty in studying herbs according to Western pharmaceutical standards. These standards favor isolating a single active ingredient; however, herbs may contain several active ingredients that work together to produce a specific effect.

Although large gaps in research remain, many clinical trials of herbs used as medication are under way. Since arriving at the OAM in 1995, Dr. Carole Hudgings has overseen the collection of more than 60,000 research citations on complementary and alternative health practices, including 2,500 clinical trials that have been compiled in a computer database. ■

Forms of herbal preparations

Herbs are available in various forms, depending on their medicinal purpose and the body system involved; they may be bought individually or in mixtures formulated for specific conditions. They may be prepared as tinctures, extracts, capsules, tablets, lozenges, teas, juices, vapor treatments, or bath products. Some are applied topically with a poultice or compress; others, rubbed into the skin as an oil, ointment, or salve.

Tinctures and extracts

An herb placed in alcohol or liquid glycerin is known as a tincture or an extract. (Tinctures contain more alcohol than extracts.) The alcohol draws out the active properties of the herb, concentrates it, and helps preserve it. Alcohol is easily absorbed by the body, and its cost is minimal. The full taste of the herb comes through in the alcohol and can be strong or unpleasant. Alcohol-based tinctures and extracts have an indefinite shelf life.

Liquid glycerin extracts called *glycerites* are an alternative to alcohol extracts. Glycerites are generally sweet to the taste and feel warm on the tongue. Glycerin is processed in the body as a fat, not a sugar, which is important to patients who must limit sugar intake, such as diabetics. Patients should be aware that taking more than 1 oz (30 ml) of glycerin can have a laxative effect. What's more, glycerin may not be an efficient solvent for some herbs that contain resins and gums; these herbs require alcohol for extraction.

> 66 *Tinctures or extracts may be taken as drops in a tea, diluted in spring water, used in a compress, or applied during body massage.* 99

Extracts should contain a minimum of 60% glycerin with 40% water to ensure preservation. The shelf life of glycerin-based extracts is shorter than that of alcohol-based extracts. An extract that contains citric acid can last for more than 2 years if stored properly.

Tinctures or extracts may be taken as drops in a tea, diluted in spring water, used in a compress, or applied during body massage. If the alcohol content of a tincture is a concern — for example, when administering the remedy to a child — a few drops may be placed in 2 oz (60 ml) of very hot water and left to stand for 5 minutes. As the tincture stands, most of the alcohol evaporates and the mixture becomes cool enough to drink.

An herbal tincture is made by filling a glass bottle or jar with herbal parts (cut fresh herbs or crumbled dry herbs), adding pure spirits such as vodka, sealing the container, and placing it in a warm area (70° to 80° F [21° to 27° C]) for 2 weeks. The mixture should be shaken daily. After 2 weeks, the herbs can be strained out and the residue squeezed out.

Extracts are also made with alcohol or water to bring out the essence of the herb. The product label should indicate which base was used. Extracts have about the same advantages and disadvantages as tinctures, but they're more concentrated and therefore more cost-effective. Because of their strong herbal taste, they're usually diluted in juice or water.

Capsules and tablets

Capsules and tablets contain the ground or powdered form of the raw herb and are much less potent than tinctures; however, they're easier to transport and generally tasteless. The capsule or tablet should be made within 24 hours of milling the herb because herbs degrade quickly. The best products use fresh herbs, which should be indicated on the label. Capsules can be a hard gel or soft gel made of animal or vegetable gelatin. Most patients find capsules easier to swallow than tablets.

> *Capsules and tablets may contain a large amount of filler, such as soy or millet powder, which makes the herb difficult to identify. Consequently, a poorer quality herb may be substituted without the patient's knowledge.*

The patient should be aware that capsules and tablets may contain a large amount of filler, such as soy or millet powder. Filler makes the herb difficult to identify in the powdered form, and a poorer quality herb may be substituted without the patient's knowledge. Tablets may also contain a binder, such as magnesium stearate or dicalcium phosphate, which may contain lead. Binders are used to help the herb absorb water and break down more readily for easy absorption by the body.

Capsules or tablets can be swallowed whole, as indicated, or they may be mixed with a spoonful of cream-style cereal or applesauce. They may also be dissolved in sweet fruit juice.

Lozenges

Herbal lozenges are nutrient-rich, naturally sweetened preparations that are dissolved in the mouth. They're available in various formulas, such as cough suppressant, decongestant, or cold-fighting. Most lozenges contain natural vitamin C. One type that has become popular is the horehound lozenge, used to relieve coughs and minor throat irritation.

Lozenges should be taken as directed by a physician or herbalist. For self-treatment, use the directions on the package.

Teas

Herbal teas, which can be made from most herbs, are used for various purposes, with formulations aimed at specific conditions or desired effects. They're generally prepared by infusion or decoction. An *infusion* is prepared by allowing a dried herb to steep in hot water for 3 to 5 minutes. A *decoction* is made by putting the herb into a rolling boil of water for 15 to 20 minutes; this method is preferable for denser plant materials, such as roots or bark. Teas may be steeped in a muslin or conventional tea bag or tea ball or used in loose form for their fragrant, aromatic flavor.

Some teas taste bitter because they contain alkaloids (for example, goldenseal root) or highly astringent tannins (for example, oak bark). Teas may be sweetened with honey if the patient is an adult or a child older than 18 months. However, honey shouldn't be used if the child is younger because of the risk of infant botulism.

> *If a nursing mother takes an adult dose of an herbal remedy, the effect will be transmitted to her child through her breast milk.*

For infants, the tea may be mixed with breast milk or formula, then put into a bottle, an eyedropper, or an empty syringe (without a needle) and gently squirted into the infant's mouth. If a nursing mother takes an adult dose of an herbal remedy, the effect will be transmitted to her child through her breast milk.

The Chinese teach that the heat of the water and the taste of the herb enhance its effectiveness. Steeping an herb in hot water draws out its therapeutic essence. When using dried herbs, 2 heaping tablespoons of the herb are generally used for every cup of tea, unless directed otherwise on the product label. The herbs should be placed in a china or glass teapot or cup (plastic or metal containers are considered unsuitable for steeping) and then immersed in 8 oz (237 ml) of freshly boiled water (for each cup) and covered.

Leaf or flower herbs are generally steeped for 5 to 10 minutes. Roots or bark are simmered or boiled for 10 minutes, then steeped for an additional 5 minutes. After steeping, the tea is strained and allowed to cool to a comfortable temperature before serving. If a tincture or extract is being placed in the tea, the cup of hot water should be allowed to sit for 5 minutes to allow the alcohol to evaporate. Teas may be served hot, cold, or iced, depending on the purpose and instructions.

When using fresh herbs, three parts of a fresh herb generally equal one part of a dry herb. Bark, root, seeds, and resins must be powdered to break down the cell walls before they're added to water. Seeds should be slightly bruised to release the volatile oils from the cells. An aromatic herb may be infused in a pot with a tight lid to decrease the loss of volatile oil through evaporation. Because roots, wood, bark, nuts, and certain seeds are tough and their cell walls strong, they should be boiled in water to release their properties.

Juices

Juices are made by washing fresh herbs under cold running water, cutting them with scissors into suitable pieces, and then running them through a juice extractor until they turn into a liquid. Juices are usually administered by placing a few drops in tea or spring water. They may also be applied externally by dabbing them on the affected part of the body. Fresh juices ideally should be taken immediately after extraction; however, they may be stored in a small glass bottle, corked tightly, and refrigerated for several days without appreciable loss of vital properties.

Vapor and inhalation treatments

Used primarily for respiratory and sinus conditions, vapor and inhalation treatments open congested sinuses and lung passages, help discharge mucus, and ease breathing. One inhalation method requires a sink and an herbal oil. The sink is filled with very hot water and 2 to 5 drops of the herbal oil are added. Hot water should be allowed to trickle into the sink to keep the water steaming. As the mixture becomes diluted, a few more drops of the herbal oil may be needed. The steam should be inhaled for 5 minutes.

Another method involves heating a large, wide pot of water, adding a handful of dried or fresh herbs, and bringing the pot to a boil. After the herbs have simmered for 5 minutes, the pot is removed from the heat and placed on a trivet to cool slightly. (If an aromatic oil is being used, the water should first be heated to just short of boiling and then removed from the heat.) With the pot on a trivet, the patient adds 4 to 5 drops of the oil, and then drapes a towel over his head to form a tent and leans over the pot, inhaling the steam for 5 minutes. *Caution:* If the vapor is too hot, it can burn the nasal passages.

Herbal baths

If the herb is in a soluble agent, such as baking soda or aloe gel, it may be dissolved in hot bath water. If the herb is an oatmeal type preparation, it may be finely milled or whirled into a powder in a blender. Fresh or dried herbs can also be bagged in a square of cheesecloth or placed in a washcloth and tied securely. The goal is maximum release of the herbal essence without having parts of the herb floating in the bath water. Full baths require about 6 oz (170 g) of dried or fresh herbs.

> 66 *Squeezing the bag of herbs in the bath water releases a rich stream of essence that may be directed to the affected body part.* 99

As the tub fills with water, the bagged herbs are placed under a forceful stream of comfortably hot water, and then dragged through the bath water to better distribute the herbal essence. Squeezing the bag releases a rich stream of essence that may be directed to the affected body part. The bag may also be gently rubbed over itching skin. *Caution:* Herbs with pointy or rough edges may be too irritating to use in this manner.

An herbal infusion can also be added to bath water. To make the infusion, 6 tablespoons (57 g) of dried or fresh herbs are soaked overnight in 3 cups (710 ml) of hot water. The next morning, the strained infusion can be poured directly into the bath water.

Poultices and compresses

A *poultice* is a moist paste made from crushed herbs that is applied directly to the affected area (or wrapped in cloth to keep it in place and then applied). Poultices are especially useful in treating bruises, wounds, and abscesses. A *compress* is made by soaking a soft cloth in a strong herbal tea, a tincture or glycerite, an oil, or aromatic water and then wringing it out and applying it to the affected area. Compresses are effective for bleeding, bruises, muscle cramps, and headaches.

Only fresh herbs should be used for poultices. One preparation method involves wrapping the herbs in a clean white cloth (such as gauze, linen, cotton, or muslin), folding the cloth several times, and then crushing the herbs to a pulp with a rolling pin. (Pulping the herb directly onto the poultice cloth helps to retain its juices and improves the effectiveness of the poultice.) Then the pulp is exposed and applied to the affected area. Wrapping the entire area with a woolen cloth or towel will trap the herbal juices and hold them in place. This type of poultice can remain in place overnight.

The herbs also may be prepared by placing them in a steamer, colander, strainer, or sieve over a pot of rapidly boiling water and allowing the steam to penetrate and wilt the herbs. After 5 minutes, the softened, warmed herbs are spread on a clean white cloth, such as loosely woven cheesecloth, and the cloth is applied to the affected area. Wrapping the poultice with a woolen cloth or towel helps retain the heat. This type of poultice can be left on for 20 minutes or overnight if the patient finds the wrap comforting and soothing.

Making a compress usually involves soaking a linen or muslin cloth in an herbal infusion, then wringing the cloth, folding it, and applying it to the affected area. The compress, which may be applied hot or cold, can be held in place by a bandage or plastic wrap.

Oils, ointments, salves, and rubs

Herbal oils are usually expressed from the peels of lemons, oranges, or other citrus fruits. Because they may be irritating to the skin, they're commonly diluted in fatty oils or water before being topically applied. Essential oils are used in massage and aromatherapy; diluted oils can be used to prevent skin irritation.

To make an oil, the fresh herbs are first washed and left to dry overnight. The herbs are then sliced (or crumbled if using dry herbs), placed in a glass bottle or jar, and covered with about 1″ [2.5 cm] of light virgin olive oil, almond oil, or sunflower oil. The container is covered tightly and allowed to stand in a very warm area, such as on a stove or in the sunshine, for 2 weeks. The oil should be strained before use.

Herbal ointments, salves, and rubs are applied topically for various conditions. Some examples are calendula ointment for broken skin and wounds; goldenseal for infections, rashes, and skin irritations; aloe vera gel for minor burns; and heat-producing herbs for muscle aches and strains. The commercial varieties are usually more appealing than homemade concoctions.

Ointments can be made in a ceramic or glass double boiler by heating 2 oz (60 ml) of vegetable lanolin or beeswax until it liquefies. When the lanolin or wax has melted, 80 to 120 drops of tincture are added and the compound is mixed together. The formula should then be poured into a glass container and refrigerated until it hardens. A strong herbal tea made from fresh or dried herbs can be used instead of a store-bought tincture.

Procedure

A visit to an herbalist begins with an evaluation that includes the patient's history. The herbalist may assess the patient's pulse and tongue to assist in diagnosis and may perform a physical assessment. Some herbalists assess the iris, a technique known as iridology, to aid in diagnosis. This procedure involves the correlation of minute markings on the iris with specific parts of the body.

Most herbalists also ask which drugs the patient is taking to avoid an interaction between the herb and any prescription or over-the-counter medications. For example, the herb St. John's wort, which is used as an antidepressant, shouldn't be taken with prescription antidepressants. What's more, the herbalist must learn which herbs the patient is already using to avoid causing a cumulative effect.

Like conventional health care practitioners, the herbalist asks whether the patient is pregnant or breast-feeding because certain herbs can induce miscarriage (abortifacient effect) or can be passed to the infant in breast milk and cause adverse reactions.

After the evaluation, the herbalist suggests individual herbs or combinations of herbs for the treatment of a particular condition. Medicinal plants may be combined to increase their therapeutic effect, alter the individual actions of each herb, or minimize or negate toxic effects of stronger herbs. As with traditional drug combinations, herbal compounds have a synergy that allows the remedy to function more effectively. The art of herbal compounding has been practiced for more than 5,000 years and is the basis of today's herbal practice.

Dosages

Dosages for herbal remedies have been established over the years, but these guidelines for quantity and frequency must be adjusted to each individual based on various factors, such as age, weight, and use of other herbs or drugs. (See *Determining herbal dosages,* page 318.)

The length of time a particular herb is used depends on whether it's used as a therapy (to relieve symptoms), a tonic (to build strength), or both. An herb that's being used therapeutically may be taken for only a brief period — typically, 1 to 4 weeks. As with other drugs, herbs should be taken at certain times of the day. Some herbs are more effective when taken in the morning; others, in the evening.

An herbal compound that's used as a tonic generally requires a longer period of use — usually 4 to 6 months or longer. For example, hawthorn berry, a cardiovascular tonic, is most effective when used for 6 to 12 consecutive months.

Some herbs work best if used with a resting cycle. For example, the patient might use an herb for 6 days followed by 1 day off, 6 weeks on and 1 week off, 6 months on and 1 month off, or some similar pattern. The theory behind a resting cycle is that each period of rest from the herb treatment allows its effect to become integrated into the patient's physiology. If the desired effect doesn't appear in the specified time, or if the patient has an adverse reaction, the dosage or herb may be changed. (See *Selected herbal therapies,* pages 319 to 341.)

Nursing perspective

Although their overall risk to public health appears to be low, some traditional herbal remedies have been associated with potentially serious adverse effects. For example, ma huang, an ingredient in numerous diet pills, contains the same active ingredient that's in the bronchodilator ephedrine and can cause irregular heartbeats, seizures, and even death.

(Text continues on page 342.)

Determining herbal dosages

Pharmacologic prescribing

Most herbal dosages are set by a method called pharmacologic prescribing, in which the amount of a botanical preparation is sufficient to induce definite, visible, strong, sustained changes in the patient. The oldest dosage method and best represented by the British herbal tradition, pharmacologic prescribing can mask symptoms if the dose is improper or used too long.

Physiologic prescribing

In physiologic prescribing, the herbalist recommends the minimum dosage of an herb required to induce a physiologic change. For example, he'd give a laxative only until a change in bowel action occurs.

Homeopathic prescribing

Homeopathic prescribing is based on the homeopathic principle of "like cures like." For example, cantharis or apis causes burning urination and kidney damage in high doses, but it's given in low doses to treat urinary tract infections and kidney disease.

Wise woman prescribing

Based on ancient wisdom, wise woman prescribing is also known as folk herbalism. Herbs are taken in large doses like foods. The herbalist avoids strong, toxic, and rare plants, choosing those that grow freely and close at hand.

Prescribing herbal extracts

The standard dosage of herbal extracts for the average adult is 6 g/day. However, this dosage is only a guideline and may be modified for patients who aren't average size.

Age and weight dosing

The age dosing guideline, useful for treating infants and younger children, is based on organ maturity — the organ's ability to metabolize, use, and eliminate herbs. The weight-to-dose guidelines are based on the principle that the herb is distributed to different parts of the body. This dosage method is useful for patients who fall outside the normal weight range, requiring either an increased or decreased dose, but it may not be reliable for very young children. It's similar to Clark's rule, which is used to verify pediatric dosages.

Selected herbal therapies

The chart below provides information on a variety of herbal remedies your patients may be taking. Included you'll find each herb's popular and Latin names, traditional and current uses, available forms, adverse effects, and precautions your patients should be aware of.

Common and scientific names	Traditional uses	Nursing considerations
Acidophilus *Lactobacillus acidophilus*	▶ Produces hydrogen peroxide and lactic acid to suppress pathogenic bacteria ▶ Used for lactose intolerance, digestive disorders, or antibiotic-induced diarrhea because it helps replace intestinal flora; also used to treat the pain of a sore mouth caused by oral candidiasis, fever blister, canker sores, hives, and acne ▶ Used intravaginally for yeast or bacterial infections, uncomplicated UTIs, and vaginosis in pregnant women in the first trimester ▶ Claimed by some to retard the growth of tumors and reduce cholesterol levels, but no data exists to support this	▶ Contraindicated if sensitive to dairy products, feverish, pregnant, or breast-feeding ▶ Contraindicated in children younger than age 3 ▶ Not to be used for longer than 2 days ▶ Flatulence common initially but decreases with continued use ▶ Refrigerated to maintain potency ▶ *Available forms:* capsules, granules, milk, powders, tablets, yogurt
Alfalfa *Medicago sativa*	▶ Used in an attempt to lower cholesterol levels and to treat asthma, hay fever, and kidney and bladder disorders, but without documented success	▶ Perennial herb; leaves and flowering tops used ▶ Reversible pancytopenia reported in a man who ingested huge amounts of alfalfa seed ▶ Latent systemic lupus erythematosus reactivated in at least two patients after ingestion of alfalfa tablets ▶ *Available forms:* tablets, capsules (containing leaves and seeds), sprouts, bulk dried leaves, teas, extracts

(continued)

Selected herbal therapies (continued)

Common and scientific names	Traditional uses	Nursing considerations
Aloe *Aloe vera* *A. barbadensis* *A. vulgaris*	▶ Used since ancient Egyptian times to treat burns, insect bites, and scrapes ▶ Promotion of wound healing as well as analgesic, anti-inflammatory, and antipruritic effects ▶ Emollient effect due to polysaccharides in gel ▶ Antibacterial and antifungal properties, although studies show conflicting results ▶ Aloe juice, or latex (obtained from cells just below epidermis of leaves), effective as potent, bitter-tasting cathartic ▶ Laxative effect stronger than senna or cascara	▶ Perennial succulent with more than 100 species; aloe gel obtained from inner part of leaves ▶ Safe and inexpensive with no adverse effects when gel used externally on minor cuts ▶ Approved internal use limited to dried latex form as a cathartic; possible GI cramping from ingestion; contraindicated in pregnancy ▶ *Available forms:* tinctures, extracts, fresh gel from whole leaves, bottled gel, dried latex, soaps, lotions
Angelica *Angelica atropurpurea* *A. archangelica*	▶ Used in folk remedies for respiratory illnesses and arthritis ▶ In Chinese herbal medicine, prepared as a tea to treat menstrual irregularity and premenstrual syndrome (*Oriental Materia Medica* states that volatile oils relax uterine muscle, while non-volatile, water-soluble compounds stimulate uterine muscle.) ▶ Volatile oil used as flavoring (particularly of alcoholic beverages such as Benedictine, Chartreuse, and gin) and scent	▶ Perennial or biennial herb; roots, leaves, and seeds used ▶ Similar in appearance to extremely poisonous water hemlock ▶ Contact dermatitis possible in fair-skinned people with topical use ▶ Severe poisoning reported from high doses ▶ Carcinogenic and mutagenic effects in laboratory animals ▶ *Available forms:* capsules, tablets, extracts (alcoholic and nonalcoholic)

Selected herbal therapies (continued)

Common and scientific names	Traditional uses	Nursing considerations
Anise *Pimpinella anisum*	▶ Cultivated since ancient times in Egypt for use as spice and fragrance ▶ Used historically to freshen breath, help breathing, relieve pain, and promote diuresis ▶ Applied externally as insect repellent and treatment for lice and scabies ▶ Used as carminative (digestive aid); antispasmodic action in higher doses ▶ Antiseptic expectorant for cough, asthma, and bronchitis ▶ Promotes iron absorption	▶ Annual herb; seeds used ▶ Occasional allergic reactions of skin, respiratory tract, and GI tract; pulmonary edema; vomiting; and seizures ▶ May interfere with contraceptives due to estrogenic activity ▶ May interfere with anticoagulants and monoamine oxidase inhibitors ▶ Not recommended for use during pregnancy because of reputed abortifacient effect ▶ *Available forms:* anise oil, seeds
Arnica *Arnica montana* *A. fulgens* *A. sororia* *A. latifolia* *A. cordifolia*	▶ Used for 400 years in Europe and America for various conditions ▶ Applied topically to reduce inflammation and pain from sprains and bruises ▶ Anti-inflammatory, analgesic, and weak antibiotic activity from active ingredients	▶ Perennial herb; all parts of plant used originally; currently, just flower heads used ▶ Cardiotoxic and hypertensive effects when taken internally ▶ Contact dermatitis possible in allergic individuals ▶ *Available forms:* tablets, gels, ointments
Basil *Ocimum basilicum*	▶ Used as an antiseptic, antimicrobial, diuretic, insect repellant, antihypertensive, digestion stimulant, and appetite stimulant ▶ Also used to treat halitosis and to cure warts	▶ Not for use in pregnant or breast-feeding women or in young children ▶ No adverse reactions reported ▶ May cause cancer in large quantities; apparently safe in amounts used in cooking ▶ *Available forms:* oil, spice

(continued)

Selected herbal therapies (continued)

Common and scientific names	Traditional uses	Nursing considerations
Boneset *Eupatorium perfoliatum*	▶ Used by Native Americans as antipyretic ▶ Reputed diuretic and laxative in small doses; emetic and cathartic in large doses ▶ Contains alkaloids known to cause liver damage after long-term use	▶ Hardy perennial herb; leaves and flowering tops used to make tea ▶ Few adverse effects reported, but long-term use discouraged ▶ *Available forms:* extract, dried leaves and flowering tops
Burdock *Arctium lappa A. minus*	▶ Traditionally used in teas to treat many illnesses, including colds, gout, arthritis, stomach ailments, and cancers; also used as a diuretic, diaphoretic, laxative, and aphrodisiac ▶ Root edible, with mild diuretic, diaphoretic, antipyretic, and antimicrobial action ▶ Used in shampoos to treat dandruff and in other skin care products	▶ Perennial or biennial herb; dried or fresh root and young leaves used ▶ Contact dermatitis possible ▶ Atropine poisoning reported when burdock root inadvertently contaminated with root of deadly nightshade, which has a similar appearance ▶ *Available forms:* liquid extract, fresh or bulk dried root
Calendula Marigold *Calendula officinalis*	▶ Long history of use; taken internally for spasms, fevers, suppressed menstruation, and cancer; used externally to heal and prevent infection of wounds ▶ Currently used topically to heal skin irritations and wounds	▶ Annual herb; flower used ▶ Nontoxic ▶ *Available forms:* extract, gel, ointment
Cascara sagrada *Ramnus purshian*	▶ Traditionally and currently used as cathartic (laxative) ▶ Active ingredient mostly absorbed from small intestine and then secreted into large intestine, where it produces irritation in about 8 hours	▶ Tree; bark aged for at least 1 year used ▶ Mild intestinal cramping possible ▶ Contraindicated during pregnancy and breast-feeding ▶ *Available forms:* extract, tablets, bulk dried bark

Selected herbal therapies *(continued)*

Common and scientific names	Traditional uses	Nursing considerations
Cayenne *Capsicum frutescens*	▶ Active ingredient capsaicin said to improve digestion by acting as GI stimulant ▶ Capsaicin ointment applied locally to reduce chronic pain due to various neuropathies, including diabetic neuropathy ▶ Rubefacient effect (reddening of skin) when applied externally; possible anti-inflammatory activity ▶ Good source of vitamin C	▶ Numerous varieties and hybrids developed; fruit used ▶ Considerable pain resulting from contact with eyes ▶ Difficult to wash off because not very soluble in water; may be removed with vinegar (except in eyes) ▶ *Available forms:* capsaicin ointment, bulk ground powder, tablets, extracts
Chamomile *Matricaria chamomilla* (German) *Anthemis nobilis* (Roman or English)	▶ Used externally in compresses as anti-inflammatory and anti-infective for various conditions of skin and mucous membranes ▶ Historically ingested as carminative, antispasmodic for GI and menstrual cramping and flatulence, and anthelmintic ▶ Anti-inflammatory and antispasmodic effects from bisabolol, the pharmacologically active chemical extracted from the essential oil ▶ Acts as a mild sedative in hot tea ▶ Also used as food flavoring, and as scent in perfumes and shampoos	▶ German chamomile, an annual, used most in United States and Europe (also most investigated); Roman chamomile a slow-growing perennial; flower heads used ▶ Allergic reactions and vomiting rare; should be used cautiously in people allergic to ragweed pollen, asters, or chrysanthemums because of reported hypersensitivity reactions ▶ Vomiting reported when dried flowers taken in large quantities ▶ *Available forms:* bulk dried flower heads, capsules, tablets, tea
Chicory *Cichorium intybus*	▶ Root used in Egyptian folk medicine to treat tachycardia ▶ Traditionally used as mild tonic with some diuretic and laxative effects ▶ Believed to have mild sedative effect that counteracts stimulant properties in coffee and tea	▶ Perennial herb; leaves used as cooked greens; roots boiled and eaten or roasted, ground, and used as additive or replacement for coffee and tea ▶ Occasional contact dermatitis

(continued)

Selected herbal therapies *(continued)*

Common and scientific names	Traditional uses	Nursing considerations
Chicory *(continued)*	▶ Possible anti-inflammatory activity from alcoholic extracts of root	▶ Considered safer than caffeine-containing beverages ▶ *Available forms:* roots, leaves, oil
Cinnamon *Cinnamomum cassia*	▶ Historically and currently used mainly as cooking spice; also used historically as digestive aid ▶ Possible antifungal and antibacterial effects	▶ Tree; bark used ▶ Contact dermatitis and stimulation of vasomotor system, causing tachycardia, increased peristalsis, tachypnea, and diaphoresis (from exposure to large amounts of cinnamon) ▶ *Available forms:* whole or ground bark
Cloves *Syzgium aromaticum*	▶ Oil traditionally used as mild anesthetic, especially for teething pain and toothaches; also used as stimulant and carminative ▶ Some anti-inflammatory and antifungal activity demonstrated ▶ Used as cooking spice	▶ Tree; dried flower bud used ▶ No adverse effects noted ▶ *Available forms:* oil of cloves, bulk dried flower buds, bulk ground powder
Comfrey *Symphytum officinale* *S. asperum*	▶ Despite reported risks, one of the most widely used herbs in the United States: as poultice to heal wounds; as tea or extract to treat gastric ulcers and respiratory ailments ▶ Promotes cell proliferation when used externally in poultices ▶ Anti-inflammatory activity reported ▶ Historically used as green vegetable in Japan	▶ Perennial herb; roots and leaves used ▶ Hepatotoxic and carcinogenic effects from alkaloids in all parts of plant (United Kingdom research association states, "No human being or animal should eat, drink, or take comfrey in any form.") ▶ *Available forms:* bulk dried root, extract

Selected herbal therapies *(continued)*

Common and scientific names	Traditional uses	Nursing considerations
Coriander *Coriandrum sativum,* *Chinese parsley*	▶ Stimulates gastric acid secretion and has spasmolytic properties. May have hypoglycemic, hypolipedemic, and antiseptic effects ▶ Used to enhance appetite, treat dyspepsia, flatulence, diarrhea, colic, coughs, chest pains, fever, bladder ailments, halitosis, postpartum complications, measles, dysentery, hemorrhoids, and toothaches ▶ Oil used in aromatherapy for soothing effect and to improve blood circulation ▶ Also used as a flavoring agent and fragrance	▶ Severe allergy symptoms, including breathing difficulty, airway tightness, and urticaria ▶ Sunscreen advised and avoiding exposure to direct sunlight ▶ Other possible complications: melena, hematemesis, and significant weight loss ▶ Available forms: capsules, seed, oil, powder and tea; also in natural deodorant products and curry powder
Cranberry *Vaccinium* *macrocarpon*	▶ Useful in combating urinary tract infections	▶ Shrubby perennial; berry used ▶ No adverse effects reported ▶ *Available forms:* juice, capsules
Dandelion *Taraxacum officinale* *Leontodon* *taraxacum*	▶ Bitter-tasting leaves used raw in salads, cooked as greens, or made into wine; roasted root used to make nonstimulant, coffeelike beverage ▶ Used for liver ailments and as antidiabetic agent, laxative, diuretic, and appetite stimulant ▶ Little proven therapeutic benefit, but greens are good source of vitamin A	▶ Perennial herb; leaves and root used ▶ Contact dermatitis in susceptible individuals ▶ *Available forms:* bulk dried leaves, bulk plain dried root, bulk roasted root, extracts, capsules, teas

(continued)

Selected herbal therapies (continued)

Common and scientific names	Traditional uses	Nursing considerations
Echinacea *Echinacea angustifolia* *E. pallida* *E. purpurea*	▷ Used historically by Native Americans to treat wounds, fever, scarlet fever, ulcers, and spider, snake, and insect bites ▷ Used today for its antiviral, antitumor, immunostimulant, and wound healing properties and to treat colds and sore throats ▷ Shown to increase breast milk production ▷ Popular herbal remedy in the central United States, where plant is indigenous	▷ Perennial herb; leaves, stem, and flowers used ▷ Acrid taste, tingling of lips and tongue from chewing plant ▷ *Available forms:* most readily available in U.S. as liquid and powder; capsules (relatively inactive), ointment (topical), extract, tincture (alcoholic and nonalcoholic bases), bulk dried flowers, tablets, tea
Elder Elderberry *Sambucus canadensis* *S. nigra*	▷ Roots and inner bark used in folk medicine to treat cancers and headaches and to induce labor ▷ Flowers and berries traditionally used as diuretic and laxative; strong purgative effect from juice ▷ Jams, jellies, and wine made from berries; extracts used as flavorings	▷ Tall shrub; flowers and berries used ▷ Use of leaves, which contain a cyanogenic glucoside, not recommended ▷ *Available forms:* berry extract
Ergot *Claviceps purpurea*	▷ Historically used by midwives to stimulate uterine contractions during labor and to prevent postpartum hemorrhage; action due to ergot alkaloid which contracts uterus and constricts endometrial blood vessels ▷ Used to treat migraines because its second major alkaloid, ergotamine, mainly constricts blood vessels of brain	▷ Fungus found in rye and rye flour ▷ Nausea, vomiting, cramps, diarrhea, drowsiness, dizziness, headache, and confusion (signs and symptoms of toxicity) ▷ Lysergic acid-like base contained in ergot alkaloids ▷ *Available forms:* commercial drugs given under physician supervision

Selected herbal therapies *(continued)*

Common and scientific names	Traditional uses	Nursing considerations
Eucalyptus *Eucalyptus globulus*	▸ Used to treat bronchitis and asthma due to its expectorant effects ▸ Essential oil and eucalyptol forms shown to dilate bronchial tubes ▸ Applied topically as antiseptic and analgesic ▸ Volatile oil from leaves used as germicide ▸ Topical combination of eucalyptus and peppermint shows promise as analgesic	▸ Tree; leaves used ▸ No adverse effects noted ▸ Oil applied topically or combined with water, boiled, and inhaled; leaves steeped and drunk as tea ▸ *Available forms:* tea, essential oil, bulk dried leaves
Fennel *Foeniculum vulgare*	▸ Volatile oil shown to have spasmolytic effect ▸ Seeds traditionally used to aid digestion, to loosen phlegm, and as flavoring and fragrance ▸ Stalks eaten as vegetable	▸ Perennial herb; stalks and dried seeds used ▸ Rare allergic response from seeds; skin irritation, vomiting, seizures, and pulmonary edema from oil (even small quantities) ▸ *Available forms:* seeds, volatile oil, capsules, tea
Feverfew *Tanacetum parthenium*	▸ Anti-inflammatory used to treat fever, migraines, menstrual irregularities, and stomachache ▸ Spasmolytic that renders the smooth walls of cerebral blood vessels less reactive to substances thought to be related to headaches such as serotonin	▸ Perennial herb; leaves used ▸ Contraindicated in people with ragweed allergy and during pregnancy ▸ Fresh leaves chewed or steeped as tea ▸ Must be taken daily for extended period ▸ *Available forms:* tablets, capsules, tea, tincture (alcoholic and nonalcoholic), bulk dried leaves, extract

(continued)

Selected herbal therapies *(continued)*

Common and scientific names	Traditional uses	Nursing considerations
Flax *Linum usitatissimum*	▶ Linseed oil from seeds used topically as demulcent and emollient and internally as laxative ▶ Diets high in flax seed effective in lowering low-density lipoprotein (LDL) and total cholesterol levels in hypercholesterolemia	▶ Annual plant; seeds and leaves used ▶ No known adverse effects
Foxglove *Digitalis purpurea*	▶ Used since Middle Ages to treat dropsy (edema caused by poorly functioning heart) ▶ Contains cardiac glycosides digitoxin and lanatoside, used today to treat heart failure and electrophysiologic cardiac abnormalities	▶ Hardy biennial; leaves used ▶ Nausea and vomiting possible ▶ All parts of plant considered poisonous because of potency of digoxin preparations ▶ *Available forms:* tablets, available by prescription only
Garlic *Allium sativum*	▶ Traditionally used since ancient times as a food, a magic substance to ward off evil spirits, and a cure for just about everything ▶ Many beneficial effects proven, such as antioxidant and antihypertensive activity; ability to lower serum cholesterol, triglyceride, and LDL levels and to increase high-density lipoprotein levels; and ability to decrease platelet aggregation; requires 5 to 10 cloves of fresh garlic per day to achieve effects	▶ Perennial bulb; bulb used ▶ Heartburn, flatulence, and other symptoms of indigestion from large quantities ▶ *Available forms:* fresh bulbs, bulk powder and granules, oils

Selected herbal therapies *(continued)*

Common and scientific names	Traditional uses	Nursing considerations
Ginger *Zingiber officinale* *Z. capitatum* *Z. zerumbet*	▶ Widely used in Asian medicine as carminative, diuretic, antiemetic, anti-inflammatory, stimulant, and as a condiment and flavoring in Asian cuisines ▶ Volatile oil shown to have cardiotonic (inotropic), antipyretic, analgesic, antitussive, carminative, prostaglandin-inhibiting, antibacterial, and antineoplastic activity in animal studies ▶ Effective as antiemetic in hyperemesis gravidarum and motion sickness	▶ Perennial; root and rhizome used ▶ No reports of severe toxicity ▶ *Available forms:* capsules containing powdered herb, tea made from rhizome, candied ginger, bulk powdered root
Ginkgo *Ginkgo biloba*	▶ Extract from leaves associated with dilation of arteries, capillaries, and veins ▶ Used to treat symptoms of Raynaud's disease, impotence, and memory loss ▶ May prevent kidney and liver damage caused by use of immunosuppressant drug cyclosporine	▶ World's oldest living tree species; leaves used ▶ GI upset or headache possible; after contact with whole plant, pulp, or seeds, severe allergic reaction (similar to that of poison ivy) possible, with symptoms ranging from erythema and pruritus to severe rectal sphincter spasm ▶ May reduce clotting time; caution advised for concomitant use with anticoagulants ▶ *Available forms:* tea (caffeinated and decaffeinated), tablets, capsules, tincture (alcoholic and nonalcoholic), bulk dried leaves, extract

(continued)

Selected herbal therapies *(continued)*

Common and scientific names	Traditional uses	Nursing considerations
Ginseng, American *Panax quinquefolius*	▶ Root used in past to treat atherosclerosis, blood and bleeding disorders, and colitis; also used as aphrodisiac ▶ Used today for adaptogenic effects (helping body adapt to stress and improving endurance and performance)	▶ Roots and leaves used ▶ Diarrhea, skin eruptions, nervousness, sleeplessness, and hypertension common ▶ *Available forms:* tea (caffeinated and decaffeinated), capsules, tincture (alcoholic and nonalcoholic), tablets, bulk dried root, extracts
Green tea *Camellia sinensis*	▶ Used to increase immunity and longevity ▶ Found to have antioxidant effects ▶ Associated with reduced incidence of pancreatic, stomach, and other cancers ▶ With heavy consumption, may reduce total cholesterol levels and delay atherosclerosis	▶ Evergreen shrub; leaves used ▶ Contraindicated in women who are pregnant or may become pregnant because caffeine content shown to have teratogenic effects in animal studies ▶ May stain teeth ▶ *Available forms:* tea (caffeinated and decaffeinated), capsules
Holly *Ilex aquifolium* *I. opaca* *I. vomitoria*	▶ Yaupon tea made from *I. vomitoria* leaves used as emetic ▶ Fruit tea used by Chinese to treat coronary disease	▶ Evergreen tree and shrub with more than 400 species; leaves and berries used ▶ Possible vomiting, diarrhea, and stupor if berries eaten in large quantities (20 to 30 may be lethal for a child) ▶ *Available forms:* traditional flower remedies, bulk dried leaves

Selected herbal therapies *(continued)*

Common and scientific names	Traditional uses	Nursing considerations
Lavender *Lavendula anguistifolia* *L. officianalis* *L. spica* *L. stoechas* *L. dentata* *L. latifolia* *L. pubescens*	▶ Used internally in folk medicine as antispasmodic, carminative, diuretic, and tonic ▶ Used externally to treat acne, migraines, and joint pain ▶ Included in commercial herbal antidiabetic mixtures ▶ Oil found effective in aromatherapy for insomnia; also used to increase mental activity, diminish fatigue, improve mood, and lessen anxiety ▶ Used as food flavoring	▶ Shrubby evergreen perennial; fresh flowering tops used ▶ Contact dermatitis in susceptible individuals ▶ *Available forms:* liquid extract, infusion, decoction, oil, bulk dried flowers
Licorice *Glycyrrhiza glabra* *G. uralensis* *G. palidiflora*	▶ Used by ancient Greeks as expectorant and carminative ▶ In Chinese herbal medicine, used as antiarrhythmic ▶ In the West, used mostly as flavoring agent in medicines, candies, and tobacco; as expectorant; and in shampoos to suppress sebum secretion ▶ Glycoside found in root	▶ Shrubby hardy perennial; roots used ▶ Toxic effects from overdose, including lethargy, flaccid weakness, dulled reflexes, sodium and fluid retention, hypertension, and one case of quadriplegia ▶ *Available forms:* liquid extract, bulk dried root, tea
Melatonin *MEL*	▶ A hormone stimulated by darkness and inhibited by light; may regulate circadian rhythms, body temperature, CV function, and reproduction ▶ Used to treat insomnia, jet lag, shift-work disorder, blind entrainment, immune system enhancement, tinnitus, depression, benzodiazepine withdrawal in geriatric patients with insomnia, cachexia, and chemotherapy-induced thrombocytopenia	▶ May cause excessive drowsiness; avoiding hazardous activities and avoiding taking with CNS depressants or alcohol advised ▶ May also cause abdominal cramps ▶ Contraindicated in those who are using immunosuppressants, have an autoimmune disease, such as multiple sclerosis, or are pregnant or breast-feeding

(continued)

Selected herbal therapies *(continued)*

Common and scientific names	Traditional uses	Nursing considerations
Melatonin *(continued)*	▶ Also used as a cancer therapy adjuvant, antiaging product, and prophylactic therapy for cluster headaches ▶ Used topically for skin protection against UV light	▶ Contraindicated in children ▶ May interfere with the therapeutic effect of many conventional drugs, such as beta-adrenergic blockers, CNS depressants, fluoxetine, and verapamil; shouldn't be taken together ▶ May increase human growth hormone levels ▶ *Available forms:* tablets, lozenges, spray
Mistletoe *Phoradendron seroninum,* *Viscum album*	*American Mistltoe:* ▶ Can cause hypertension, hypotension, and bradycardia, increased uterine and intestinal motility, depolarization of skeletal muscle, smooth muscle contraction, vasoconstriction, and cardiac arrest ▶ Used as a smooth-muscle stimulant for increasing blood pressure and uterine and intestinal contractions *European mistletoe:* ▶ May possess anticancer and immunostimulation activity ▶ Effects include hypotension, bradycardia, and sedation ▶ Used to treat hypertension, cancer, internal bleeding, major blood loss, blood purification, arteriosclerosis, epilepsy, gout, and hysteria	▶ Marketing of mistletoe and products that contain it forbidden by the FDA; use should be avoided, as safety is unproven ▶ Toxicity signs and symptoms: nausea, bradycardia, gastroenteritis, hypertension, delirium, hallucinations, and diarrhea and vomiting which can lead to serious dehydration, hypovolemic shock, and CV collapse. Rapid gastric emptying suggested if berries are ingested ▶ *Available forms:* Dried leaves, stems, flowers, fruit extract; injectable form unavailable in the United States

Selected herbal therapies (continued)

Common and scientific names	Traditional uses	Nursing considerations
Papaya *Carica papaya*	▎ Latex from unripened fruit's milky sap (called crude papain or vegetable pepsin) used as carminative, anthelmintic, and meat tenderizer ▎ Derivative of papain experimentally used by neurosurgeons to dissolve herniated intervertebral disks	▎ Small tropical tree; leaves and sap used ▎ May cause allergic reaction in susceptible people ▎ *Available forms:* tablets, bulk dried leaves
Parsley *Petroselinum crispum*	▎ Seeds used as carminative, roots as diuretic, and oil as emmenagogue ▎ Uterine stimulation and abortion caused by active ingredients in the oil ▎ Antipyretic effects ▎ Popular cooking herb; good source of vitamins A and C, iron, and calcium	▎ Biennial herb; leaves, roots, and seeds used ▎ Headache, dizziness, seizures, renal damage, and allergic reactions (from oil) ▎ Oil, juice, and seeds contraindicated during pregnancy ▎ *Available forms:* bulk dried leaves, extract
Passion flower *Passiflora incarnata*	▎ Extract long used as sedative and sleep aid ▎ Edible fruit used commercially to produce juice	▎ Woody vine; roots, stems, leaves, flowers, and fruit used ▎ CNS depression possible from large doses of extract ▎ *Available forms:* extract, bulk dried flowers, capsules
Pau d'Arco *Tabebuia impetiginosa*	▎ Tea used to treat cancer, ulcers, diabetes, rheumatism, and other ills ▎ Falsely touted as a cure for acquired immunodeficiency syndrome ▎ Despite demonstrated antineoplastic activity in humans, not useful because of severe adverse effects at effective plasma levels	▎ Evergreen tree; inner bark used ▎ Nausea, vomiting, anemia, and bleeding tendency possible ▎ *Available forms:* dietary supplement, bulk dried bark, extract (alcoholic and nonalcoholic), tea (marketed as ipe roxo, lapacho colorado, lapacho morado, and taheebo tea)

(continued)

Selected herbal therapies *(continued)*

Common and scientific names	Traditional uses	Nursing considerations
Pepper (black) *piper nigrum*	▶ Stimulates thermal receptors and increases secretion of saliva and gastric mucus; may have diaphoretic, insecticidal, and antimicrobial effects ▶ Used to treat constipation, gonorrhea, dyspepsia, colic, cholera, diarrhea, scarlatina, bronchitis, flatulence, nausea, vertigo, and arthritic conditions ▶ Used externally to treat neuralgia and scabies ▶ Also used as a spice	▶ Obtained from berries of Piper nigrum; green fruit sun-dried or roasted after shell is removed ▶ May cause eye irritation if inhaled or allowed in the eyes. May also cause tremors, numbness, nausea, gastric pain, skin irritation, sweating, mucus membrane irritation, and salivation. ▶ Contraindicated in those who are pregnant or hyper-sensitive to black pepper ▶ *Available forms:* dried berries, powder, ointment
Peppermint *Mentha x piperita*	▶ Used in traditional medicine worldwide as aromatic, antispasmodic, and antiseptic ▶ Oil used as spasmolytic for indigestion and irritable bowel; also used as digestive aid ▶ Menthol, primary component of volatile oil, widely used as flavoring in commercial cough and cold preparations to mask unpleasant taste	▶ Perennial herb in mint family; leaves and flowering tops used ▶ Contact dermatitis, flushing, and headache possible ▶ Often confused with spearmint, which doesn't contain menthol ▶ Contraindicated for infants and very young children ▶ *Available forms:* tea, peppermint oil, bulk dry leaves
Rose hip *Rosa canina*	▶ Used to treat diarrhea, colds and flu, vitamin C deficiency, gastric spasms and inflammation, edema, gout, arthritis, sciatica, diabetes, metabolic disorders of uric acid metabolism, lower urinary tract and gallbladder ailments, gallstones, kidney stones, and inadequate peripheral circulation	▶ Caution urged for those with asthma, who should stop use immediately and seek medical advice if wheezing or shortness of breath occurs ▶ Taken with vitamin C 2 hours before or 4 hours after taking antacids

Selected herbal therapies *(continued)*

Common and scientific names	Traditional uses	Nursing considerations
Rose hip *(continued)*	▶ Also used as a diuretic, laxative, astringent, and booster of immune function during exhaustion ▶ Used recently to treat osteogenesis imperfecta in children	▶ Pregnant, breast-feeding, or asthmatic patients restricted to amounts found in foods ▶ Possible adverse reactions, including insomnia, headache, fatigue, flushing, nausea, vomiting, abdominal cramps, esophagitis, gastroesophageal reflux, diarrhea, kidney stones, severe respiratory allergies, itching, prickly sensations, and anaphylaxis ▶ Interacts with the following drugs: aluminum-containing antacids, aspirin, barbiturates, estrogens, oral contraceptives, tetracyclines, iron, warfarin, milk or cream, and Echinacea ▶ *Available forms:* capsules, tablets, powder, tea
Rue *Ruta graveolens* *R. montana* *R. bracteosa*	▶ Used in folk medicine as antispasmodic, sedative, and emmenagogue ▶ Extracts shown to have antispasmodic effects on smooth muscle ▶ Large doses of extract used as abortifacient ▶ Commonly used as insect repellent	▶ Shrubby perennial with unpleasant odor and bitter taste; leaves, volatile oil, and extract used ▶ Redness, swelling, and blistering possible from skin contact with fresh leaves ▶ Photosensitivity resulting in severe sunburn from external or internal use ▶ Violent gastric pain, vomiting, and death possible from abortifacient doses ▶ *Available forms:* no commercial preparations currently available

(continued)

Selected herbal therapies *(continued)*

Common and scientific names	Traditional uses	Nursing considerations
Saffron *Crocus sativus, nagakeshara*	▶ Used to stimulate digestion and to treat amenorrhea, atherosclerosis, bronchitis, sore throat, headache, vomiting, and fever ▶ Also used as an abortifacient and a sedative	▶ Contraindicated in pregnant or breast-feeding women except as a food ingredient ▶ Possible adverse reactions with overdose (doses greater than 5 g): central paralysis, dizziness, stupor, vomiting, intestinal colic, bloody diarrhea, and hemorrhaging of skin on the nose, lips, and eyelids; may be lethal at doses above 12g; treated with gastric lavage and use of activated charcoal ▶ *Available forms:* dried stigmas or styles, powder
Sage *Saliva officinalis*	▶ Traditionally used as carminative, tonic, antispasmodic, antiseptic, astringent, and mouthwash and gargle for oral inflammations; to dry up the milk of nursing mothers; and to treat dysmenorrhea, diarrhea, gastritis, sore throat, and excessive sweating ▶ Estrogenic and hypoglycemic effects shown ▶ Antispasmodic and antisecretory effects demonstrated in lab animals ▶ Used as cooking herb and as a fragrance in soaps and perfumes	▶ Small shrubby perennial; leaves and flowering tops used ▶ Stomatitis and dry mouth with local irritation possible ▶ Conflicting reports on safety of sage because of presence of thujone, the poisonous ingredient in wormwood ▶ *Available forms:* bulk dried leaves, extract

Selected herbal therapies *(continued)*

Common and scientific names	Traditional uses	Nursing considerations
Sassafras *Sassafras albidum*	▶ Used by Native Americans and modern herbalists as a spring tonic, stimulant, antispasmodic, and diaphoretic ▶ Used externally to treat insect bites, rheumatism, gout, sprains, swelling, and skin eruptions ▶ Used to flavor toothpaste, root beer, and tobacco	▶ Tree; root bark used ▶ Vomiting, stupor, hallucinations, diaphoresis, dermatitis, and abortion possible from small amounts of oil ▶ Carcinogenic in rats and mice; banned for use as drug or food product by FDA ▶ *Available forms:* bulk dried root, extract
Saw palmetto *Serenoa repens* *S. serrulata*	▶ Traditionally used to manage prostate problems, increase sperm production and sexual vigor, increase breast size, and promote diuresis ▶ May be useful in managing benign prostatic hyperplasia because of confirmed estrogenic and antiprogesterone effects	▶ Fan palm; berries used ▶ Headache and diarrhea after ingesting large amounts (rare) ▶ Contraindicated during pregnancy because of potential hormonal effects ▶ *Available forms:* bulk dried berries, capsules, tablets, extract (alcoholic and nonalcoholic)
Senna *Cassis senna* *C. autifolia* *C. alexandrina*	▶ Active glycosides used as potent cathartics in many laxatives ▶ Concentrate obtained from pod said to cause less abdominal pain than other forms	▶ Perennial shrubs; dried leaflets used ▶ Diarrhea, nausea, and cramping possible ▶ *Available forms:* tea, syrup, Senokot tablets, bulk dried leaves, capsules, fluidextract
Soy *Glycine max, soya*	▶ Antioxidant and phytoestrogenic properties to the isoflavones in soy; may reduce the risk of hormone-dependent cancers, such as breast and prostate cancers	▶ Products containing soy contraindicated in those with soy hypersensitivity ▶ Not for use with estrogen, raloxifene, and tamoxifen due to possible decreased effects; or with calcium, iron, or zinc due to possible decreased absorption (should be taken several hours apart)

(continued)

Selected herbal therapies *(continued)*

Common and scientific names	Traditional uses	Nursing considerations
Soy *(continued)*	▶ Significant decrease in total cholesterol, HDL, and LDL levels from soy-based diet; claim officially supported by the FDA ▶ Used to treat cancers, CV disease, menopausal symptoms, and osteoporosis ▶ Also used as a detoxicant, circulatory stimulant, and protein supplement	▶ May cause asthma, allergic reaction, or occasional GI effects ▶ *Available forms:* soy protein or isoflavone supplements in powder, capsules, or tablets, beans, flour, many food items
Spearmint *Mentha spicata*	▶ Used historically to treat indigestion, nausea, and excessive gas; used today to flavor medicines, foods, and beverages ▶ Less effective than peppermint as a carminative	▶ Hardy perennial in mint family; leaves and flowering tops used ▶ No adverse effects noted ▶ *Available forms:* bulk dried leaves
St. John's wort *Hypericum perforatum*	▶ Used as anti-inflammatory, diuretic and, recently, to treat anxiety and depression ▶ Plant pigment, hypericin, shown to be a powerful MAO inhibitor with antiviral activity; now being investigated as treatment for HIV infection	▶ Tops, flowers used ▶ Commonly causes photosensitivity resulting in rash; exposure precautions needed for fair-skinned people to avoid dermatitis, severe burning and, possibly, blisters ▶ Contraindicated during pregnancy because of uterotonic effects in animals ▶ Concomitant use with prescribed antidepressants not recommended ▶ *Available forms:* teas, tablets, capsules, tincture (alcoholic and nonalcoholic), oil extract for topical use, bulk dried leaves

Selected herbal therapies *(continued)*

Common and scientific names	Traditional uses	Nursing considerations
Valerian *Valeriana officinalis*	▶ Used as sedative for centuries ▶ Mild sedative properties confirmed in humans	▶ Herbaceous perennial; fresh or dried rhizome used ▶ Can increase morning drowsiness ▶ Potential for additive effects with CNS depressants ▶ Headache, excitability, uneasiness, and cardiac disturbances possible ▶ *Available forms:* tea, tincture, extract, bulk dried root
White willow *Salix alba*	▶ Used since ancient times to treat pain, fever, and inflammation ▶ Ingredient, salicin, converted in body to salicylic acid (used in aspirin) ▶ Especially useful in treating arthritis	▶ Deciduous tree; bark used ▶ Tinnitus, nausea, and vomiting possible ▶ *Available forms:* dry bark, liquid extract
Wintergreen *Gaultheria procumbens*	▶ Tea used to treat cold symptoms, relieve pain, and aid digestion ▶ Used as topical analgesic, astringent, and rubefacient ▶ Widely used today as topical ointment for muscular and rheumatic pain and as flavoring agent ▶ Topical analgesic effects from methyl salicylate, major ingredient	▶ Perennial shrub; oil distilled from leaves ▶ Vomiting and death possible from large doses taken internally ▶ Salicylate poisoning (tinnitus, nausea, and vomiting) possible even when used externally ▶ *Available forms:* ointments, oil

(continued)

Selected herbal therapies *(continued)*

Common and scientific names	Traditional uses	Nursing considerations
Witch hazel *Hamamelis virginiana*	▶ Traditionally used topically to treat skin itching and inflammation, eye inflammation, and hemorrhoids; also taken internally for hemorrhaging ▶ Currently used topically for astringent properties: to soothe hemorrhoids, shrink varicose veins, treat bruises and sprains and, as a gargle, to relieve oral inflammations ▶ Some hemostatic effects	▶ Deciduous bush or small tree; bark, dried leaves, and twigs used ▶ Few adverse effects ▶ Internal use not recommended ▶ *Available forms:* crude leaf and bark, fluidextract, witch hazel water
Yerba maté *Ilex paraguariensis,* Bartholomew's tea	▶ Used as a CNS stimulant for drowsiness or fatigue and as a mild analgesic for headaches caused by fatigue ▶ Also used as a diuretic and appetite suppressant ▶ Claims not validated scientifically	▶ Several methylxanthines contained in leaves, chiefly caffeine (0.2% to 2.0%) and theophylline; overstimulation possible when herb is combined with other caffeine-containing products or with grapefruit juice, which interacts with caffeine metabolism and can increase caffeine levels ▶ Contraindicated in those with cardiovascular disease, such as hypertension, or ischemic heart disease, or chronic liver disease, and in pregnant or breast-feeding women ▶ To avoid additive effect, shouldn't be taken with other CNS stimulants or diuretics; can cause sleeplessness, restlessness, irritability, and anxiety ▶ Liver toxicity and bladder and esophageal cancer possible

Selected herbal therapies (continued)

Common and scientific names	Traditional uses	Nursing considerations
Yerba maté *(continued)*		▶ Among withdrawal symptoms: headache and sleep disturbances ▶ *Available forms:* dried leaves, liquid extract
Yohimbe *Pausinystalia yohimba*	▶ Traditionally used to treat angina and hypertension and smoked for hallucinogenic effects ▶ Principle alkaloid, yohimbine (purified from bark), used as aphrodisiac in traditional and modern medicine ▶ Yohimbine an alpha-adrenergic blocker, which works by dilating blood vessels, and an MAO inhibitor	▶ West African tree; bark used ▶ Severe hypotension, abdominal distress, and weakness when taken in high doses ▶ Contraindicated in people with diabetes or kidney or liver disease ▶ May activate psychoses in schizophrenic patients ▶ Contraindicated for use with other MAO inhibitors or with tyramine-containing foods, such as liver, cheese, and red wine ▶ *Available forms:* available in the United States by prescription only
Yucca Spanish-bayonet *Yucca aloifolia* Our-Lord's-candle *Y. whipplei* Mohave yucca *Y. schidigera* Joshua tree *Y. brevifolia* Soapweed *Y. glauca*	▶ Used to treat arthritis, hypertension, and elevated cholesterol levels ▶ Currently used commercially as foaming agent for carbonated beverages, flavorings, and in drug synthesis research ▶ Roots used to make soap and shampoos	▶ Tree with about 40 species; leaves and roots used ▶ Relatively nontoxic, even orally ▶ *Available forms:* extract

▶ If your patient is taking an herbal remedy—or considering taking one—make sure he understands the potential risks involved in self-treatment. These include misdiagnosing his ailment, taking the wrong herb, worsening his condition by delaying conventional treatment, having the herbal drug counteract or interact with prescribed medical treatment, and aggravating other disorders.

▶ Make sure your patient is aware of the actions and adverse effects of the herb he'll be taking *before* he begins taking it. Possible signs of sensitivity or an adverse reaction include headache, upset stomach, and rash. In addition, some patients are predisposed to react to particular herbs. For example, a patient with depressive symptoms shouldn't take certain herbs that treat insomnia, because they can heighten symptoms of depression. This warning may appear on the herbal remedy package, but the lack of federal regulation means there is no guarantee that remedies will carry adequate warnings.

▶ Advise your patient to discontinue using any herb if he develops an adverse reaction, such as headache, an upset stomach, or a rash.

▶ Inform him that if his responses to an herb are favorable but too intense, he should decrease the dose or stop taking the herb altogether. For example, a laxative that's administered for constipation may cause the patient to develop diarrhea. Obviously, he should stop taking the laxative in this case.

▶ If the patient experiences an adverse reaction, find out if he has been taking the herb too often or using it for too long. Sometimes symptoms are related to incorrect dosage. For example, chamomile taken orally daily over an extended period may cause an allergy to ragweed. Also, eating black licorice in large quantities on a daily basis can lead to high blood pressure.

Selected references

Abascal, K., and Yarnell, E. "Herbs for Treating Periodontal Disease," *Alternative and Complementary Therapies.* 7(4):216-20, August 2001.

Angier, B. *Field Guide to Medicinal Wild Plants.* Harrisburg, Pa.: Stackpole Books, 1978.

Butler, K. *Consumer's Guide to Alternative Medicine.* Buffalo, N.Y.: Prometheus Books, 1992.

Facts and Comparisons: The Review of Natural Products. St. Louis: Facts and Comparisons, 2002.

Foster, S., and Tyler, V.E. *Tyler's Honest Herbal: A Sensible Guide to the Use of Herbs and Related Remedies,* 4th ed. New York: The Haworth Herbal Press, 1999.

Gruenwald, J., et al. *PDR for Herbal Medicines,* 2nd ed. Montvale, N.J.: Medical Economics Co., 2000.

Guidelines for the Assessment of Herbal Medicines. Geneva: World Health Organization, 1991.

Jellin, J.M., et al. *Natural Medicines Comprehensive Database,* 3rd ed. Stockton, Calif.: Therapeutic Research Faculty, 2000. *www.naturaldatabase.com.*

Kuhn, M.A, et al. *Herbal Therapy & Supplements: A Scientific and Traditional Approach.* Philadelphia: Lippincott Williams & Wilkins, 2000.

Martindale, The Extra Pharmacopoeia, 32nd ed. London: Pharmaceutical Press, 1999.

McGuffin, M. et al. *American Herbal Products Association's Botanical Safety Handbook.* Boca Raton: CRC Press, 1997.

McKenry, L.M., and Salerno, E. *Mosby's Pharmacology in Nursing,* 21st ed. St. Louis: Mosby–Year Book, Inc., 2001.

National Cancer Institute. "Mistletoe Extract." *www.cancer.gov/ cancer_information/doc.aspx?viewid=1894C4CD-AA87-4F84-8EE4-9A815CE7F90E.*

Pittler, M.H., and Ernst, E. "The Efficacy of Kava Extract for Anxiety: Systematic Review and Meta-Analysis," *Journal of Clinical Psychopharmacology* 20:84-89, February 2000.

"Protectants," in *Drug Facts and Comparisons.* St. Louis: Facts and Comparisons, 2002.

Robbers, J.E., and Tyler, V.E. *Tyler's Herbs of Choice: The Therapeutic Use of Phytomedicinals,* Revised 1st ed. New York: The Haworth Herbal Press, 1999.

Rosenfeld, I. *Dr. Rosenfeld's Guide to Alternative Medicine: What Works, What Doesn't, and What's Right for You.* New York: Random House, 1996.

Weiner, J.A., and Weiner, M.A. *Herbs that Heal: Prescription for Herbal Healing.* Mill Valley, Calif.: Quantum Books, 1994.

Zand, J.A., et al.(eds.). "Preparing Herbal Treatments," in *Smart Medicine for a Healthier Child: A Practical A-to-Z Reference to Natural and Conventional Treatments for Infants and Children.* Garden City, N.Y.: Avery Publishing Group, 1994.

9

Diet and nutrition therapies

For centuries, food has been used to heal the body and maintain optimum health. Hippocrates, the father of modern medicine, recognized the healing properties of food when he said, "Let food be your medicine." However, mainstream Western medicine largely ignored the role of food in maintaining health and combating illness until recently. Today, diet and nutrition are once again in the spotlight. It seems as though every day the news media report stories on the benefits of a particular food or nutrient (such as broccoli and oat bran) or the hazards of another (such as caffeine and saturated fats). Although the results sometimes contradict each other, nutrition researchers have proved one fact conclusively: The food we eat *does* affect our health — in the West, primarily in a negative way.

> ❝ *Whereas people in the past suffered diseases associated with nutritional deficiencies, modern man's illnesses are associated with nutritional excesses.* ❞

The eating habits of people in technologically advanced societies have changed dramatically in the past century. Whereas people in the past suffered diseases associated with nutritional *deficiencies*, modern man's illnesses are associated with nutritional *excesses*. Nutritionists now believe that the "modern affluent diet," characterized by a high intake of processed, refined, and high-fat foods and an inadequate intake of whole grains, fruits, and vegetables, is responsible — either directly or indirectly — for the high incidence in the West of chronic degenerative illnesses, such as heart disease, diabetes, arthritis, and certain types of cancer.

Modern affluent diet

Why do so many Americans and others in affluent societies have such an unhealthy diet? Affluence itself is part of the problem. People today have more money but less time than their ancestors had. As a result, they consume large quantities of packaged convenience food, "fast food," and processed snack products that weren't even an option 50 years ago. These foods tend to be high in fats, salt, sugar, refined carbohydrates, partially hydrogenated vegetable oils, additives, and preservatives — substances known to have harmful effects when consumed in excess.

Advances in technology have also had a major effect on the way Americans eat. Changes in food production, processing, and storage typically involve the addition of chemicals and the depletion of food nutrients. Americans also consume more calories and get less exercise than they did a few generations ago; as a result, about one-third of all Americans are now classified as obese.

> *❝About 2,000 additives — including artificial colorings and flavors, stabilizers, sweeteners, preservatives, and antibiotics — are currently approved by the FDA for use in the foods we eat. Many of them are believed to be carcinogenic.❞*

The link between the modern diet and the increase in certain diseases has been established in several well-publicized studies during the past decade. These studies, comparing different population groups, showed that people who adopt a modern Western diet tend to develop the modern Western diseases previously mentioned. For example, Native Americans have a much higher incidence of diabetes since changing from their traditional diet to the typical American diet. And Japanese women who live in the United States have twice the incidence of breast cancer as those who live in Japan.

Harmful substances

Nutritionists generally agree that the most harmful substances in the modern diet are additives, refined sugars and starches, saturated fat, and hydrogenated oils. (See *Common food additives.*)

Additives

About 2,000 additives — including artificial colorings and flavors, stabilizers, sweeteners, preservatives, and antibiotics — are approved by the Food and Drug Administration for use in food. Many are believed to be carcinogenic. Some additives have also been linked to hyperactivity and learning disorders in children. Drugs may also contain some food additives.

Refined sugars and starches

Refined foods, such as white sugar and white flour, go through extensive processing, which strips them of their nutrients. Some nutrition experts believe a diet high in such refined carbohydrates contributes to nutritional deficiencies and overall poor health.

Sugar is a hidden ingredient in many processed foods and beverages. (Even a serving of pork and beans contains 1 cup of sugar!) Excessive consumption of refined sugars may increase the risk of heart disease (by increasing triglyceride levels) and obesity, promote dental decay, and contribute to decreased immune functioning. Research has also linked refined sugar to behavioral problems, hyperactivity, and poor scholastic achievement in children.

Saturated fat

Commonly referred to as the "bad" fat, saturated fat is the kind found in animal foods and tropical oils (coconut and palm). This type of fat is believed to elevate levels of low-density lipoproteins, thus increasing the risk of heart disease.

Hydrogenated oils

The partially hydrogenated oils found in many processed foods contain manmade molecules called trans-fatty acids, which may impair the metabolism of the essential fatty acids normally found in the body. This impaired metabolic function may af-

Common food additives

Some nutritionists and alternative practitioners believe that common food additives, which appear in many of the foods we eat, may contribute to symptoms of common disorders. Here you'll find some of the most common additives along with the symptoms they may be associated with.

▶ Aspartame—This artificial sweetener, known by the brand names NutraSweet and Equal, may cause rash, headaches, nausea, tetany, insomnia, changes in taste perception, blurred vision, depression, and seizures in susceptible individuals.

▶ Monosodium glutamate (MSG)—A flavor enhancer commonly known by its initials, MSG is found in many fast foods, processed foods, and packaged foods. In people with MSG sensitivity, it may cause headache, flushing, chest tightness, heart palpitations, and nausea—a combination of symptoms sometimes called "Chinese restaurant syndrome," because many people experience them after eating Chinese food.

▶ Nitrites—These common preservatives are used to prevent spoilage in cured meats, such as bacon and smoked sausages. In the body, nitrites combine with naturally occurring stomach chemicals to form cancer-causing nitrosamines. They may also be associated with birth defects. People with nitrate sensitivity commonly experience headaches and blurred vision.

▶ Saccharin—An artificial sweetener used in many soft drinks, saccharin is found in the familiar pink packets with the brand name Sweet 'n Low. Saccharin may cause headache and nausea in susceptible people; it may also be carcinogenic.

▶ Sulfur dioxide, sodium bisulfite, and sulfites—These additives are used as preservatives, especially in dried fruits, shrimp, and frozen potatoes. Sulfites are also found in most wines. Rash, headache, flushing, and palpitations have appeared in asthma patients and those with sulfa allergies.

▶ Yellow Dye No. 6—This dye, used in candy and carbonated beverages, is thought to cause chromosomal damage as well as allergic reactions. It's banned in Norway and Sweden.

▶ Citrus Red Dye No. 2—This dye, used to color the skins of oranges, is associated with chromosomal damage and may have some carcinogenic properties.

fect hormone synthesis and immune system function. These oils also contain by-products of oxygen metabolism called free radicals. These free radicals can damage tissues and promote cancer and may contribute to cholesterol's role in atherosclerosis. Hydrogenated oils are believed to alter liver function and damage the coronary arteries, which may contribute to heart disease.

Alternative diets

Alternative approaches to diet and nutrition are quite varied. Some aren't therapies at all, but rather a change in diet aimed at improving health or preventing disease. For example, many healthy people have begun consuming foods, vitamins, and supplements, such as broccoli and ginseng, believed to have beneficial effects or adopting a vegetarian, Asian, or Mediterranean diet, all of which are believed to offer protection against chronic illnesses. (See *Orthomolecular therapy.*)

Actual therapies include "fad" diets that focus on consumption of a specific food (such as grapefruit) for its perceived benefits; the use of megadoses of vitamins for therapeutic purposes (known as orthomolecular medicine); diets aimed at combating specific diseases, such as cancer and cardiovascular disease; fasting to cleanse the body; and juice therapy to nourish and cleanse the body.

In this chapter, we'll focus on the so-called "healing food" — both actual food and substances found in food — that are believed to enhance health, diets aimed at fighting specific diseases, fasting, and juice therapy.

Healing food chemicals

Dietary remedies have been a component of ancient cultures, such as India's Ayurvedic system and traditional Chinese medicine, for thousands of years. Indeed, the first healing medicines were herbs that people consumed as food. Today, science is taking a closer look at the "healing" properties of certain food chemicals and finding that many of them may actually help prevent disease.

> *All the chemicals in food work better together than as isolated ingredients and thus provide greater benefit when consumed from food than from supplements.*

All of the chemicals in food work better together than as isolated ingredients and thus provide greater benefit when

Orthomolecular therapy

The idea that high doses of certain vitamins can be used to treat disease dates back to the work of two Canadian psychiatrists in the 1950s, who proposed the theory that schizophrenia was caused by a biochemical defect that could be corrected with huge doses of vitamins B_3 and C. Their interest in these vitamins was spurred by a report that patients with pellagra, a deficiency of vitamin B_3, exhibited the same symptoms as schizophrenic patients.

In 1968, Nobel laureate Linus Pauling coined the term "orthomolecular" (from the Greek root "ortho," meaning "correct" or "proper") to refer to this concept of treating disease with the "proper" amount of nutrients that are normally present in the body. Expanding on the work of the two psychiatrists, Pauling suggested that orthomolecular medicine might be effective in treating nonpsychiatric disorders as well.

Although the American Psychiatric Association later criticized the psychiatrists' studies and rejected the use of megavitamin therapy, Pauling continued his work in this field and in the mid-1970s published several studies claiming that megadoses of vitamin C caused tumor regression in some patients with cancer. The Mayo Clinic then conducted its own studies on vitamin C but found no effect on cancer. Despite the skepticism of other scientists, Pauling continued to advocate the use of vitamin C as an adjunctive treatment to build up cancer patients' immunity and as a means of preventing or minimizing symptoms of the common cold and flu.

Recent studies encouraging

In recent years, mainstream science has begun taking a closer look at megavitamin therapy. Today, niacin is an accepted treatment for hypercholesterolemia and vitamin E is known to speed the healing of burns and wounds. Studies in the past 2 decades have found evidence that megavitamin therapy may benefit patients with other conditions as well:

▶ Acquired immunodeficiency syndrome—Increased CD4+ T-cell counts were reported in patients infected with human immunodeficiency virus who received high doses of betacarotene.

▶ Asthma—I.V. magnesium sulfate was found to relieve respiratory failure in asthmatic patients who failed to respond to conventional drug therapy.

▶ Cardiovascular disease—Vitamin E appears to reduce the risk of postoperative thromboembolism, and magnesium has shown anticoagulant effects in patients with preeclampsia and heart attacks.

(continued)

Orthomolecular therapy (continued)

▶ Mental and neurologic disorders — Folic acid may improve the recovery of depressed and schizophrenic patients, and vitamin C may enhance the effects of antipsychotic drugs.

▶ Cancer — Studies done in the early 1990s seem to support Pauling's theory on vitamin C. When given as an adjunctive therapy, vitamin C has been found to enhance the effectiveness of conventional therapies and reduce the toxicity associated with chemotherapy.

Keep in mind that these studies, for the most part, have focused on vitamins used as adjuncts to, not replacements for, conventional therapy.

consumed from food than from supplements. Among the most powerful of these substances are the antioxidants, carotenoids, phytoestrogens, flavonoids, and polyphenols.

In addition, newly recognized plant chemicals called phytochemicals, found by the thousands in fruits and vegetables, are currently under intense scrutiny by nutrition researchers. They aren't nutrients per se but compounds that interact with one another in complex but complementary ways to protect plants from damage due to excessive light and pollution. Scientists theorize that phytochemicals that act as antioxidants in plants may provide similar benefits in humans. The National Science Institute recently launched a multimillion-dollar study of these substances, which initial research suggests may be useful in combating cancer.

Antioxidants

Antioxidants are chemicals or other agents that inhibit or retard oxidation. They include vitamins A, C, E, the trace mineral selenium, and the carotenoids (especially betacarotene). These substances have been in the news frequently because of their ability to destroy disease-causing free radicals, highly reactive and unstable compounds that form when the body metabolizes oxygen. Free radicals, which the body produces increasingly with age, are believed to promote tumor growth and may contribute to atherosclerosis.

The protective mechanisms of antioxidants continue to be studied. Vitamin E has shown some promise in reducing the risk of heart disease. There's evidence that selenium may protect against prostate, lung, colon, and esophageal malignancies. In other studies, combinations of antioxidants have suggested benefits in such conditions as breast, stomach, lung, colon, and prostate cancers and cataracts; they may also retard aging.

Food sources

Groups such as the American Heart Association and the American Cancer Society believe that it's too soon to recommend dietary supplements containing antioxidants. Until the Food and Nutrition Board of the National Academy of Sciences issues a report listing recommended intake of these nutrients, the best source of antioxidants is a well-balanced diet.

Good whole food sources of antioxidants are dark orange, yellow, red, and green fruits and vegetables. Betacarotene, the most important of the carotenoids, is found in cruciferous (broccoli, cauliflower, Brussels sprouts, cabbage, kale, turnips) and dark green leafy vegetables (collard greens, spinach, arugula), yellow-to-red vegetables (sweet potatoes, carrots, squash, red peppers) and yellow or orange fruits (cantaloupes, oranges, peaches, apricots, citrus fruits). Recent studies at Tufts University showed that blueberries are also an excellent source of antioxidants. Selenium can be found in Brazil nuts, unrefined grains, and seafood.

These fruits and vegetables are sometimes called "healing foods," "super foods," or "power foods" because they contain numerous groups of chemicals that may help prevent disease and promote health. For example, the cruciferous vegetables contain indoles and isothiocyanates, families of phytochemicals that may halt the action of carcinogens in the body, including those from tobacco smoke and pollution. Brussels sprouts contain glucosinolate, a substance that can disarm aflatoxin (a group of naturally occurring toxic by-products produced by the fungus *Aspergillus flavus*). (See *Healing foods: A closer look,* pages 352 and 353.)

Carotenoids

Carotenoids are plant pigments found primarily in vegetables and fungi. They aren't vitamins but some of them — such as

Healing foods: A closer look

"Healing foods," including fruits, vegetables, legumes, grains, nuts, and seeds, contain combinations of phytochemicals that scientists believe may enhance health and ultimately prolong life. For each group of phytochemicals that appears below, you'll find the benefits that they're believed to bestow and the foods that contain them.

Phyto-chemicals	Potential benefits	Food sources
Antioxidants Vitamins A, C, E, the trace mineral selenium, carotenoids and flavonoids	▶ Help prevent heart attack and stroke ▶ May halt the actions of carcinogens in the body ▶ Work to limit the formation of free radicals or neutralize them before they can damage the body	▶ Yellow to red vegetables (beets, carrots, peppers, sweet potatoes, tomatoes, winter squash) ▶ Leafy green vegetables (collard and mustard greens, kale, watercress) ▶ Nuts ▶ Yellow or orange fruits (apricots, melons, nectarines, pineapples) ▶ Citrus fruits ▶ Unrefined grains ▶ Seafood ▶ Garlic, leeks, shallots
Carotenoids Plant pigments that occur in vegetables, fungi, and some crustacea	▶ Help protect the eyes against damage from excessive light ▶ Decrease the risk of prostate cancer ▶ Some converted to vitamins (betacarotene into vitamin A) ▶ Antioxidant potential in most	▶ Cruciferous vegetables (broccoli, Brussels sprouts, cabbage, cauliflower, kale) ▶ Red and yellow fruits and vegetables (apricots, carrots, red and yellow bell peppers, sweet potatoes) ▶ Green leafy vegetables (kale, spinach) ▶ Sea vegetables (blue green algae, kelp)

Healing foods: A closer look (continued)

Phyto-chemicals	Potential benefits	Food sources
Flavonoids Plant compounds responsible for the color in fruits and vegetables	▶ May prevent different types of cancer ▶ May prevent blood clots and plaque formation in arteries ▶ Work to minimize collagen destruction in inflammatory conditions, such as periodontal disease and rheumatoid arthritis ▶ Act as antioxidants	▶ Red wine ▶ Tea ▶ Most fruits and vegetables (apples, blueberries, carrots, grapes, onions, squash, tomatoes) ▶ Soy products (soy milk, tofu) ▶ Seeds (sesame, sunflower) ▶ Nuts (almonds, peanuts)
Phytoestrogens Hormonelike substances of plant origin	▶ Help prevent hormone-related cancers ▶ May enhance immunity ▶ Reduce platelet aggregation ▶ Act as estrogen agonists or antagonists in humans	▶ Whole grains (barley, corn, oats, wheat) ▶ Legumes (chickpeas, lentils, split peas, lima beans, broad beans) ▶ Soy (miso, soy flour, soy milk, tempeh, tofu)
Polyphenols Plant compounds linked to the "French Paradox"	▶ May prevent heart disease ▶ May prevent cancers ▶ Antioxidant and anticoagulant effects under investigation	▶ Red wine ▶ Tea ▶ Apples, grapes, strawberries ▶ Onions ▶ Yams

betacarotene — are converted to vitamin A in the body. Other carotenoids that show promise are lutein and lycopene. Lutein, found naturally in the pigment of the macula, is believed to protect the eyes against damage from excessive light. Lycopene, the carotenoid that provides the red color in tomatoes, may be associated with a decreased risk of prostate cancer.

Food sources
Prime food sources of carotenoids are the cruciferous vegetables, such as broccoli, cauliflower, cabbage, and kale. Red and yellow fruits and vegetables, such as apricots, carrots, and peppers, are also good sources. In addition, carotenoids are found in kelp and in green leafy vegetables, such as spinach.

> 66 *The phystoestrogens in soy products may be the reason that Japanese women, whose diets are high in soy, are four times less likely to develop breast cancer, an estrogen-driven disease, than American women.* 99

Phytoestrogens
Phytoestrogens are a specific group of hormone-like plant chemicals that act as either estrogen antagonists or agonists. Approximately 20 compounds make up this group. Isoflavones, a class of phytoestrogens found in soy products, actually bind to estrogen receptors, preventing the body's own estrogen from doing so. As a result, these compounds may help prevent hormone-related cancers, such as breast cancer and prostate cancer. (This may be the reason that Japanese women, whose diets are high in soy products, are four times less likely to develop breast cancer, an estrogen-driven disease, than American women. However, when Japanese women adopt a Western diet, their incidence of breast cancer increases.) Phytoestrogens may also enhance immunity and reduce platelet aggregation.

Food sources
Soy products (tofu, miso, tempeh, soy milk) are an excellent source of phytoestrogens. Other good sources include legumes (chickpeas, lentils, split peas) and whole grains (barley, corn, oats, wheat).

Flavonoids
Flavonoids are a class of phytochemicals that are responsible for the colors of fruits and vegetables. They appear to have anticarcinogenic, antiallergenic, and anti-inflammatory properties. By acting as antioxidants, flavonoids may prevent blood clots, clogged arteries, and some cancers. The more than 4,000 different flavonoids provide different benefits. Those

found in berries act as potent antioxidants and appear to minimize the destruction of collagen (the body protein responsible for holding together body tissues) that results from inflammatory conditions, such as rheumatoid arthritis and periodontal disease. Others, such as quercetin, modify the allergic response by inhibiting the release of histamine.

Food sources
High concentrations of flavonoids are found in blueberries, grapes, citrus fruits, apples, broccoli, cabbage, squash, yams, tomatoes, eggplant, and peppers. They're also found in red wine and green and black tea.

Polyphenols
Polyphenols are a group of phytochemicals that are responsible for the brightly colored pigments in many fruits and vegetables. These antioxidants, found in red wine tea (not the herbal variety) and other foods, are being investigated for their potential ability to prevent heart disease and cancer. Some researchers believe that polyphenols are the substance in red wine responsible for the "French paradox" — the fact that French people have a low rate of heart disease despite their high-fat diet. (See *The French paradox.*)

The French paradox

Health experts have been baffled for years about why the French, with their diet of high-fat sauces and cheeses such as brie, have a much lower incidence of heart disease than Americans. Some researchers believe the key to this puzzle — known as the French paradox — lies in the red wine that French people drink. Regular (but moderate) wine consumption seems to slow the oxidation of low-density lipoproteins and inhibit the blood from clotting. Scientists are now zeroing in on polyphenols as the phytochemicals in grapes responsible for these effects.

Not everyone accepts red wine as the answer to the French paradox. Some scientists point out that the French have a healthier lifestyle than Americans in several respects: They exercise more, eat smaller portions, don't eat between meals, eat more fruits and vegetables, and have cheese or fruit for dessert, rather than pastries and ice cream.

> 66 *Green tea, hailed as a general tonic by Andrew Weil and others, is believed to lower cholesterol, improve lipid metabolism, and have significant anticancer and antibacterial effects.* 99

Researchers have recently been taking a closer look at the health benefits of tea. Dutch studies between 1970 and 1985 found that men who drank more than four cups of tea daily had a much lower incidence of stroke than men who drank only two cups a day. Green tea, made from unfermented tea leaves, is receiving a lot of attention from Andrew Weil and others. According to Weil, who advocates drinking it as a general tonic, green tea contains compounds called catechins that lower cholesterol, improve lipid metabolism, and have "significant" anticancer and antibacterial effects.

Food sources
Aside from red wine and green, black, or oolong tea, polyphenols are found in onions, apples, grapes, strawberries, nuts, yams, and chocolate.

Miscellaneous health-enhancing substances
Numerous other nutrients and chemicals, such as those listed below, have been touted for their health benefits:

▶ *Boron*—a trace mineral required for calcium metabolism. Good sources are fruits, vegetables, and nuts. High doses of boron are said to relieve symptoms of menopause and reduce the risk of developing osteoporosis, but there's no scientific evidence to corroborate these claims. Possible adverse effects include diarrhea, nausea, and vomiting.

▶ *DHEA*—a hormone made in the adrenal gland that's converted to testosterone (in males) and estrogen (in females). Proponents say DHEA, sold in supplement form, slows the aging process, improves mood and libido, and helps in weight loss. Critics say there's insufficient research to warrant using DHEA as a supplement, especially by pregnant women and teenagers (because of the sex hormone effects). DHEA has also been linked to an increased risk of prostate and ovarian cancers.

▶ *Glucosamine sulfate*—a synthetic version of glucosamine, a naturally occurring body substance that plays an important role in maintaining and repairing joint cartilage. Advocates claim that this supplement can be used instead of aspirin and nonsteroidal inflammatory drugs to relieve the pain of osteoarthritis. Possible adverse effects include nausea, heartburn, and indigestion. Evidence of glucosamine's effectiveness and long-term safety in humans is inconclusive.

▶ *Lecithin* — a substance that helps transport fats and cholesterol throughout the body. According to advocates, lecithin supplements can lower cholesterol levels, prevent heart attacks, and improve memory. The component of lecithin that's supposed to be beneficial, choline, is found in eggs, legumes, and organ meats. Excessive doses can cause nausea, dizziness, and possible depression.

▶ *Melatonin* — a hormone secreted by the pineal gland. Because melatonin is the substance that makes humans sleepy at night, it's currently being touted as a sleep aid. Proponents say it also prevents jet lag, strengthens bones, lowers blood pressure and cholesterol levels, and enhances immune system functioning — all claims that haven't been proven. Some researchers have raised questions about melatonin's long-term safety as a supplement.

Vegetarianism

Vegetarianism is the practice of avoiding animal flesh and fish in the diet. More than a simple dietary option, vegetarianism is a complex and varied lifestyle choice. Some, like Seventh Day Adventists and vegans, adhere to the diet for ideological reasons, while others may adopt it strictly for nutritional benefits.

There are many subcategories of vegetarians: ovolactovegetarians eat only dairy and egg products, lactovegetarians eat dairy but no egg products, vegans avoid all animal-derived products, fruitarians eat only fruits and nuts, and living foodists eat only germinated seeds, cereals, sprouts, vegetables, fruits, berries and nuts. The macrobiotic diet (see "Macrobiotic diet," page 371) is sometimes incorrectly included under the heading of vegetarianism, but since it includes fish, it isn't truly vegetarian.

Differentiating among vegetarians is significant as it demonstrates the varying degrees of nutrition available in the subcategories. For instance, an ovolacto vegetarian will generally derive more protein, calcium, and B_{12} from his diet than a vegan. This isn't to suggest that those adopting a living food or vegan diet may not get adequate nutrition; rather, they must be more conscientious in their dietary choices to ensure proper nutrition.

Therapeutic uses

Vegetarianism is employed as both a lifestyle choice and as a specific treatment plan. Patients with cancer, cardiovascular disease, cerebrovascular disease, chronic renal failure, type 2 diabetes (noninsulin-dependent diabetes), obesity, ocular macular degeneration, and rheumatoid arthritis have all been shown to benefit from either the vegetarian diet in general or one of its subcategories.

RESEARCH SUMMARY Dean Ornish, a cardiologist and an advocate of a low-fat vegan diet, has established the efficacy of the diet in reversing cardiovascular disease. His groundbreaking study first appeared in *JAMA* in 1983, and in *Lancet* in 1990.

Another important dietary study, the China Project, shows a connection between diet and the risk of developing disease. Researchers studied over 10,000 Chinese, in both villages and urban settings, who maintained the same diet, lifestyle, and locality of residence for their entire lives. The first survey was taken in 1983 to 1984, the second in 1989 to 1990. One of the main conclusions derived from the study is that the vegetarian diet, and a vegan diet in particular, leads to fewer risks of cancer, obesity, and cardiovascular disease.

Another group frequently studied are members of the Seventh Day Adventist Church. Approximately 50% of church members practice vegetarianism as part of their religion, thus presenting an opportunity to study the long-term effects of the vegetarian diet. Loma Linda University in California and the Sydney Adventist Hospital in Australia have done most of the research on this group. Their conclusions support the vegetarian diet for prevention of coronary heart disease, diabetes mellitus, hypertension, arthritis, and some forms of cancer. ■

Procedure

Because vegetarianism is a lifestyle rather than a specific medication, there's no specific procedure. Rather, there are general dietary guidelines for the particular health conditions previously cited.

Complications

Vegetarianism is a safe and effective adjunct treatment for many conditions. However, in certain subgroups such as vegans, fruitarians, and living food vegetarians, it's prudent to check for deficiencies in specific nutrients, such as B_{12}, iron, calcium, zinc, and protein. Ovolacto- and lactovegetarians don't seem to have these deficiencies. The adverse effect of increased intestinal gas production is common at the onset of adoption of a vegetarian diet.

As in the nonvegetarian pregnant woman, it's important to observe overall health and to ascertain if the woman is supplementing her diet with vitamins, minerals, and other nutrients. This will give the clinician an idea of the diet's nutritional status. In a pregnant woman who appears less healthy, check for iron, fatty acid, and B_{12} deficiencies. Vitamin B_{12} deficiencies during pregnancy may lead to myelination dysfunction in the neonate or other neurologic problems that may resolve with the administration of B_{12} to the newborn. These same considerations should be addressed with the lactating vegetarian mother.

In a child's early developmental years, a strict vegetarian diet, such as vegan, living food, or fruitarian may not provide sufficient fatty acids, protein, and specific nutrients. In some instances, rickets, osteoporosis, anemia, and growth retardation have occurred. Supplementation with vitamins and minerals may avert these conditions.

As in the nonvegetarian child, the overall health of a vegetarian child depends on the quality of nutrition. Like their nonvegetarian counterparts, vegetarian children may resist eating vegetables. Creative parents can usually overcome these objections by encouraging the child to take part in grocery shopping and meal preparation. Calcium may become a critical issue with the vegan subtype, while adequate fatty acids may be more of concern with the raw or living food vegetarian than with the ovolacto or lactovegetarian. There's conflicting information concerning the growth and maturation of a vegetarian child; however, a lower body mass index is found consistently. The growth and maturation status of the vegetarian population have been within the normal to low range.

There are conflicting results in the various studies of bone mineral density (BMD) in vegetarian and nonvegetarian premenopausal and postmenopausal women. Some results find that

Vegetarian food pyramid

In 1999, the Department of Nutrition at Loma Linda University in California presented an alternative food pyramid for vegetarians as a guide for a healthier diet. The pyramid consists of a six levels. On the bottom level are whole grains (40%) and legumes (60%). The second level from the bottom recommends fruits (40%) and vegetables (60%); the third level contains nuts and seeds. The final three levels — vegetable oils, dairy products and eggs, and sweets — are considered optional. This new framework can help you advise vegetarians how to balance the various components of their diet.

the BMD at the spine is similar between vegetarians and omnivores, but that the BMD at the hip can be significantly lower in vegetarians. In other studies, which used the Wilcoxon signed-rank test, there was no significant difference in bone measurements between vegetarians and omnivores at any sites except the skull. Differentiating between vegans and lactovegetarians, there was no significant difference in BMD. Calcium supplementation is essential in the vegetarian female at this life stage.

Nursing perspective

▶ It's important to determine three factors about vegetarian patients: the type of vegetarianism the patient practices; whether the diet was adopted for ideological or health reasons; and whether the patient supplements his diet. This information gives the clinician a better idea of the nutritional value of the diet.

▶ Some vegetarians adhere to the diet for religious reasons and are less concerned about the nutritional value. Some subgroups, such as vegans and living food vegetarians, may be reluctant to take food supplementation for ideological reasons. Suggest the addition of kelp, an easily obtainable seaweed and a source of B_{12}, to these patients.

▶ Some adolescents adopt a vegetarian lifestyle as a passing fad, while others adopt it to lose weight. This particular group is often unaware of the need for beans, grains, and vegetables in their diets. They may frequently subsist on simple carbohydrates, convenience foods, and dairy products. Diets and sup-

plementation should be reviewed carefully for adequate protein, calcium, and iron. (See *Vegetarian food pyramid*.)

Anticancer diets

Despite the many new treatments for cancer that have appeared in recent years, the mortality rates for many types of
cancer haven't declined significantly, if at all. According to the
American Cancer Society (ACS), cancer still accounts for one
out of every five deaths in the United States. As a result, many
patients are turning to alternative dietary programs in an attempt to deal with cancer from a nutritional standpoint rather
than (or as an adjunct to) the customary pharmaceutical and
surgical approaches.

> 66 *The rationale behind most of the anticancer diets is that if
> diet can contribute to cancer, a conclusion that the scientific
> establishment increasingly supports, then dietary changes
> may help eliminate it.* 99

The rationale behind most of the diet therapies discussed
below is that if diet can contribute to cancer, a conclusion that
the scientific establishment increasingly supports, then dietary changes may help eliminate it. Most of these diets emphasize an increased consumption of fruits and vegetables,
whole grains, and legumes and a decreased intake of high-fat,
processed, refined, and "junk" food. This aspect of the plan is
similar to the recommendations proposed by the federal government and mainstream organizations such as the ACS. However, the diets also espouse certain unconventional practices,
such as the use of megavitamin supplements and detoxification procedures (such as coffee enemas); some also encourage
the use of specific foods and forbid others.

Most oncologists question the effectiveness of dietary
changes once a person already has cancer, but the proponents
of these diets believe that the food a person eats (or doesn't
eat) *after* diagnosis is just as important as those he eats *before*. At present, none of the diets discussed below are recommended by either the ACS or the National Cancer Institute
(NCI). In most cases, the patients who use them have failed to

respond to conventional treatments and feel they have nowhere else to turn.

Hoxsey treatment

Derived from an herbal preparation originally used to treat cancer in horses, the Hoxsey treatment is one of the oldest and most controversial alternative therapies for cancer in the United States. The plan consists of powerful herbal remedies (used internally and externally), a dietary program, and vitamin and mineral supplements. The herbal formulas at the center of the plan originated in the 1840s with an American farmer, John Hoxsey, who noticed that one of his horses with a leg tumor recovered after grazing on certain plants and grasses. Hoxsey concocted a salve out of the plants, which he gave to other farmers, and bequeathed the formula to his heirs.

Despite strong opposition from the ACS, which placed the Hoxsey treatment on its list of unproved methods in 1968, this regimen has been used as a cancer treatment for nearly 100 years. Hoxsey himself never claimed to understand what caused cancer or how his preparations worked. Cancers that are said to respond best to this treatment include lymphoma, melanoma, and external skin cancer.

Basic elements

Hoxsey's great-grandson, Harry Hoxsey, began trying the herbal preparations on humans with cancer. Between the 1920s and 1940s, he opened Hoxsey Cancer Clinics in Dallas with branches in 17 states. The cornerstone of the Hoxsey treatment is an herbal paste that is applied externally (and used primarily for skin cancers) and an herbal tonic taken internally. Other components of the Hoxsey regimen, which is still offered in a Tijuana clinic, include:
- assorted vitamins and calcium supplements
- douches and laxatives
- avoidance of pork, tomatoes, salt, sugar, artificial sweeteners, vinegar, alcohol, refined flour, alcohol, and carbonated drinks
- attitudinal counseling.

Hoxsey therapists claim they can cure 80% of patients but, as with many other alternative therapies, these claims are based on anecdotal evidence rather than clinical trials.

RESEARCH SUMMARY At least one respected researcher has found a scientific basis for the salve. Frederick Mohs, creator of the Mohs chemosurgical technique for skin cancer excision, reported that Hoxsey's paste contained ingredients that cured most basal cell skin carcinomas. One of the ingredients, bloodroot *(Sanguinaria canadensis)*, has been used by Native Americans to treat tumors and warts.

According to the 1994 report to the National Institutes of Health (NIH), *Alternative Medicine: Expanding Medical Horizons,* some of the principal herbs in the tonic — pokeweed root, burdock root, buckthorn bark, barberry, stillingia root, and prickly ash — have been shown to have anticancer and immunostimulatory effects. The report cites a 1979 study showing that pokeweed root *(Phytolacca americana)* stimulates the production of two cytokines that stimulate the immune system — interleukin-1 and tumor necrosis factor. The report says that although pokeweed is poisonous, "it apparently has been used without serious toxicity problems since the mid-18th century."

The NIH report also cites a 1984 study on burdock root's reported ability to reduce cell mutations and a 1989 World Health Organization report on this plant's reported ability to inhibit human immunodeficiency virus. The report concludes: "Among numerous anecdotal accounts of its effectiveness, some are hard to dismiss out of hand; [the treatment] therefore warrants investigation." ■

Complications
The Hoxsey diet may provoke allergic reaction in susceptible individuals. Also, topical application of the herbal salve may cause skin irritation, necessitating an end to treatment.

Nursing perspective
Patients on the Hoxsey diet should avoid tomatoes, alcohol, carbonated beverages, vinegar, and processed flour because they can negate the effects of the tonic.

Gerson diet
The Gerson diet is one of a number of "metabolic" therapies that include a combination of diet, nutritional supplements, detoxification, and enzyme therapy aimed at fighting disease by rebuilding the immune system. It is essentially a low-

sodium vegan regimen, consisting of large quantities of fruits and vegetables in the form of freshly squeezed juice along with assorted supplements, detoxification with coffee enemas or colonic irrigation, sodium restriction, and potassium supplements. Aluminum cookware and utensils are to be avoided.

Initially used to treat tuberculosis, the central theory of the diet's founder, German-born physician Max Gerson, is that disease results primarily from an accumulation of toxic substances in the body. Gerson believed that these toxins (chemicals found in food, water, and the environment) poison the liver and weaken the immune system, making people more prone to cancer and other diseases.

> ❝ Gerson came to believe that cancer was a degenerative disease stemming from impaired metabolism and that proper liver function was crucial to proper metabolic functioning. ❞

Gerson began experimenting with diet in an attempt to relieve his own migraine headaches; after succeeding, he tried dietary changes to treat various diseases in his patients (including famed physician Albert Schweitzer). Gerson gained recognition in Germany for successfully treating tuberculosis of the skin (lupus vulgaris) with a low-salt diet. He continued experimenting with different diet combinations for various diseases (including asthma, arthritis, and cancer); by the time he emigrated to the United States in 1936, he was concentrating on experimenting with diets for the treatment of cancer.

Gerson came to believe that cancer was a degenerative disease stemming from impaired metabolism and that proper liver function was crucial to proper metabolic functioning. He also placed great importance on maintaining a proper balance of sodium and potassium, believing that an imbalance (excessive sodium levels) helped create an internal environment conducive to tumor growth. Gerson believed that his stringent treatment program reversed the conditions that were necessary to sustain such growth.

Basic elements

Gerson's program included the following measures, among others:

▶ a low-salt, low-fat, high-potassium diet consisting of three vegetarian meals daily prepared from organic foods

▶ 8 oz (237 ml) of freshly prepared fruit or vegetable juice every hour for 13 hours each day (for the first 4 weeks) to bombard the body with nutrients and correct the sodium-potassium imbalance; the juice must be prepared in a special press to reduce enzyme breakdown, and potassium is added to each glass

▶ supplements of pepsin, potassium iodine (Lugol's solution), niacin, pancreatin (a digestive enzyme from bovine pancreas), and thyroid hormone

▶ coffee enemas daily to promote the release of toxins from the liver

▶ avoidance of all processed, canned, bottled, and frozen foods as well as foods cooked in aluminum pots

▶ limited dairy products and permanent avoidance of salt, berries, pineapple, pickles, nuts, mushrooms, soybeans, oil, coffee, chocolate, refined sugar and flour.

The plan originally included raw calves' liver juice as well, but that aspect was discontinued in 1989 after some patients developed bacterial infections. Reported side effects of treatment include nausea as the toxins are flushed out of the system and hypersensitivity to treatment components.

Mexican clinic. In 1977, Gerson's daughter founded the Gerson Institute, based in Bonita, California. The Institute oversees a clinic in Tijuana, Mexico, that offers the Gerson treatment to about 600 patients a year. In addition, the Institute offers a training program to licensed medical professionals consisting of four phases including a two-week internship.

After an initial treatment period at the clinic, patients continue the regimen at home for about 1½ years until their immune systems are theoretically sufficiently restored. The Institute claims success in treating not only certain types of cancer, but also heart disease, arthritis, and chronic fatigue syndrome. Its newsletter and Web site regularly offer testimonials from patients who say they've been cured, including several medical physicians.

Although the fundamental aspects of Gerson's diet—increased intake of fruits and vegetables, decreased intake of sodium and fat—are consistent with accepted theories about reducing cancer risk, the medical establishment on the whole doesn't accept Gerson's theory that diet and detoxification can cause tumor regression. It's especially critical of the use of coffee enemas. (See *Coffee enemas.*)

RESEARCH SUMMARY In 1959, the NCI reviewed the 50 case histories presented in Gerson's book, *A Cancer Therapy: Results of 50 Cases,* and concluded that Gerson's data failed to meet the basic criteria for evaluating clinical benefit. A number of more recent studies by British and Austrian researchers attempting to assess the diet's effectiveness have produced inconclusive results.

Coffee enemas

Although they may sound strange today, coffee enemas weren't an unusual treatment 50 years ago, when Max Gerson made them a part of his diet to combat cancer. In fact, mainstream surgeons gave them to clients to treat shock and postoperative bleeding.

Gerson believed that patients with cancer were "poisoned" by food additives and pesticides and thus needed to be "detoxified." The rationale behind coffee enemas was that they stimulated the liver to secrete more bile, thus helping to rid the GI tract of waste products. (The idea that impacted feces in the colon produced pathogenic toxins was a common belief at the turn of the century.)

Although the medical establishment rejects the use of coffee enemas as a treatment for cancer, they continue to be used at the Gerson Clinic in Mexico and have been incorporated into several other alternative cancer regimens. Proponents say that in addition to detoxifying the body, coffee enemas help to destroy free radicals, the harmful end-products of metabolism that are believed to contribute to the development of cancer. They're also said to reduce the pain associated with cancer, thus allowing clients to take fewer narcotics.

Critics of coffee enemas say that there has never been any scientific evidence that the "toxins" that proponents describe actually exist. They also point out that regular use of such enemas can result in electrolyte disturbances and nutritional deficiencies.

The British team visited the Gerson Clinic in Mexico in 1989 and studied 27 case histories. Twenty were deemed not assessable; of the remaining 7, 3 showed evidence of tumor regression, 1 was stable, and 3 showed cancer progression. The researchers cited subjective benefits to the patients and concluded that, in light of the patients' poor prognoses, the therapy might be a "way forward." The Austrian study, which involved use of a modified Gerson plan as an adjunctive treatment for cancer, reported subjective benefits, including pain relief and less severe adverse effects from chemotherapy. ■

Complications
Excessive intake of potassium can result in renal failure, arrhythmias, and sudden death. Vitamin toxicity may also occur. Coffee enemas disrupt the GI system's natural balance of flora and can cause dehydration, fatigue, and malaise. They've also been linked to dangerous electrolyte imbalances.

Nursing perspective
▶ If your patient is on the Gerson diet, advise him to have regular blood tests to check for potassium imbalance and vitamin toxicity.
▶ Teach your patient the signs and symptoms of dehydration, such as decreased urinary output, dark urine, and increased thirst and skin turgor.

Kelley regimen
An offshoot of the Gerson diet, the Kelley regimen is a metabolic therapy that became one of the most well-known alternative cancer treatments in the 1970s. It was developed by an orthodontist, William Kelley, after he was told he had terminal pancreatic cancer in the early 1960s. After receiving his diagnosis (which was never confirmed by a biopsy), Kelley studied the medical literature to try to determine what causes cancer.

He concluded that pollutants and an unhealthy diet impaired the body's ability to metabolize protein, which could lead to tumor growth; he believed that this metabolic problem stemmed from a deficiency of pancreatic enzymes, which were the body's first line of defense against malignant tumors. Kelley began experimenting with doses of vitamins, minerals, and enzymes to develop a corrective diet. He eventually claimed to have cured himself (and his wife and two of his children) with his diet and created a mail-order business to sell his special enzymes to the public.

Basic elements

Kelley's plan included some elements of the Gerson plan, such as juices, coffee enemas, and nutritional supplements (including pancreatic enzymes). But Kelley eventually came to believe that no single diet was right for all patients. He developed different plans for different people, based on their metabolic profile; some were put on a vegetarian diet, others were told to eat lots of red meat, and others were given a mixed diet.

The plan also advocated consumption of mostly raw foods (including raw liver), decreased protein intake, elimination of refined foods and additives, regular fasting and colonic irrigation, osteopathic or chiropractic manipulation to provide neurologic stimulation, and a positive spiritual attitude.

Gonzalez offshoot. In the 1970s, after a restraining order prohibited him from treating nondental disorders, Kelley became more cautious about promoting his plan as a cancer treatment, saying it was merely intended as a nutritional program to enhance health. Nevertheless, the Kelley regimen has been adopted and modified by a number of followers, including Nicholas Gonzalez, a New York immunologist.

Gonzalez became interested in Kelley's program after studying his case histories and discovering that some of Kelley's patients with pancreatic cancer survived for an average of 10 years compared with the average survival rate of less than 1 year with conventional treatment. Gonzalez presented 50 of these case histories in a 1987 book, *One Man Alone: An Investigation of Nutrition, Cancer, and William Donald Kelley* (no longer in print).

Like Kelley, Gonzalez tailors each patient's diet to his individual needs, incorporating the following elements:

▶ intensive (more than 100 capsules daily) nutritional supplementation, including pancreatic enzymes
▶ hydrochloric acid to aid digestion
▶ raw beef organs and glands
▶ detoxification with coffee enemas.

RESEARCH SUMMARY In the early 1990s, the Congressional Office of Technology Assessment asked a panel of six physicians —

three mainstream oncologists and three oncologists who were open to unconventional therapies — to review the 50 Kelley case histories that Gonzalez presented in his book. The results generally reflected the physicians' medical approaches. The mainstream physicians found Gonzalez's findings unconvincing, saying the patients' improvements could be attributed to earlier conventional treatments, while the more sympathetic physicians found the patient outcomes encouraging and worthy of further study. In many of the cases, the physicians found insufficient documentation, such as failure to confirm metastasis by biopsy.

Eleven patients with inoperable pancreatic cancer participated in a pilot study of the Gonzalez Regimen in 1999. The results were promising and prompted the National Center for Complementary and Alternative Medicine to sponsor a $1.4 million clinical trial. ■

Complications

The intensive nutritional supplements required by the Kelley plan could result in vitamin toxicity and electrolyte imbalances. The raw meats required could expose the patient to bacteria and viruses. Coffee enemas disrupt the GI system's natural balance of flora and can lead to dehydration, fatigue, and malaise. They've also been associated with dangerous electrolyte imbalances.

Nursing perspective

Nearly all patients with cancer have distinct nutritional deficiencies, which can impair optimal immune function. They are also prone to poor digestion and appetite.

▶ If your patient is receiving the Kelley treatment, advise him to have blood tests periodically to check for vitamin toxicity and electrolyte imbalances.

▶ Teach your patient about signs and symptoms of electrolyte imbalances.

Livingston treatment

The Livingston treatment, a combination of dietary regimen and immunotherapy, is based on laboratory studies performed in the 1940s by Virginia Livingston, a medical doctor and researcher. During microscopic examination of diseased tissues, Livingston identified a new bacterium that appeared in various sizes and shapes in the tissue of patients with scleroderma, tuberculosis, leprosy, and all types of cancer. She concluded that this microorganism, which she named *Progenitor cryptocides,* was present in all human beings at birth and normally remained dormant. However, when a person's immune system became weakened (from poor diet, chemical toxins, emotional stress, old age, or genetic predisposition), the microbe could cause cancer.

Livingston developed a vaccine against *P. cryptocides* (derived from a culture of the patient's own bacteria) and began administering it at a clinic she established in California in the 1950s. The vaccine is aimed at increasing the body's resistance to *P. cryptocides* and eliminating the internal conditions that allow it to thrive. Livingston died in 1990. That same year, the clinic was ordered by California officials to stop treating patients with cancer due to the treatment's lack of proven safety and efficacy. The clinic appealed to state health officials for an extension and continues to operate in San Diego.

Basic elements

Because she believed that diet played a role in weakening the immune system, Livingston's treatment regimen contained dietary features similar to those of the metabolic plans described above. Its primary elements include:

▶ a modified Gerson diet, including coffee enemas

▶ megadoses of vitamins, minerals, and digestive enzymes

▶ bacille Calmette-Guérin vaccine to stimulate the immune system

▶ injections every 3 to 5 days

▶ long-term use of antibiotics

▶ a ban on caffeine, alcohol, refined sugar and flour, and all processed foods.

RESEARCH SUMMARY According to the University of Pennsylvania's OncoLink Web site, "there is no scientific evidence to confirm [Livingston's] theories of cancer or to justify her treatments." This report claims that other researchers have been unable to confirm the existence of *P. cryptocides* and that cultures she submitted to a private organization for study identified her microorganism as *Staphylococcus epidermidis.* Conversely, another study, conducted at the East Virginia School, found the vaccine useful in reversing the immune-suppressed condition of patients with cancer. ■

Complications

Coffee enemas and long-term use of antibiotics can destroy the body's natural flora; enemas can also lead to dehydration, fatigue, malaise, and electrolyte imbalances. As with the other diets, megadoses of vitamins and other supplements can lead to vitamin toxicity. The vaccines can lead to sepsis or anaphylaxis.

Nursing perspective

▶ If your patient is on the Livingston regimen, inform him that he may experience reactions to the vaccine, including soreness or redness at the injection site, mild fever, and muscle or joint pain.

▶ Be alert for superinfections, such as yeast infections, from the long-term use of antibiotics.

▶ Tell your patient what adverse reactions he may experience from the prescribed antibiotic.

▶ Teach your patient the signs and symptoms of dehydration, such as decreased urinary output, dark urine, and increased thirst and skin turgor.

▶ Teach your patient about the signs and symptoms of electrolyte imbalances.

Macrobiotic diet

The macrobiotic diet (from the Greek "macro," meaning great or large, and "bios," meaning life — hence, "the great view of life") originated in Japan in the middle of the 20th century, not as a cure for any disease but as a lifestyle aimed at enhancing physical and spiritual well-being. It consists primarily of whole-grain cereals, such as wheat, barley, buckwheat, and brown rice, as well as fresh organic vegetables, beans, and nuts. The central concept of this diet is "balance equals health" — a belief that optimal health is the natural result of eating, thinking, and living in balance. The concept of balance extends not only to the selection of foods, but also to their preparation, in an attempt to achieve a harmonious combination of textures, colors, and flavors.

Today, the macrobiotic diet plan is one of the most widely practiced alternative nutritional regimens in the United States, used by healthy people to maintain good health and by patients with serious illnesses, such as cancer, who haven't been helped by conventional therapy or who are combining the diet with conventional medical treatments. Here, we will focus on its use as a cancer therapy.

Basic elements

The original macrobiotic diet was developed by a Japanese teacher, George Ohsawa (1893-1966), who reportedly recovered from a serious illness by changing from the refined diet that had been gaining popularity in Japan to the traditional Japanese diet consisting primarily of brown rice, sea vegetables, and miso soup (made from soybeans). Ohsawa believed that a simple diet was the key to good health. His plan proceeded in 10 stages, from least stringent (30% vegetables, 15% fruits and salads, 30% animal products, 10% grains, 10% soups, 5% desserts, and few beverages) to most stringent (60% grains, 30% vegetables, 10% soups).

> 66 *Proponents view the macrobiotic plan not simply as a diet but as a 'commonsense approach to daily living'.* 99

In the 1970s, Michio Kushi, one of Ohsawa's students, took the helm of the macrobiotic movement in the United States. He replaced the 10-stage program with the standard macrobiotic diet practiced today. (See *Basic elements of the macrobiotic diet.*) This essentially vegan regimen emphasizes the intake of complex carbohydrates, high-fiber foods, unsaturated fats, and unrefined foods. Proponents view the plan not simply as a diet but as a "commonsense approach to daily living."

By the early 1980s, a number of books (including *The Cancer Prevention Diet* by Kushi) were beginning to claim that the macrobiotic diet could be used not only to enhance well-being but also to prevent cancer and even induce remission. Since then, numerous reports have appeared in the popular media claiming cancer cures after patients switched to the macrobiotic diet.

Underlying principles. Proponents believe that cancer is the result of prolonged exposure to dietary and environmental "toxins," a sedentary lifestyle, and other social and personal factors, most of which are attributable to the patient's own

Basic elements of the macrobiotic diet

The standard macrobiotic diet is adjusted for each individual, depending on a number of factors, such as season, geography, and personal factors. Its basic elements include the following:

▶ 50% to 60% organically grown, cooked whole grains (brown rice, barley, bulgur, millet, oats, corn, rye, wheat, buckwheat, and limited partially processed grains)

▶ 25% to 30% organically grown, mostly cooked vegetables, classified as those that should be eaten frequently (cabbage, broccoli, cauliflower, bok choy, carrots, pumpkin, collard and dandelion greens, and most types of squash, among others); those that should be eaten occasionally (mushrooms, celery, cucumbers, iceberg lettuce, snow peas, string beans); and those that should be avoided completely (tomatoes, potatoes, eggplant, zucchini, spinach, asparagus, peppers, avocadoes, beets)

▶ 5% to 10% (1 or 2 bowls daily) soups made of vegetables, seaweed, grains, or beans, seasoned with miso or tamari soy sauce

▶ 5% to 10% beans (chickpeas, lentils, azuki beans), bean products (tofu, tempeh), and sea vegetables (wakame, hiziki, kombu, nori)

▶ occasional intake ("if needed or desired") of fresh white fish (flounder, haddock, scrod, snapper, sole, cod, trout, halibut); organically grown, local fruits (dry or cooked); seeds and nuts; vinegars

▶ nonstimulating teas or plain water (no ice)

▶ avoidance of meat and poultry, animal fat, eggs, dairy products, refined sugar, chocolate, tropical fruits, soda, coffee and caffeinated tea, hot spices, alcohol, and all refined, processed, chemically treated, canned, frozen, or irradiated foods.

The recommended cooking methods are boiling, steaming, pressure cooking, nishime (waterless cooking), water sautéing, pressing, and pickling. Foods must be cooked over gas or in a wood-burning stove, and utensils must be made of natural materials. Copper and aluminum pots should be avoided.

When used to treat cancer, the diet is modified according to the principles of *yin* and *yang* that are central to Oriental medicine. First, the cancer is classified as primarily yin or yang, depending on where in the body the primary tumor occurs. Then different foods and cooking styles are recommended, based on this classification.

unhealthful practices. Macrobiotic counselors use traditional Chinese medicine's concepts of yin and yang to explain cancer development and to provide a framework for cancer treatment.

They maintain that the primary factor responsible for cancer is the consumption of foods that are too yin (expansive) or too yang (contractive). Extremely yin foods include dairy products, tropical fruits, refined sugar, coffee, and alcohol; extremely yang foods include meat, poultry, fish, salty foods, cheese, and eggs. Whole-grain foods are considered ideal — neither too yin nor too yang.

Cancers are also classified as predominantly yin or yang (or a combination), depending on where the primary tumor originated. Tumors located in peripheral or upper areas (esophagus, breast, upper stomach, and outer parts of brain) as well as lymphoma and leukemia are considered yin; those in deeper or lower regions (colon, rectum, pancreas, prostate, ovaries, bone, inner parts of brain) are considered yang. Once the cancer is classified, the diet is modified appropriately — for example, by emphasizing yang foods for yin cancers, and vice versa — to bring yin and yang back into balance within the body. Additional measures include engaging in regular exercise; avoiding electromagnetic radiation, chemical fumes, and synthetic fabrics; and maintaining a positive attitude.

RESEARCH SUMMARY In his book, Kushi says cancers of the breast, colon, cervix, pancreas, liver, bone, and skin have responded best to macrobiotics. Despite substantial anecdotal evidence, to date there's no clinical data in support of these claims.

Most mainstream physicians and nutritionists are skeptical about claims that the macrobiotic diet (or any other diet) can cure cancer or other diseases. However, Dr. Barrie Cassileth, a founding member of the OAM's Advisory Council and currently affiliated with Harvard Medical School, says that certain aspects of the diet "have merit if not carried to extremes." Like other low-fat diets, she says, the macrobiotic diet can lower weight, blood pressure, and cholesterol levels and may help prevent heart disease and possibly certain cancers. However, like other vegetarian diets, it requires the use of supplements to make up for certain nutritional deficiencies.

A 1993 editorial in the *Journal of the American College of Nutrition* suggests that the macrobiotic diet may be worth examining as a treatment for cancer *because* of its nutritional inadequacy, noting that "a nutritional regimen clearly deficient in growth-promoting substances might actually be helpful in controlling otherwise untreatable diseases." ■

Complications

Although the standard macrobiotic diet allows small amounts of fish, people who forego all dairy products and meats may develop frank deficiencies of calcium, vitamin B_{12}, and vitamin D. To replace minerals, sea vegetables are used in cooking. Sesame seeds, used as a condiment, are also high in calcium. For children, who need vitamin D for proper growth and development, Kushi advocates fish liver oils, exposure to sunlight, and other foods that contain the vitamin. For teenagers and adults, he advises exposure to sunlight and no supplements unless deficiencies develop.

Nursing perspective

If your patient is on a macrobiotic diet, suggest that he have blood tests periodically to check for anemia (from protein deficiency) and vitamin and iron deficiencies.

Diets for cardiovascular disease

According to the National Center for Health Statistics, cardiovascular disease is the leading cause of death and disability in the United States, killing nearly as many people as all other diseases combined. Nearly 3% of the population have clinical coronary artery disease, and 30% of the adult population have high blood pressure, a risk factor for stroke and heart disease.

Researchers have known for years that a low-fat diet may play a key role in preventing cardiovascular disease but, until recently, the medical community hadn't considered diet a viable treatment for chronic heart conditions. In the 1970s, when Nathan Pritikin first proposed that a low-fat, low-cholesterol diet, combined with exercise, could reduce the symptoms of heart disease, he was ridiculed by the medical community. A decade later, when Dean Ornish made the same claim, he was taken more seriously for two reasons: He was a medical physician, and he had "before" and "after" angiograms of arterial blockages to prove his contentions. The Pritikin and Ornish plans are discussed below.

Pritikin program

The Pritikin program, named after its founder, is essentially a dietary regimen combined with regular exercise. The diet is very low in fat (less than 10% of daily calories), low in cholesterol, and high in complex carbohydrates. The program also calls for 45 minutes of walking daily.

> *Although the medical community rejected Pritikin's basic theory for years, today the American Heart Association and the medical community as a whole have accepted the link between diet, exercise, and heart disease.*

Nathan Pritikin, a layman, began to study heart disease in the early 1960s, when his cardiologist told him he was at high risk for death from myocardial infarction (MI). He developed a low-fat diet similar to that of the people of Uganda, who had practically no incidence of MI-related death. After a few years on the diet, Pritikin's symptoms abated and he decided that the diet had saved his life. In the late 1960s, he founded his clinic in Santa Monica to treat other patients with heart disease.

Although the medical community rejected Pritikin's basic theory for years, today the American Heart Association and the medical community as a whole have accepted the link between diet, exercise, and heart disease. The Pritikin Longevity Center, now run by Pritikin's son, Robert, offers a 26-day program to initiate patients to the plan and teach them how to prepare meals and exercise.

Basic elements

The Pritikin program consists of a diet that's high in complex carbohydrates and fiber, low in cholesterol, and extremely low in fat. The diet allows 3½ oz (99 g) of animal protein (lean chicken or fish) as well as two glasses of skim milk daily. The program also calls for a 45-minute walk every day.

RESEARCH SUMMARY A 1983 report in the *Journal of Cardiac Rehabilitation* documented the results of a 5-year follow-up study of 64 patients with heart disease who participated in the

Pritikin program in lieu of undergoing bypass surgery. According to the report, 80% of the participants still hadn't had the surgery 5 years later. A 1990 analysis of 4,587 participants in the Pritikin residential program showed an average decrease of 23% in total and low-density lipoprotein cholesterol and a 33% drop in triglyceride levels.

The Pritikin diet has also shown promise in controlling newly diagnosed cases of type 2 diabetes without drugs. ∎

Complications

Unlike some more restrictive diets, the Pritikin diet provides adequate protein; however, it might result in a deficiency of iron or other nutrients.

Nursing perspective

▶ Because this diet is extremely low in fats, suggest that your patient take a multivitamin while on the plan to ensure that he receives enough vitamins and other nutrients.

▶ Some people who have been on the plan for 1 or 2 years have noted the appearance of white vertical ridges on the nails, which may be a sign of an iron or vitamin deficiency. Suggest that your patient have his blood tested periodically to detect such deficiencies. He may require supplements.

▶ People who are allergic to gluten, the protein portion of grains, would have difficulty maintaining the Pritikin diet because of its emphasis on whole grains.

Ornish program

Even more restrictive than the Pritikin program, the Ornish program evolved from a series of studies done in the late 1970s and early 1980s by Dean Ornish, an assistant clinical professor of medicine at the University of California, San Francisco. In what came to be known as the Lifestyle Heart Trial, Ornish studied the effects of diet and lifestyle modification on patients with confirmed heart disease. Early studies showed that after only 30 days on the program, patients showed a marked reduction in cholesterol levels, blood pressure, and the frequency of angina as well as increased blood flow to the heart and an improved capacity for exercise. A longer, 1-year study confirmed the early results.

Ornish's program consists of three components: a low-fat vegetarian diet, regular exercise, and stress management techniques. Because Ornish is a medical physician and had before-and-after angiograms to support his contentions, the medical community has been more receptive to his program than to the ideas of Pritikin, a layman. Ornish's findings have also received much attention in the popular media.

Basic elements

Ornish's diet provides about 1,800 calories per day: 75% from carbohydrates and less than 10% from fats. It allows no meat, fish, or poultry (unlike the Pritikin diet, which allows some chicken or fish); no caffeine, nuts, seeds, or fat (even for cooking); and no egg yolks or dairy products, except for a cup of nonfat milk or yogurt daily. The diet allows 2 oz (60 ml) of alcohol daily.

The plan also calls for at least 1 hour of walking three times per week, regular meditation or yoga to reduce stress, and support group sessions for emotional support.

RESEARCH SUMMARY Ornish's 1-year randomized, controlled study of patients with partially blocked arteries followed 28 patients who were put on the Ornish program and 20 who received conventional care. After 1 year, those on the Ornish regimen reported significant decreases in angina frequency (91%), duration (42%), and severity (28%). In contrast, the control group receiving usual care reported significant increases in these three parameters. Angiograms showed an overall reduction of arterial blockages in patients on the Ornish plan and a progression of blockages in the control group.

In the late 1980s, a 3-year British study of patients with blocked arteries and high cholesterol showed that those on a fat-restricted diet (allowing up to 27% fat) suffered only one-third as many heart attacks, strokes, and deaths as those who were allowed to eat their usual diet. ■

Complications

Some nutrition experts believe the Ornish diet is too low in fats and protein and might lead to nutritional deficiencies. However, the plan's benefits in reversing atherosclerosis may outweigh any perceived drawbacks for patients with heart disease.

Nursing perspective

If your patient is on the Ornish plan, suggest that he have blood tests done periodically to detect anemia or iron and vitamin deficiencies. He may require supplements.

Coenzyme Q10

The vitamin supplement coenzyme Q10 (Co Q10) is believed to improve the heart's ability to recover from disease and stress. Co Q10 is a lipid-soluble benzoquinone that's structurally related to vitamin K. It's found in every cell in the body, and acts as a free radical scavenger and membrane stabilizer. It's also an important cofactor in electron transport in the mitochondria.

In 1957, Dr. Frederick Crane from Wisconsin first isolated Co Q10 from beef heart mitochondria. The pharmaceutical company Merck was able to synthesize Co Q10 in 1958. It was first used for medicinal purposes in the mid-1960s in Japan in the treatment of heart failure.

RESEARCH SUMMARY Patients with heart failure have significantly lower levels of Co Q10 in heart muscle cells than healthy people. This fact alone doesn't prove that Co Q10 supplements will help treat heart failure; however, it has prompted medical researchers to try using Co Q10 as a treatment for heart failure. Several double-blind studies have found that Co Q10 supplements, when taken along with conventional medication, can markedly improve symptoms and objective measurements of heart function. ■

Therapeutic uses

Co Q10 is used to treat ischemic heart disease, hypertension, and heart failure. It's also used in the treatment of acquired immunodeficiency syndrome (AIDS), muscular dystrophy, and chronic fatigue syndrome. Co Q10 is used to protect against doxorubicin cardiotoxicity and to protect the myocardium during invasive cardiac surgery. It may also stimulate the production of blood cells. Low levels of Co Q10 have been found in patients with breast cancer, periodontal diseases, diabetes, and heart disease.

RESEARCH SUMMARY Co Q10 has been studied in many countries. Its use was studied in the treatment of over 2,600 patients with heart failure in Italy (Baggio et al.). Co Q10 proved to be a safe and effective treatment for heart failure. A randomized, double-blind trial of 144 patients who had suffered an acute myocardial infarction in India was done with Co Q10. The Co Q10 group showed significant reduction in angina, arrhythmias, and left ventricular dysfunction as well as noninfarction and cardiac deaths. ■

Procedure
Co Q10 is for oral use. The typical dosage is 30 to 300 mg daily with dosages above 100 mg taken in divided doses, two to three times per day.

Complications
Adverse effects associated with the use of Co Q10, though rare, include epigastric discomfort, loss of appetite, nausea, and diarrhea. Beta-adrenergic blockers may inhibit Co Q10-dependent enzymes. Hydroxymethylglutaryl coenzyme A (HMG-CoA) reductase inhibitors and gemfibrozil may decrease levels of Co Q10. Co Q10 may decrease insulin requirements in patients with type 1 diabetes mellitus. International normalized ratio may decrease when warfarin is used with Co Q10. Oral hypoglycemics decrease serum Co Q10 levels, whereas food maximizes its absorption.

Those with a hypersensitivity to Co Q10 and patients who are pregnant or breast-feeding should avoid use.

Nursing perspective
▶ Monitor vital signs and electrocardiogram results as needed.

▶ Warn your patient not to treat signs and symptoms of heart failure — such as increasing shortness of breath, edema, or chest pain — with Co Q10 before seeking appropriate medical evaluation because doing so may delay diagnosis of a potentially serious medical condition.

▶ Advise your patient who has heart failure that Co Q10 shouldn't replace conventional drug therapy. Encourage him to discuss use of Co Q10 with his health care provider so treatment may be properly monitored.

▶ If your patient is pregnant or breast-feeding, advise her not to use Co Q10.

▶ If your patient is diabetic, alert him to the signs and symptoms of hypoglycemia and hyperglycemia, and instruct him to monitor his blood glucose level.

▶ Instruct your patient to inform his health care provider if he's taking a cholesterol lowering or heart drug, an anticoagulant, or insulin.

▶ Tell your patient to remind his prescriber and pharmacist of any herbal or dietary supplement he's taking when obtaining a new prescription.

▶ Advise your patient to consult his health care provider before using an herbal preparation because a treatment with proven efficacy may be available.

> ❝ *Fasts theoretically provide a resting period for the digestive system. While it rests, the excretion of toxins continues and no new toxins are being introduced to the body.* ❞

Fasting

Proponents of fasting, the restriction of dietary intake to liquids, say that fasting is a way of ridding the body of toxins while promoting healing. Because the body expends a great deal of energy breaking down food, fasts — usually lasting from 2 to 5 days — theoretically provide a resting period for the body. While the digestive system rests, the excretion of toxins continues and no new toxins are being introduced to the body. In addition to its healing effects on the body, proponents claim fasting can also promote mental and spiritual well-being.

Fasting has been practiced in many cultures for centuries. Ancient cultures used fasts not for weight loss or detoxification, but as a means of self-deprivation for religious purposes. Today, Islam and Judaism still require fasting on certain holidays.

All fasting regimens allow fluids — water, juices, or herbal teas. Many naturopathic physicians recommend fasting, usually twice a year for 5 days, as part of a regular health maintenance program. Some recommend a vegetable juice fast, while others consider juice a food and recommend water only. (See "Juice therapy," page 383.)

Therapeutic uses

Advocates believe that fasting enables the body to cleanse the liver, kidneys, and colon; flush out toxins; and purify the blood. They say that the energy the body saves during a fast can be redirected to other functions, such as revitalizing the immune system. Some of the conditions they suggest may benefit from fasting include hypertension, arthritis, food allergies (identification and elimination), inflammatory diseases, and headaches.

RESEARCH SUMMARY A 13-month Norwegian study on patients with rheumatoid arthritis showed a significant improvement in patients who fasted for 7 to 10 days and then followed a special vegetarian diet. The therapeutic benefits exceeded what might have been expected from elimination of food allergens alone. However, there's only a small amount of evidence to relate findings to all patients with rheumatoid arthritis. ■

Procedure

Therapeutic fasting regimens vary according to the philosophy of the practitioner and the purpose of the fast. The patient usually must undergo some form of preparation before beginning the fast, such as eating raw fruits and vegetables or drinking certain fluids for a prescribed amount of time. For example, he may be instructed to drink a specified amount of water along with pure juices and two to three cups of herbal tea each day.

The practitioner will determine the duration and type (water or juice) of fast that is appropriate for the patient. Most practitioners recommend a 2- to 3-day fast, although longer fasts are sometimes used. Those who prefer a water fast usually recommend drinking at least three glasses of distilled or spring water daily. Those who prefer a juice fast say that it's less stressful to the body. They say that pure water fasting can release toxins too quickly, resulting in headaches, and that juice provides necessary nutrients and prevents low blood glucose levels. Vegetable juices are preferable to fruit juices, which contain large amounts of sugar.

Reintroducing food

Patients coming off a fast should eat frequent small meals rather than a heavy meal because the GI system needs time to replenish digestive juices. Patients should also avoid eating highly refined or spicy foods to prevent diarrhea, vomiting, or abdominal pain. The longer the fast, the more consideration and care are needed in reintroducing food. Water fasts are usually broken with fruit or vegetable juices; solid foods are reintroduced gradually. Juice fasts are usually followed by a 2-day diet of fresh raw fruits and vegetables.

Complications
Rather than enhancing the immune system, fasting may impair it by depriving the body of essential nutrients, according to mainstream physicians. In addition, when blood glucose levels decline, the body starts breaking down muscle to provide energy. This muscle breakdown results in increased production of ammonia and nitrogen, leaving the patient weak, tired, and nauseated.

Other adverse effects may include dry skin or skin eruptions, headaches, dizziness, irritability, coated tongue, foul-smelling stools, body aches, and mucous discharge. (Fasting advocates say these symptoms are signs that toxins are leaving the body.) More serious complications, such as cardiac arrhythmias (from electrolyte imbalances), anemia, hypotension, and bradycardia, have also been reported. The longer the fast, the more dangerous it becomes.

Nursing perspective
▶ Urge patients to consult their physicians before beginning any type of fast. This is especially important for patients with health problems and those taking prescribed medications. Dosage requirements may change during a fast.
▶ Fasting is contraindicated for patients with diabetes, eating disorders, epilepsy, kidney disease, severe bronchial asthma, stomach ulcers, ulcerative colitis, tuberculosis, or malnutrition. It's also not recommended for children, elderly people, or women who are pregnant or breast-feeding.
▶ If you're caring for a patient who is fasting, advise him to notify his physician if he experiences any adverse reactions, especially potentially life-threatening ones such as an irregular heartbeat.

Juice therapy
According to advocates of juice therapy, drinking the fresh, raw juice of vegetables and fruits is an effective method of nourishing and detoxifying the body, stimulating the immune system, and even treating certain health problems. Juice therapy is commonly used as a component of, or complement to,

fasting, but it can also serve as a dietary supplement during times of stress or as part of a regular health maintenance program.

> 66 *Proponents say that juices have certain advantages over raw fruits and vegetables because they require less energy to digest and are more easily absorbed in the body.* 99

Proponents say that juices have certain advantages over raw fruits and vegetables because they require less energy to digest and are more easily absorbed in the body. What's more, the breakdown of fiber that occurs in the juicing process allows the body to absorb ingredients that would otherwise be excreted. Critics and most nutritionists, on the other hand, say that fiber is an essential and beneficial component of raw produce that's necessary for proper bowel function and elimination.

Therapeutic uses

Because they contain the same health-enhancing phytochemicals that fresh fruits and vegetables contain, juices provide similar health benefits — such as protection against chronic degenerative diseases — with regular use. However, specific juices are also believed to have medicinal attributes that make them useful in treating certain conditions, such as the following:

▶ citrus — iron deficiency (from vitamin C)
▶ apple — laxative effect (from sorbitol)
▶ lemon — appetite-stimulating effect
▶ cherry — treatment of gout
▶ pineapple — anti-inflammatory effects (from enzyme bromelain)
▶ cranberry, blueberry — prevention of urinary tract infections.

Juices can be a useful source of nutrition for patients who are weak or have difficulty eating, such as those with cancer or acquired immunodeficiency syndrome.

Equipment

Because juicing advocates recommend fresh-squeezed juice made from organic produce, a juice extractor is necessary.

Fresh juice should also become more widely available in health food, specialty, and grocery stores and juice bars.

Procedure

Whenever possible, organically grown produce should be used to ensure the optimal nutritional benefit and prevent ingestion of pesticides and other chemicals. (Bananas, strawberries, green beans, and apples tend to have high pesticide residues.) If this isn't possible, the produce should be washed using a vegetable brush. (A dilute dishwashing liquid or a vegetable wash solution, available in grocery stores, can be used.)

Many different juice recipes are available; some use a variety of fruits or vegetables to provide specific health benefits. For example, an iron-rich juice made with beets, carrots, green pepper, and apples could benefit an anemic person. Juices made from green vegetables (such as dandelion greens, spinach, celery, and alfalfa sprouts) are believed to promote detoxification. Fresh apple or carrot juice may be added to dilute or sweeten a green drink.

Juicers are widely available. Generally, a juicer with a heavy, strong motor is best, especially when juicing root vegetables. Other things to consider when purchasing a juicer are ease of cleaning, the size of the feed hole, and the store's refund policy.

Most produce can be placed in the juicer with the leaves, stems, and skin intact. However, certain precautions should be followed when juicing some fruits and vegetables. (See *Juicing precautions,* page 386.) After juicing, the fresh juice should be consumed immediately to prevent loss of nutrients. Some juicing advocates recommend drinking fruit and vegetable juices several hours apart to minimize gas and enhance digestion.

Complications

Some juices are strong stimulants to the liver and gallbladder and may have a laxative effect.

Nursing perspective

▶ Infants, young children, elderly people, and patients with diabetes shouldn't use juice therapy unless under the care of a physician.

Juicing precautions

If your patient is on a juice therapy regimen, make sure he's aware of the following precautions associated with certain fruits and vegetables:

▶ Remove the rinds of oranges and grapefruit because they are bitter and contain toxic substances.

▶ Don't use the core of the apple because the seeds contain cyanide. (Most other seeds are safe to use.)

▶ Remove carrot and rhubarb greens before juicing because they contain toxic substances.

▶ Always remove the skins of tropical fruits, such as papayas, kiwis, and mangos, because they may contain harmful fungicides and pesticides that are illegal to use in the United States and Canada but permitted in foreign countries.

▶ Very sweet juices (such as those made from grapes, pears, apples, and carrots) can cause bloating and gas and may be hard to digest. Diluting them with equal parts water or a less-sweet juice is advisable.

▶ When juicing potatoes, avoid those with a green tint, because this indicates the presence of the chemical solanine, which may cause abdominal pain, vomiting, and diarrhea.

▶ To prevent GI discomfort, consume green juices gradually and in moderation.

▶ Juice fasts aren't recommended for women who are pregnant or breast-feeding.

▶ Juices may be contraindicated for patients with hyperglycemia or hypoglycemia.

▶ Patients should avoid fruits or vegetables to which they're allergic.

▶ Inform your patient that juices aren't considered a substitute for whole fruits and vegetables but should be considered a supplement to a regular diet.

▶ Make sure your patient understands that frozen, canned, or bottled juices aren't recommended for juice therapy because they contain preservatives and other chemicals that decrease nutritional value. Also, the high temperatures that are part of the pasteurizing process destroy the enzymes in the juice. To ensure optimal benefits, individuals should make their own juice with fresh, organic fruits and vegetables.

▶ Advise your patient to be suspicious of marketers who promise miraculous cures or rejuvenation from juice.

Enzyme therapy

Enzymes are protein molecules that act as catalysts or initiators for most of the biochemical reactions that occur in the body. Without these initiators, cells and tissues would be unable to perform all the biochemical reactions required to meet the body's needs.

Enzymes are essential for digestion, tissue repair, and cellular energy. Digestive enzymes break down food for energy, while other enzymes convert this energy for use by the body. Still other types of enzymes may help coagulate blood, help the lungs expel carbon dioxide, and help convert nutrients to make new tissue for muscles, nerve cells, bones, and skin. Vitamins, minerals, and hormones couldn't do their work without enzymes.

The enzymes used for digestion are produced by the salivary glands, stomach, pancreas, and small intestine; at each step in the process, certain enzymes break down specific types of food. The four main categories of digestive enzymes are amylase, protease, lipase, and cellulase. *Amylase* breaks down carbohydrates and is found in saliva and digestive and pancreatic juices. *Protease* helps digest protein and is found in pancreatic and stomach juices. *Lipase* aids in fat digestion and is found in stomach and pancreatic juices. *Cellulase* digests fiber and must be consumed from plants because the body is unable to make it.

Conventional medical doctors prescribe enzyme replacement therapy to treat specific enzyme deficiencies, such as lactase deficiency, and chronic diseases that affect the digestive process, such as cystic fibrosis. However, alternative therapy practitioners believe that enzyme supplements can be used to treat conditions that are unrelated to enzyme deficiencies. They believe that taking enzyme supplements strengthen the digestive system and that a properly functioning digestive system can help prevent and remedy a variety of acute and chronic health problems. Enzyme therapy makes use of both pancreatic and plant-derived enzymes.

Therapeutic uses

Proponents of enzyme therapy say that pancreatic enzyme supplements are useful in treating viral disorders (by digesting the virus's protein coating) and cancer (by dissolving the cancer cells' outer coating, allowing white blood cells to destroy them). There have also been reports of improvement in patients with multiple sclerosis. Some athletes take pancreatic enzymes after an injury to promote inflammation and thus accelerate healing.

Plant enzymes are said to relieve digestive disorders, sore throats, hay fever, and candidiasis. Practitioners may also prescribe specific enzymes to assist in protein, carbohydrate, or fat digestion, depending on an individual's health needs.

RESEARCH SUMMARY There's no scientific evidence to support the use of enzyme supplements to treat serious diseases, such as cancer or multiple sclerosis. Both consumer groups and the Food and Drug Administration have condemned companies that tout enzyme supplements as cures for such diseases. ■

Procedure

Enzymes are given with meals if the purpose is to aid digestion. When used for other problems, they're given between meals so they won't be used for breaking down food. Enzyme therapy practitioners also encourage patients to eat a whole food diet with large amounts of raw fruits and vegetables because cooking can destroy plant enzymes.

The strength of some enzymes may be reported using different units. Caution the patient to compare potency of different brands with the amount per capsule.

Complications

Enzyme therapy may cause adverse GI reactions, such as nausea, vomiting, diarrhea, or obstruction.

Nursing perspective

▶ Patients with pancreatitis, acute exacerbation of chronic pancreatic disease, or a known hypersensitivity to pork protein should avoid pancreatic enzyme therapy.

▶ If your patient is considering taking enzyme supplements for a disorder unrelated to enzyme deficiency, advise him that there's no scientific support for such treatment.

Selected references

Adams, C. *Living Among Meat Eaters: The Vegetarian's Survival Handbook.* New York: Three Rivers Press, 2001.

"Alternative Medicine," *Harvard Health Letter* 25(11):1, September 2000.

Alternative Medicine: Expanding Medical Horizons. A report to the National Institutes of Health on Alternative Medical Systems and Practices in the United States. Prepared under the auspices of the Workshop on Alternative Medicine, Chantilly, Va., September 14-16, 1992. NIH pub. 94-066. Washington, D.C.: U.S. Government Printing Office, 1994.

Balch, P.A., and Balch, J.F., *Prescription for Nutritional Healing: A-to-Z Guide to Supplements,* 3rd ed. Garden City Park, N.Y.: Avery Publishing Group, 2000.

Calabresi, P. "Medical Alternatives to Alternative Medicine," *Cancer* 86(10):1887-889, November 1999.

Challem, J., ed. *FAQs: All About Carotenoids: Beta-carotene, Leutein and Lycopene.* New York: Avery Penguin Putnam, 1999.

Dunne, L. *Nutrition Almanac,* 5th ed. New York: McGraw-Hill Book Co., 2002.

"Flavonoids, the Next New Thing?" *Harvard Health Letter* 26(2):6, December 2000.

Gerson, M.B. *A Cancer Therapy: Results of Fifty Cases: A Summary of 30 Years of Clinical Experimentation.* Barrytown, N.Y.: Station Hill Press, 1997.

Jensen, B. *Dr. Jensen's Guide to Body Chemistry and Nutrition.* Los Angeles: Keats Publishing, 2000.

King, L.A., and Carr, B.R. "Phytoestrogens: Fact and Fiction," *Patient Care* 33(6):127-28, 130-32, 134, 143, March 1999.

Kushi, M., and Jack, A. *The Cancer Prevention Diet,* rev. ed. New York: St. Martin Press, 1993.

LeMarchand, L., et al. "Intake of Flavonoids and Lung Cancer," *Journal of the National Cancer Institute* 92(2):154-60, January 2000.

Micozzi, M. *Fundamentals of Complementary and Alternative Medicines,* 2nd ed. St. Louis: Mosby–Year Book, Inc., 2001.

Morita, K., et al. "A Desmutagenic Factor Isolated from Burdock," *Mutation Research* 129(1):25-31, October 1984.

Muirhead, G. "CAM Strategies to Promote Wellness," *Patient Care* 33(18):143-45, 149-50, 155-58 passim., November 1999.

Muller, H., et al. "Fasting Followed by Vegetarian Diet in Patients with Rheumatoid Arthritis: A Systematic Review," *Scandanavian Journal of Rheumatology* 30(1):1-10, 2001.

Pelletier, K.R. *The Best Alternative Medicine: What Works? What Does Not?* New York: Simon and Schuster, 2000.

"Phytoestrogens," *Harvard Women's Health Watch* 7(3):4-5, November 1999.

Pritikin, N., and McGrady, P. *The Pritikin Program for Diet and Exercise.* New York: Bantam Books, 1984.

Pritikin, R. *The Pritikin Weight Loss Breakthrough: Five Easy Steps to Outsmart Your Fat Instinct.* New York: Dutton, 1998.

Rosenfeld, I. *Dr. Rosenfeld's Guide to Alternative Medicine: What Works, What Doesn't, and What's Right for You.* New York: Random House, 1996.

Ulene, A., ed. *The NutriBase Nutrition Facts Desk Reference,* 2nd ed. New York: Avery, 2001.

World Health Organization. *Diet, Nutrition, and the Prevention of Chronic Diseases. Report of a WHO Study Group* (Technical Report Series 797). Geneva: World Health Organization, 1990.

Internet resources

Alternative Therapies in Health and Medicine: *www.alternative-therapies.com*

HealthWorld on Line: *www.healthy.net*

Journal of Alternative and Complementary Medicine (available online with subscription): *www.catchword.com/titles/1075535.html*

National Center for Complementary and Alternative Medicine: *www.nccam.nih.gov*

Quack Watch: *www.quackwatch.com*

10

Pharmacologic and biological therapies

A lternative pharmacologic and biological treatments differ from other types of alternative and complementary therapies in that they use active biological or chemical compounds and are generally invasive. The substances used range from the essential oils used in aromatherapy to shark cartilage and antineoplastons used to treat cancer.

Points of view regarding these treatments' safety and efficacy vary widely. Proponents see them as nontoxic, natural compounds that offer hope for patients with life-threatening diseases that mainstream medicine has been unable to conquer, such as cancer and acquired immunodeficiency syndrome (AIDS). Critics, including the medical community, regard them as questionable remedies with no reliable scientific evidence proving their effectiveness, especially as "cures" for cancer or AIDS. In addition, they fear that these treatments will deter seriously ill patients from seeking conventional medical care, which could result in disease progression.

Most pharmacologic and biological therapies are taught in postgraduate seminars. The American College for Advancement in Medicine and the American Academy of Environmental Medicine offer courses in a number of them.

The role of the nurse trained in pharmacologic and biological therapies is to administer the therapies, assist other trained persons in administering them, counsel patients who are using the therapies, and inform those interested in the therapies.

Apitherapy

Products derived from honeybees — including bee venom and raw honey — have been used for therapeutic purposes since ancient times. The Greek physician Hippocrates is said to have treated joint problems with bee venom. Today, proponents of apitherapy claim that this type of therapy can be used to treat a wide range of disorders, including arthritis and multiple sclerosis.

The most popular form of apitherapy used today is bee venom, administered either by injection or live bee stings, to treat chronic inflammatory disorders such as arthritis. Proponents claim that the venom works by stimulating the immune system: The inflammation that occurs at the injection site triggers the production of anti-inflammatory substances that help relieve the pain and swelling from the venom and, simultaneously, the pain and inflammation from the arthritis. Other bee products available as pills or capsules are bee pollen, raw honey, royal jelly, beeswax, and propolis (the "glue" used to cement the hive).

The American Apitherapy Society in Red Bank, New Jersey, collects and disseminates information on this treatment and provides a forum for researchers to present their findings in a quarterly newsletter.

Therapeutic uses

Apitherapy advocates claim that bee venom can alleviate low back pain, the chronic pain associated with arthritis, tendinitis, fibromyalgia, migraine headaches, and the symptoms of multiple sclerosis and dermatologic conditions, such as psoriasis and eczema. It's also used to desensitize people to bee stings. Bee pollen and raw honey are said to increase energy and endurance when ingested. In China, raw honey is applied to burns as an analgesic and antiseptic. Other claims made for bee pollen are that it can fight infection, relieve allergies, and slow the aging process.

Propolis is used orally for tuberculosis and infections and for its anti-inflammatory effects. It's also used topically for cleaning wounds. Beeswax is reported to help lower lipids and relieve ulcers. It's a common ingredient in soaps, cosmetics, and foods. Both propolis and beeswax are used in skin care products.

> ❝ Presumably based on its effects on the queen bee, proponents and marketers of royal jelly claim it can increase energy and stimulate immune function in humans. ❞

Royal jelly is the substance that worker bees secrete and then feed to a female bee, which then becomes queen. After ingesting the royal jelly, the queen becomes twice as large as the other bees, is able to lay 2,000 eggs per day, and her life span increases from 3 months to 5 years. Presumably based on these effects on the queen bee, proponents and marketers of royal jelly claim it can increase energy and stimulate immune function in humans.

RESEARCH SUMMARY Most of the evidence in support of bee products for therapeutic purposes consists of anecdotal reports collected by the American Apitherapy Society, rather than the results of controlled scientific experiments. The medical community doesn't accept such reports as proof of efficacy. ■

Procedure
Some apitherapists inject venom using a hypodermic needle, but most prefer to use live bee stings. This treatment involves repeated bee stings administered at specific sites (depending on the condition) for a given time period — for example, 4 to 8 weeks for arthritis. Some practitioners use electrophoresis or ultrasonophoresis to administer the venom. Other bee products are usually taken orally as capsules, pills, powder, or liquid.

Complications
Bee pollen and royal jelly can cause life-threatening allergic reactions in sensitive individuals. There have also been reports of infants developing botulism after eating raw honey. Bee venom can cause inflammation, itching, and swelling as well as nausea, vomiting, headache, hypotension, and anaphylaxis.

Nursing perspective

▶ If your patient is considering using bee products, caution him about the possibility of allergic reactions.

▶ Inform your patient that bee pollen may contain bee feces and larvae, fungi, and bacteria.

▶ Bee venom is usually from honeybees. Avoid confusion with venom from other related insects.

Aromatherapy

Used since ancient times to heal the body, mind, and spirit, aromatherapy refers to the inhalation or application of essential oils distilled from various plants. These essential oils are extremely concentrated and therefore not administered orally; to do so would tax the liver's ability to metabolize them. Those who use aromatherapy today say it's effective in reducing stress, preventing disease, and even treating certain illnesses, both physical and psychological.

The therapy as we know it today dates back to the work of French chemist René-Maurice Gattefosse in the 1930s. Gattefosse began to study the healing effects of plant oils after burning his hand in his family's perfume factory. He plunged his hand in a container of lavender oil for relief and found that his wound healed quickly and without a scar. This incident sparked his interest in plant oils' possible therapeutic effects, a field he called *aromatherapy*.

Today, aromatherapy is still popular in Europe, where essential oils are inhaled, massaged into the skin, or placed in bath water for specific therapeutic purposes. Specific oils are believed to have either relaxing or stimulating effects. When absorbed by body tissues, they're thought to interact with hormones and enzymes to produce changes in blood pressure, pulse rate, and other physiologic functions. (See *Understanding aromatherapy.*)

Aromatherapy may be self-administered or administered by a practitioner trained in the field. In the United States, where interest in aromatherapy has skyrocketed in the past decade, several organizations train and certify aromatherapists, including the Pacific Institute of Aromatherapy in San Rafael, California, and the National Association of Holistic Aromatherapy in St. Louis, Missouri. These organizations can also pro-

Understanding aromatherapy

Scientists know that humans have an acute sense of smell and that particular smells can evoke vivid memories. But can smells affect physiologic function? Aromatherapists believe they can — through their effects on the limbic system, the part of the brain associated with emotion and memory.

Odors stimulate receptors in the nose, which convert the odors to nerve impulses that are then sent to the limbic system. There, the nerve impulses trigger memories associated with those odors. According to aromatherapy researchers, the emotions that are evoked — joy, sadness, anger, anxiety — can then affect heart rate, blood pressure, breathing, brain wave activity, and the release of hormones that regulate insulin production, body temperature, stress, metabolism, and hunger.

Because the limbic system also affects the nervous system, odors can also stimulate the release of neurotransmitters and endorphins in the brain, affecting emotional well-being.

vide information to interested laymen and health care providers, referrals to aromatherapists, and sources for obtaining essential oils.

Because there's no scientific evidence indicating that aromatherapy prevents or cures disease, it's typically used strictly as a complementary therapy. Nurses trained in aromatherapy may recommend specific oils as adjuncts to conventional therapies, teach patients how to use them, and provide treatments themselves.

Therapeutic uses

Aromatherapists use specific oils — either alone or in conjunction with other therapies such as massage or herbal therapy — to treat specific ailments. Proponents claim that aside from creating pleasant sensations and promoting relaxation, aromatherapy can be used to treat bacterial and viral infections, anxiety, pain, muscle disorders, arthritis, herpes simplex, herpes zoster, skin disorders (such as acne), premenstrual syndrome, headaches, and indigestion. (See *Therapeutic effects of essential oils,* page 396.) Many essential oils

Therapeutic effects of essential oils

This chart lists some popular essential oils and the traditional indications for which practitioners use them.

Essential oil	Traditional therapeutic uses
Chamomile (*Anthemis nobilis*)	▶ Anti-inflammatory, antifungal, and antibacterial effects ▶ Relieving mental or physical stress ▶ Balancing body and mind
Eucalyptus (*Eucalyptus radiata*)	▶ Antiviral and expectorant effects ▶ Relieving nausea and motion sickness ▶ Clearing the sinuses ▶ Soothing irritable bowel ▶ Stimulant effect
Geranium (*Pelargonium x asperum*)	▶ Antiviral and antifungal effects ▶ Stimulating metabolism in the skin ▶ Improving cell generation ▶ Improving circulation ▶ Relieving pain ▶ Improving vital organ function
Lavender (*Lavandula augustifolia*)	▶ Anti-inflammatory and antibacterial effects ▶ Treating burns, insect bites, and minor injuries ▶ Soothing stomachache and colic ▶ Relieving toothache and teething pain ▶ Relieving mental or physical stress
Peppermint (*Mentha piperita*)	▶ Antibacterial and antiviral effects ▶ Decongestant and expectorant effects ▶ Relieving nausea and motion sickness ▶ Soothing irritable bowel ▶ Stimulant effect
Rosemary (*Rosmarinus officinalis*)	▶ Antibacterial, antifungal, and antiviral effects ▶ Restoring energy and alleviating stress ▶ Improving cell regeneration
Tea tree (*Melaleuca alternifolia*)	▶ Anti-inflammatory, antibacterial, and antiviral effects ▶ Treating burns, insect bites, and minor injuries ▶ Calming, sedative effects

slightly lower the pH of the blood. This may create an environment that inhibits the growth of bacteria and partially explain how they work.

RESEARCH SUMMARY Claims that aromatherapy can prevent or treat specific diseases aren't supported by scientific evidence. ■

Equipment
In addition to the appropriate essential oil, aromatherapy may require other supplies, depending on the administration method being used. Massage requires a carrier oil and, for a full-body massage, a massage table. Inhalation requires a bowl of hot water and a large towel. An aromatherapy bath requires a tub filled with warm water. Diffusion requires a micromist or candle diffuser or a ceramic ring that can be placed on a light bulb.

Procedure
Massage involves diluting the essential oil in the appropriate carrier oil and applying it to the exposed body part or the entire body using massage techniques. Bergamot, lemon, orange, grapefruit, and other citrus oils shouldn't be applied before exposure to the sun.

For inhalation therapy, the patient leans over a bowl of steaming water that contains a few drops of the essential oil, keeping his face far enough from the water's surface to avoid a burn injury. With the towel draped over his head and the bowl to concentrate the steam, the patient inhales the vapors for a few minutes.

For a bath, the patient adds a few drops of essential oil to the surface of the bath water and then soaks in the tub for 10 to 20 minutes, inhaling the vapors as he soaks.

Diffusion involves placing a few drops of the essential oil in the diffuser and turning on the heat source to diffuse microparticles of the oil into the air. The patient should be at least 3′ (1 m) away from the diffuser. The average treatment time is 30 minutes.

Complications
Basil, fennel, lemon grass, rosemary, and verbena oils may cause irritation in people with sensitive skin. Very high doses (10 to 20 ml) of certain oils (wintergreen, sage, aniseed,

thyme, lemon, fennel, clove, cinnamon, camphor, and cedar wood) can result in nonlethal poisoning.

Nursing perspective

▶ Aromatherapy is contraindicated during pregnancy because many essential oils can pose a toxic risk to the mother and fetus or, rarely, even trigger spontaneous abortion.

▶ Aromatherapy should be used with caution in infants and children under age 5 because many essential oils are toxic to this age-group. Among these are oils with a high level of terpene, such as rosemary and eucalyptus.

▶ Inform your patients that origanum, sage, savory, thyme, and wintergreen oils are *not* safe for home use.

▶ Advise patients to avoid applying cinnamon or clove oil on the skin and to stop using basil, fennel, lemon grass, rosemary, and verbena oils if skin irritations develop.

▶ Caution patients to keep essential oils away from the eyes and mucous membranes to avoid irritation. If contact occurs, the patient should flush copiously with water; if flushing doesn't relieve the pain, he should seek medical attention.

▶ Instruct patients not to ingest essential oils.

Chelation therapy

Chelation therapy is a chemical process that removes metallic or mineral toxins (such as lead, mercury, copper, iron, arsenic, aluminum, and calcium) from the body by binding them to another substance for elimination. That substance is an amino acid called ethylenediaminetetraacetic acid (EDTA). Administered I.V. by a physician, the EDTA bonds with specific metals and minerals in the body and transports them to the urine for excretion.

> *Proponents claim that chelation therapy can reverse atherosclerosis and possibly prevent the need for angioplasty and bypass surgery.*

Although chelation therapy is an accepted treatment for lead poisoning and other heavy metal toxicities, alternative medicine practitioners claim that it can be used to treat other medical problems, especially coronary artery disease. They believe that EDTA binds to the calcium in arterial plaque and that this compound is then excreted in the urine. In this way, proponents claim, chelation therapy can reverse atherosclerosis and possibly prevent the need for angioplasty and bypass surgery.

In addition, proponents say, EDTA acts as an antioxidant protecting the blood vessels and body tissues from inflammation caused by free radical damage. As a result, they believe it can relieve the pain associated with chronic inflammatory diseases, such as arthritis, lupus, and scleroderma, and even slow the aging process.

In the United States, hundreds of thousands of people currently undergo chelation therapy every year, and more than 1,000 physicians support the use of this therapy for cardiovascular disease (some even use it themselves). The average cost for a course of 20 to 30 treatments is $5,000. The American College for Advancement in Medicine (ACAM) in Laguna Hills, California, has established standards of practice and guidelines for EDTA chelation therapy. Other allied organizations are the American Board of Chelation Therapy in Chicago and the American Holistic Medical Association in Raleigh, North Carolina.

Therapeutic uses

When combined with specialized nutritional supplements, exercise, weight normalization, and dietary changes, proponents claim that EDTA chelation therapy is an effective method of preventing or treating conditions related to atherosclerosis, such as coronary artery disease, myocardial infarction (MI), angina, cerebrovascular accident (CVA), and peripheral vascular disease, and may ultimately prevent associated conditions, such as gangrene and senility.

In addition, this therapy is thought to promote revascularization of the brain after a CVA, of the heart after MI, and of the peripheral circulation in patients with peripheral vascular disease. Through all of its biochemical effects, EDTA may also improve metabolic function.

RESEARCH SUMMARY As with many of the therapies in this book, proponents point to studies they say prove the treatment's effectiveness, while mainstream critics condemn the studies as anecdotal and unscientific.

Many chelationists belong to the ACAM. Their Web site and brochure describing chelation therapy make several claims including "every single study of the use of chelation therapy for atherosclerosis which has been published, without exception, has described an improvement in blood flow and symptoms." In December 1998, this and other claims precipitated the Federal Trade Commission to secure a consent agreement barring ACAM from making unsubstantiated claims of the efficacy of chelation therapy in atherosclerosis or other diseases of the circulatory system.

Dr. George Wyse of the University of Calgary, Alberta, Canada, conducted a 6-monitor trial of chelation therapy for patients with chest pain. He found no benefit, and his results were presented in March 2001, at the meeting of the American College of Cardiology.

The Food and Drug Administration (FDA) hasn't approved EDTA for use in anything other than heavy metal poisoning. The American Heart Association remains skeptical. ■

Equipment

Administration of chelation therapy requires venous access equipment for the placement of a peripheral line and needles or needleless devices and syringes for the administration of EDTA. A prescribed flush solution is needed to clear the line after EDTA administration.

Procedure

EDTA chelation therapy should be administered by a licensed physician as outlined in the protocols of the ACAM. A nurse may insert a peripheral venous access line for EDTA administration. The dosage of EDTA must be individualized for each patient according to age, sex, weight, and renal function.

Chelation therapy is administered on an outpatient basis. The patient reclines in a chair as the infusion is administered. (Vitamins and minerals are usually added to the EDTA solution.) Many studies have been performed to investigate the possibility of oral chelation therapy. However, to date this administration form has been unsuccessful because only 5% to 10% of the EDTA is absorbed orally (whereas 100% of I.V. EDTA is absorbed).

A typical course of treatment involves 20 to 30 sessions, 1 to 3 per week, each lasting about 3½ hours. Most physicians who administer chelation therapy for cardiovascular disease also recommend that patients undertake a whole-foods, low-fat diet and an exercise program.

Complications
Adverse effects of EDTA chelation therapy may include hypotension, hypoglycemia, headache, rash, fatigue, and thrombophlebitis. Years ago there were reports of kidney and bone marrow damage, cardiac arrhythmias, I.V. site irritation, anemia, and even death. However, proponents say those effects resulted from excessive dosages of EDTA and that the lower dosages recommended by the ACAM today are safe.

Nursing perspective
▶ EDTA chelation therapy should be instituted only after consultation with a physician to avoid interference with any pre-existing conditions or interactions with current medications.
▶ EDTA chelation therapy is contraindicated in children, pregnant women, and patients with renal failure or severe heart failure.

Colonic irrigation
Advocates of colonic irrigation (also know as colonic hydrotherapy or colonic therapy) believe that over time, pathogenic fungi, bacteria, mucus, and other debris accumulate in the colon leading to skin problems, constipation, and a lack of energy. Colonic therapy is a procedure designed to help improve the elimination of this toxic build-up by removing fecal matter from the colon walls and diluting the concentration of bacteria in the large intestine. This reduces proliferation of pathogenic bacteria and maintains proper levels of beneficial microflora. Once the colon is free of debris, the patient should notice changes in energy level, skin tone, weight, and stress level. In addition, a patient may no longer suffer from constipation or experience painful abdominal cramping or bloating. Enhanced absorption of vitamins and minerals is also noticed following a detoxification program using colonic therapy. The concept of colonic irrigation is based on the premise that intestinal waste products are a major contributor to disease and can poison the body if not removed.

Therapeutic uses

One of the main uses for colonic irrigation is the treatment of chronic constipation. Inflammatory conditions of the colon can also be addressed using colonic therapy. Patients suffering from bloating, stomachache, or abdominal pain may also find relief using colonic therapy. Other conditions for which colonic therapy is used include acne, psoriasis, and eczema.

Patients with arthritis also seem to benefit from using colonic therapy. Some patients with arthritis are thought to have increased bowel permeability, leading to a toxic condition in the GI tract in which toxins are continually reabsorbed into the blood. Once in the blood, these toxins attack the joints, leading to inflammation and stress.

Another major use for colonic therapy is in patients with cancer. These patients tend to have deficient levels of various minerals, vitamins, and essential fatty acids. They may also suffer from constipation due to use of potent narcotic analgesics. Therefore, removing intestinal debris by colonic irrigation may lead to increased absorption of vitamins, minerals, and other key nutrients. Additionally, it may relieve constipation, allowing for enhanced elimination of toxins released from tumor cells.

RESEARCH SUMMARY The literature contains several reports of colonic irrigation. However, most don't focus on validating the therapy in patients with bowel-related complications or diseases. Rather, they emphasize adverse effects and complications that can occur. A 1997 study showed positive results in patients with fecal soiling and fecal incontinence, with the majority of patients in both groups claiming improvement in quality of life. ■

Equipment

Administration of a colonic irrigation requires a small sterile plastic hose (speculum) for delivery of solution, a colonic irrigation machine, and sterilized, distilled, or purified water.

Procedure

The day before the colonic irrigation, the patient is instructed to eat two salads. In the dinner salad, the patient adds 1 tablespoon of cooked corn in order to determine bowel transit time. The patient is also advised to avoid rice, pasta, and bread the day before and the day of the colonic irrigation and not to eat any food for at least 2 hours before the treatment.

With the patient lying on his side, a small plastic hose is gently inserted into the patient's rectum. This hose is connected to the colonic irrigation machine, which has controls for water temperature and volume. Water that has been filtered to remove bacteria, heavy metals, and chlorine begins to flow into the patient's rectum and throughout the colon. The volume of water, varied according to the patient's tolerance, induces peristaltic contractions of the colon, which expel the fecal matter into another hose leading back to the irrigation machine. This clear tube allows inspection of colon contents. The patient may experience a feeling of warmth during the session due to the presence of toxins in the fecal matter. During the irrigation, the therapist gently massages different areas of the abdomen to help dislodge and loosen areas of impaction. A session usually lasts 30 to 45 minutes. Most patients require a series of colonic irrigations to dislodge all of the fecal matter.

Complications

If the therapist uses too much water, the treatment may be uncomfortable or painful. If the therapist uses too little water, the patient's bowel is forced to work harder to achieve peristalsis.

Overdistention of the colon during the procedure or an improperly inserted hose can cause perforation of the intestinal wall. A 1999 case report cited an incidence of perineal gangrene following a perforation of the bowel during colonic therapy.

An outbreak of amebiasis occurred in the early 1980s in a Colorado chiropractic clinic, most likely due to incomplete cleaning of the irrigation machine between patients.

A patient with cancer wishing to have a colonic irrigation performed should use caution. Colonic irrigation in a patient who's weak may weaken him further. Close monitoring by an experienced health care provider is necessary.

Nursing perspective

▶ No certification is required to perform colonic irrigation. Selecting an experienced physician or practitioner of alternative medicine to properly monitor the colonic therapy is important.

▶ Patients with diverticulitis, ulcerative colitis, Crohn's disease, severe hemorrhoids, tumors of the large intestine or rectum, excessive acidity in intestinal tract, or bowel perforation shouldn't undergo colonic irrigation. No data exists regarding the safety of colonic irrigations in pediatric, maternal, and geriatric populations.

▶ Colonic irrigation is considered a legal medical practice in the United States. However, most third-party insurance payers don't reimburse patients for receiving colonic irrigations.

Detoxification

Detoxification, or cleansing, is being used increasingly as a therapeutic modality to support and improve health. Our bodies are exposed to a vast array of toxic chemicals, called xenobiotics, which are ubiquitous in our environment. Xenobiotics are easily absorbed by the body through the skin, lungs, or the mucosal lining of the GI tract. Chronic health problems can develop if detoxification doesn't take place and these toxins are allowed to circulate within the body. Excretion of toxins is a difficult process; however, the more water-soluble the toxin, the easier it is to remove.

The liver plays an important role in the removal of toxins because it transforms fat-soluble toxins into excretable, water-soluble metabolites. The enzymatic (phase I) and conjugation (phase II) reactions are liver processes responsible for detoxification. Phase I reactions activate the body's enzymes to enhance their accessibility to phase II. Phase II facilitates conversion of toxins to a water-soluble form for excretion in urine or stool. The proper functioning of the bowel is also paramount to successful detoxification.

Therapeutic uses

Many chronic health problems can be traced to compromised digestive and detoxification function. Exposure to toxins, intestinal permeability defects, and parasitic infections are common conditions associated with GI dysfunction. The liver's capacity for detoxification can become impaired due to excessive exposure to toxins as well as deficiencies in nutrients. Common signs and symptoms of toxicity include weakness, headaches, neurologic disturbances, multiple chemical sensitivities, immune dysfunction, abdominal pain, bloating, inflammatory bowel disorders, liver disorders, and chronic skin disorders.

RESEARCH
SUMMARY Toxicity overload is becoming epidemic and is responsible for a host of chronic degenerative diseases. Reducing exposure to toxins, improving digestion, replacing intestinal pathogens with healthy bacteria, and supporting detoxification with appropriate methods all decrease the toxic burden and promote healing and optimal health. ■

Equipment

No special equipment is needed for detoxification therapy.

Procedure

Treatment modalities generally include three categories of procedures: reducing exposures to toxins, enhancing GI function, and supporting the detoxification process.

Reducing toxin exposure decreases the body's overall burden of toxins directly by avoiding the addition of new toxins and, indirectly by improving the body's ability to defend itself. Lifestyle, environmental, and dietary factors all affect the body's total toxic load. The use of alcohol, caffeine, and prescription drugs is a lifestyle factor that increases the toxic burden. Environmental factors include exposure to volatile organic compounds, such as solvents and formaldehyde, which are found in products ranging from automotive fuel to household cleaners and building materials. Food is the most common source of exposure; about 3,000 chemicals are used by the food industry for various types of food processing. Another 12,000 chemicals are used in food packaging materials. Numerous studies have found pesticide residues in a significant percentage of food samples. Organically grown and unprocessed or minimally processed foods may be an option to reduce toxin exposure. Avoiding exposure may necessitate significant changes in lifestyle and the environment.

Enhancing GI function improves digestion and, consequently, increases absorption of nutrients. GI function is inadequate if the proper digestive enzymes and pH are unbalanced. Enzymes, such as lipase, amylase, pancreatin, pepsin, and protease, may be inactive in those patients with gastric or pancreatic hypofunction. This inactivity can lead to malabsorption of nutrients, food intolerance, and food allergy. Foods that aren't completely digested can putrefy in the intestine, producing toxins. Using plant enzymes can assist in promoting digestion and absorption of nutrients in those individuals with imbalances of GI pH.

Lifestyle factors also influence digestive function. Thorough chewing of food is imperative to adequate digestion because it provides mechanical breakdown of food and the necessary surface area for enzymatic activity to take place. Normal digestive secretions and motility may be impaired by depression and anxiety. Raw foods promote digestion because of their naturally occurring enzymes.

Fiber is essential for the maintenance of normal GI function. Soluble fiber is fermented by colonic microflora, resulting in the production of short chain fatty acids such as butyric acid, which is essential for normal colonic functioning. Dietary fiber helps to bind to toxins and aids with elimination through the bowel. Oral use of bentonite clay has also been shown to help bind toxins and prevent their systemic absorption.

The GI tract is considered one of the largest immune systems of the body. After all, faulty bowel mucosa compromises not only digestive and absorptive functions, but also vital immune functions. Defects of permeability can be caused by intestinal parasites, dysbiosis, impaired digestion, pancreatic insufficiency, food allergies, and the use of alcohol or nonsteroidal anti-inflammatory drugs.

Through competitive inhibition, normal bowel flora help prevent intestinal pathogens from forming. Probiotics such as *Lactobacillus* and *Bifidobacteria* species contribute to a healthy intestinal environment by maintaining optimum pH and producing important nutrients and enzymes. However, because many intestinal pathogens produce toxins, which place an additional burden on the immune system, elimination of the pathogens is necessary for a healthy intestinal tract. Preparations to restore balance to the intestinal flora include formulas containing plant extracts from *Artemisia annua*, allicin, berberine, *Hydrastis canadensis*, and *Allium sativa*. Enemas or colonic irrigations may be advised to facilitate toxin removal.

Glutathione, superoxide dismutase, catalase, betacarotene, vitamin E, selenium, and N-acetylcysteine are all essential to detoxification. Vitamin and mineral co-factors required for cytochrome P-450 reactions include riboflavin, niacin, magnesium, iron, and several trace minerals. Cruciferous vegetables and quercetin have also been shown to support phase I detoxification. Phase II detoxification is promoted by usage of calcium D-glucarate, which is a natural ingredient in certain fruits and vegetables and results in increased elimination of toxins.

Other helpful agents include amino acids, such as glycine, cysteine, glutamine, methionine, taurine, glutamic acid, and aspartic acid. Dietary supplementation may help to replace depleted supplies of nutrients needed for detoxification.

Dietary support to encourage hepatic detoxification includes emphasis on freshly prepared natural, organic, unrefined, and unprocessed foods containing a minimum of additives and chemical residues. Fresh vegetables and fruits, whole grains, and unrefined starches should constitute a significant portion of the diet. Red meats, animal fats, sugar and other simple and refined carbohydrates, salt, alcohol, and caffeine should be consumed in moderation or, preferably, avoided. Elimination of allergenic foods can facilitate mucosal healing and decrease the body's total load of toxins.

The total effect of toxins and resulting tissue damage tends to accumulate over time, leading to a cascade of illnesses. A comprehensive approach is needed to address reduction of toxin exposure, healing of the GI tract, and support of hepatic detoxification.

Complications

As the toxin load of the body decreases, the patient may experience headaches, fatigue, irritability, body aches, and strong cravings for foods removed from the diet.

Nursing perspective

▶ Patients with serious medical concerns should consult with their physicians before making dietary, lifestyle, or medication changes.

▶ Caution your patient that detoxification should be carried out only under the guidance of a qualified medical practitioner.

Light therapies

Although sunlight has been used for healing purposes since ancient times, Western scientists have only recently begun to explore how exposure to light affects human functioning. In the 1970s, scientists first proposed the theory that the winter depression that plagued people in northern climates was due to insufficient exposure to sunlight — a condition now known as seasonal affective disorder (SAD). Since then, light therapy has become an accepted treatment for people with SAD.

Today, alternative medicine proponents claim that light from various sources can be used to treat a host of other disorders, from bulimia and psoriasis to various types of cancer. Types of alternative light therapy include ultraviolet (UV) light therapy, colored light therapy, photodynamic therapy, syntonic optometry, and cold laser therapy. (See *Alternative light therapies: A closer look.*)

Therapeutic uses

Proponents of alternative light therapies claim that they've benefited patients with Alzheimer's disease, arthritis, hypertension, bulimia, depression, digestive disorders, headache, hyperactivity in children, immune disorders, symptoms of AIDS, insomnia, menstrual disorders, chronic pain, respiratory problems, sexual dysfunction, psoriasis and other skin problems, and breast, colon, and rectal cancers.

RESEARCH SUMMARY There's no scientific evidence for the safety or effectiveness of light therapy in treating anything other than SAD and jaundice in neonates. However, clinical trials sponsored by the National Institutes of Health are currently being conducted by Columbia Clinical Chronobiology Program at Columbia University. These trials include two nondrug treatments for chronic depression, light therapy for depression during pregnancy, and three nondrug treatments for SAD. ■

Equipment

The type of alternative light therapy used will determine the equipment required. For UV light therapy, the patient must go to a facility that's equipped with a UV light therapy machine. This machine applies different wavelengths of ultraviolet light (UVA, UVB, and UVC) to treat the disorder. Colored light therapy can be administered at home with a portable machine that applies different colored lights, patterns, and strobe effects to different parts of the body. Syntonic optometry requires the use of a machine that emits the light. Photodynamic therapy requires specific color dyes.

Procedure

Most light therapies require the patient to sit in a darkened room while the machine used for the particular therapy applies the appropriate light to the designated part of the body. For SAD, full spectrum fluorescent lighting at approximately

Alternative light therapies: A closer look

The following alternative light therapies use various forms of artificial light for therapeutic effects.

Ultraviolet light therapy

Various wavelengths of ultraviolet (UV) light are used to treat specific disorders. For example, UVA-1 is used for systemic lupus erythematosus, and psoralen UVA (commonly called PUVA) is used for pigmentation disorders such as vitiligo (in theory by drawing pigment-producing cells to the skin surface) and psoriasis (by preventing disease cells from dividing). UV light is also used for premenstrual syndrome, high cholesterol, and cancer.

Colored-light therapy

Practitioners of colored-light therapy believe that different colors of light affect specific diseases, perhaps by altering the production of brain chemicals. For example, opaque white or violet light is believed to induce relaxation, thus helping to relieve pain and induce sleep. Monochromatic red light is used to treat headaches, allergies, sore throats, sinus problems, endocrine and GI problems, diabetes, dysmenorrhea, and impotence. Sometimes a flashing pattern of light is used.

Photodynamic therapy

In this therapy for basal and squamous cell skin cancer, an injectable dye that absorbs light is injected directly into the malignant tumor, where it absorbs different wavelengths of external light. The combination of the light and the dye is thought to produce a chemical reaction that causes the cancer cells to die.

Syntonic optometry

In this form of light therapy, colored lights are directed at the patient's eyes in an attempt to influence brain function. The patient sits in a darkened room, where a device called a Lumatron emits rapid flashes of colored lights. The light signals travel from the eyes to the brain, where they're believed to normalize autonomic nervous system function. This therapy is currently used to treat headaches and traumatic brain injuries.

Cold laser therapy

Also called soft or low-level laser therapy, cold laser therapy uses a laser beam to induce enzymatic and bioelectric reactions in tissue. This is believed to stimulate a healing process that begins at the cellular level. Cold laser therapy has been used in pain management, skin problems, trauma, and dentistry.

3,000 lux (a unit of lighting) is required. The patient must sit 3 feet from the light for a minimum of 30 minutes in the early morning and early evening (60 minutes total/day). For optimal results, the lights should be placed directly in front of the patient or directly overhead.

Complications
Proponents say that light therapies are safe for all age-groups.

Nursing perspective
Because the only conclusive research available on light therapy concerns natural light from the sun, alternative light therapies shouldn't be used in place of treatment by a physician. A delay in treatment for any of the illnesses mentioned above could have detrimental effects.

Live cell therapy

In live cell therapy, live whole cells or extracts derived from living cells of animal organs or embryos are administered in their natural, undenatured form either sublingually or by injection to improve or rejuvenate the function of targeted organs. Live cell therapy is promoted as a treatment for a wide range of specific conditions and also as a panacea to slow the effects of aging and degeneration.

Proponents of live cell therapy claim that the idea goes back thousands of years, referring to similar therapies found in the Kama Sutra, the Papyrus of Eber, and the writings of Hippocrates. The modern introduction of this therapy is credited to Paul Niehans, a Swiss endocrinologist. In 1931, Dr. Niehans was called in to care for a patient whose parathyroid gland had been inadvertently removed during goiter surgery. Hoping to provide temporary relief from the resulting convulsions, he administered a preparation of freshly macerated oxen parathyroid gland with the intention of providing some hormonal effect. This impromptu preparation provided more than temporary relief; the patient made a rapid and complete recovery.

Dr. Niehans' theories were based on results seen in the work of Nobel laureate biologist Alexis Carrel. Starting in 1912, Dr. Carrel had performed experiments showing that when spleen cells from young, healthy sheep were placed in close proximity to old senescent cells, the older cells would revitalize. Dr. Niehans believed that his injection of live parathyroid cells rejuvenated the remaining injured parathyroid cells, thereby restoring their function. He went on to administer over 45,000 live cell therapy injections over the next 42 years from his clinic in Switzerland. Similar treatments, using substances extracted from pituitary, adrenal, ovary, testes, or other glands, were common in the United States during the same period.

> 66 Dr. Niehans theorized that once ingested, these extract cells migrate to the area of greatest injury in the body, line up with the damaged cells, then start replicating to replace and rejuvenate damaged tissue. 99

Reliance on live tissue extracts diminished with the availability of synthetic hormones and vitamin isolates. Use of live cell therapies further diminished as new research suggested that the benefits of these treatments resulted from their high vitamin, mineral, or hormonal content. However, effects such as the disappearance of chronic conditions remain unexplained. A therapy very similar to live cell therapy, called protomorphogen therapy, in which oral medications made from dried glandular or tissue extracts are administered orally, is still in widespread use among practitioners of nutritional medicine.

Early live cell therapy was based on the simple theory that administering an extract of a specific organ will improve that organ's function. Some products have a general effect; for example, mesenchyme extracts, derived from undifferentiated bovine embryonic connective tissue, are used for any condition involving tissues derived from mesenchyme cells — that is, bone, tendons, connective tissue, and the central nervous system. Dr. Niehans theorized that once ingested, these extract cells migrate to the area of greatest injury in the body, line up with the damaged cells, then start replicating to replace and rejuvenate damaged tissue.

Proprietary products currently on the market no longer contain live cells. Rather, they contain protein extracts from living cells that have been carefully extracted, purified, and preserved. These undenatured, or "live," proteins contain an array of still undefined growth factors and other cellular products that apparently stimulate the cells in similar tissue. The number of live cell products currently sold is limited, but if current trends are predictive, their availability and variety will grow. Current products include thymus, mesenchyme, adrenal, pancreas, liver, brain, and shark cartilage.

The product to be used is chosen according to the traditional model of Dr. Niehans' live cell therapy. Thymus extracts are used to increase and balance immune system activity. Mesenchyme extracts are used to stimulate repair and improve function in all mesenchyme-derived tissues. Adrenal extracts are given to improve adrenal function, liver extracts to improve liver function.

Therapeutic uses

Live cell therapy is recommended for a wide range of diseases and injuries, and products are frequently used in combination. For example, liver cirrhosis due to hepatitis C might be treated by using a combination of three products: thymus to rebalance immune function and decrease the damage the immune system causes the liver, liver extracts to increase liver function, and mesenchyme to repair liver damage.

RESEARCH SUMMARY Recently published studies suggest that live cell products are useful in treating liver disease, multiple sclerosis, chronic fatigue syndrome, and a range of other problems. However, these articles were often sponsored by the manufacturer and were peer reviewed.

Berbari, et al. (1999) reported on the antiangiogenic effects of shark cartilage extract. Oral administration of the extract decreased wound angiogenesis. This is significant, as it was the first report published that demonstrated this phenomenon. Antiangiogenic effect would be valuable in treating a number of disease processes, including metastatic progression of tumors, age-related macular degeneration, rheumatoid arthritis, and skin disorders such as psoriasis, hypertrophic scarring, and keloids. ■

Procedure

Live cell products are typically dispensed in 7-ml vials shipped frozen from the distributor and thawed one at a time just prior to use. A pretreatment test injection screens for allergic reaction. The extracts are administered either by I.M. injection or sublingually. Typical dosing protocols call for the administration of two vials per week during acute treatment and as few as one vial per month for long-term maintenance.

Complications

Care must be taken regarding the source, transport, and storage. The Canadian facility Aeterna, which manufactures the NatCell and CarTCell lines, complies with Canadian pharmaceutical guidelines. Obvious concern for sanitary practice and contamination-free products exists.

No adverse effects have been reported. Cell therapy isn't recommended for those with severe kidney disease, liver failure, or acute infections and inflammatory diseases. Patients who show an allergic reaction to the test injection shouldn't receive the treatment.

Nursing perspective

▶ Clinical experience with these products is still limited. Caution should be used in treating anyone who has suffered from any infections, including dental problems, tonsillitis, or appendicitis; be sure to get a complete history.

▶ Also take a complete drug history. Sedatives or similar drugs may weaken the effects of therapy.

▶ Note dates of any vaccinations, especially those received within 6 to 8 weeks of therapy.

Neural therapy

Neural therapy involves the injection of local anesthetics — most commonly procaine and lidocaine — into various parts of the body to restore the proper flow of electrical energy in the body and thus promote healing. Although not widely used in the United States, neural therapy is popular in Germany and South America, where it's most often used to relieve chronic pain.

> ❝ Huneke believed that interference fields in one area could cause problems in other areas of the body and that injections of anesthetics could destroy the interference fields and allow healing to proceed. ❞

An unusual discovery by German physician Ferdinand Huneke in 1940 laid the foundation for neural therapy. When Huneke injected procaine (Novocain) into a patient's stiff shoulder, the injection had no effect on the shoulder pain, but an old scar on the patient's leg began to itch. Thinking there might be some relation between the itching and the shoulder injection, Huneke then injected the scar with Novocain, and the patient's shoulder pain immediately disappeared.

From this incident, Huneke began to develop his theory of "interference fields," disruptions in the flow of electrical energy that he believed were responsible for chronic illnesses. He believed that interference fields in one area could cause problems in other areas of the body, as the shoulder incident had shown, and that injections of anesthetics could destroy the interference fields and allow healing to proceed.

The American Academy of Neural Therapy in Seattle, Wash., trains physicians in neural therapy techniques and provides referrals to trained practitioners. A board certification program is currently under development.

Therapeutic uses
Neural therapists believe this treatment is useful for dozens of conditions. (See *Indications for neural therapy*.)

RESEARCH SUMMARY Neural therapists say that this therapy isn't conducive to double-blind studies because not all patients with the same symptoms are treated the same way. The studies that have been done, mainly in Europe, are by proponents and generally don't meet the standards of the medical and scientific communities. ■

Equipment
Neural therapy requires a sterile anesthetic for injection (usually procaine), gloves, needle and syringe, alcohol pads, and a receptacle in which to dispose of the contaminated items.

Procedure
Neural therapy is administered by a clinician who has had postgraduate training in the field. Qualified clinicians may include physicians, osteopaths, dentists, naturopaths, chiropractors, and acupuncturists. After the clinician has located the patient's interference fields through a detailed medical history, he injects the anesthetic into the appropriate area. This can include acupuncture points, peripheral nerves, glands, scars,

Indications for neural therapy

Neural therapy practitioners believe that dozens of medical problems can be alleviated by neural therapy, including:

- allergies
- arteriosclerosis
- arthritis
- asthma
- back pain
- bladder problems
- chronic pain
- circulatory problems
- colitis
- depression
- dizziness
- emphysema
- gallbladder disease
- glaucoma
- headaches
- heart disease
- infertility
- kidney disease
- liver disease
- muscle injuries
- peptic ulcers
- skin disorders
- thyroid disorders.

According to practitioners, neural therapy isn't beneficial in treating cancer, metabolic disorders, genetic diseases, nutritional deficiencies, psychiatric disorders (other than depression), or end-stage chronic diseases.

or "trigger points"—areas that experience sharp pain when pressed. The number of treatments depends on the condition being treated.

Complications
There are no reports of complications from neural therapy.

Nursing perspective
▶ Neural therapy is contraindicated in patients who have cancer, coagulation disorders, renal failure, myasthenia gravis, or diabetes mellitus and in those allergic to local anesthetics or their derivatives.
▶ Neural therapy shouldn't be administered to patients receiving morphine, anticoagulants, or antiarrhythmic therapy.

Reconstructive therapy

Reconstructive therapy, also known as prolotherapy, is a technique that stimulates the body's own healing capability to regenerate ligaments and tendons, thus restoring function to injured joints. It involves injecting the fibro-osseous junction at an area of ligament or tendon tears with a solution that stimulates fibroblast proliferation. The goal of reconstructive therapy is to complete an incomplete healing process and to restore normal connective tissue length and strength in the affected area in order to restore adequate skeletal support as well as affect the pain cycle.

The solution used is a combination of a natural proliferant (a substance that irritates the tissue) and a local anesthetic that provides a biochemical stimulus to the area. By inducing inflammation, the solution triggers the body's natural healing mechanism. The swelling causes more blood to flow to the area, which produces new collagen to rebuild the tissue within and around the joint. Light exercises allow the new tissue to align correctly with the joint. The result is that the treated joint is stronger than the original joint, providing more support and strength and lowering the potential of future injury.

> ❝ *Recent research shows tissue from prereconstructive and postreconstructive therapy to be histologically undifferentiated. The developing tissue is actually new ligament being created over old ligament rather than scar tissue.* ❞

Reconstructive therapy has been used for centuries to treat chronic joint pain. Hippocrates used cautery of the anterior/inferior shoulder capsule to create scar tissue for chronic dislocations in javelin throwers. In 1937, Earl Gedney began using a technique called sclerotherapy. The term was originally applied to denote the use of a sclerosing agent to aid in the development of scar tissue that tightened damaged ligaments. Recent research, however, shows tissue from prereconstructive and postreconstructive therapy to be histologically undifferentiated. The developing tissue is actually new ligament being created over old ligament rather than scar tissue. The term has thus been change to prolotherapy or proliferation therapy.

Dr. George Hackett began using prolotherapy in the 1940s. In 1956, he published a book on his procedure, which involved injecting a proliferating agent into torn vertebral ligaments for the treatment of lower back pain. Then, in the 1970s, Dr. M.J. Ongley developed the now commonly used solution called P2SG — a combination of phenol, glucose, and glycerin.

The rationale behind reconstructive treatment of low back pain and sciatica is based on the traditional orthopedic principle of stabilization of weakened joints and ligaments. Stretched or torn ligaments and tendons generally don't heal on their own because they lack the influx of good blood supply that is present in uninjured areas of the body. Modern anti-inflammatory drugs further limit the blood flow by blocking the inflammation process that generates the fibroblast cells necessary to the formation of fibrous connective tissue that lays down the collagen. If the ligaments and tendons don't repair fully, an underlying weakness in the tissues occurs. The instability of the underlying ligaments or tendons causes the surrounding muscle to tighten reflexively in order to stabilize the joint, thus creating pain.

Reconstructive therapy is recommended by its proponents as an economical and less risky alternative to surgery that not only gives lasting relief from pain, but also increases endurance and aids in preventing future injury.

Reconstructive therapy has been practiced for more than 40 years in the United States but is still considered an alternative treatment. There are approximately 250 physicians who are certified and offer it in the United States. Treatments are usually covered by private insurance but aren't covered by Medicare.

Therapeutic uses

Reconstructive therapy is used to treat back pain, herniated discs, sciatica, back fractures, arthritis, fibromyalgia, carpal tunnel syndrome, and repetitive use syndrome. The treatment is used for shoulder pain and a variety of joint problems: dislocations, a sensation of deep aching or pulling pain in a joint, and grinding, popping, or clicking in a joint. It's used to treat ligament or tendon sprains or incomplete tears. It's also used to treat shooting pains, tingling or numbness, when chiropractic adjustments fail to provide lasting relief, and when muscle relaxants, arthritis medication, cortisone shots, or nerve blocks fail to resolve the problem within six weeks.

RESEARCH SUMMARY Several studies indicate that reconstructive therapy is effective in treating joint pain. Results of several double-blind studies show that 88% of patients treated with reconstructive therapy improve. Two studies performed by the Department of Orthopedic Surgery at the University of Iowa, in 1983 and 1985, demonstrated similar positive results; joints treated with reconstructive therapy were stronger than the original joints. Studies show that both ligaments and tendons can increase up to 40% in strength and size with this therapy.

Other studies have demonstrated increased collagen fiber diameter and cellularity on biopsy of injected areas. Disability, range of motion, and pain levels all improved significantly in patients injected after 5 or more years of chronic pain. In human knees with reproducible ligamental laxity, as measured by a computerized knee analysis device, a statistically significant reduction in ligamental laxity was demonstrated.

Randomized, double-blind control studies have demonstrated statistically significant improvements in low back pain and disability rating. Typically, when a patient doesn't improve with the therapy, one or more coexisting conditions, such as infection or use of cortisone, are inhibiting the body's healing process. ■

Procedure

A structural evaluation is performed and a treatment plan designed. A trained physician uses a 22- to 27-gauge needle 2 to 3 inches in length, depending on the area of the body being treated, to inject a proliferative solution into the fibro-osseous junction where damaged ligaments and tendons surround a joint. The most commonly used solution is P25G, which is a combination of glucose, glycerin, phenol, lidocaine or procaine, and sterile water. Several other solution combinations are available. Sodium morrhuate or straight dextrose is also used, but more caution is required with straight dextrose due to increased infections and concerns with patients with diabetes.

A fibrosis process begins approximately 15 hours after injection of the solution into the tissues. The fibrous tissue is firm by 7 days and progresses to adult compact bundles in about 18 days. The tissue formation is permanent, and rearrangement into tendinous and ligamentous structure results in the stabilization of previously unstable joints. Treatment also includes joint positioning, proper nutrition, active and passive exercise, and soft tissue massage.

The American Osteopathic Academy of Sclerotherapy states that maximum benefits are derived when the patient regains full strength and endurance and all other symptoms have been resolved, all examinations returned normal, and the examining physicians note that all ligaments, tendons, and joints have become firm. Reconstructive therapy normally requires between

6 and 12 treatments, sometimes more, depending on the severity of the damaged joint. Treatments are given weekly or every other week.

It is important to emphasize that reconstructive therapy isn't a pain management treatment; rather, it is a strengthening and regeneration treatment. With strengthening, pain is typically reduced.

Complications

When performed correctly, reconstructive therapy carries a low risk of adverse effects. Some patients experience sensitivity to the solution in the form of swelling, headache, nausea, and tiredness. The reaction rarely lasts longer than 2 to 4 days after the injection. There's minor risk of infection and hemorrhage.

Nursing perspective

▶ Reconstructive therapy isn't generally used to treat acute injuries.

▶ Treatment is usually performed at least 4 to 6 weeks after the initial injury.

▶ Before treatment, check the patient's history for allergies to the solution ingredients. Make certain that any medications your patient is currently taking won't conflict with the treatments.

▶ Advise your patient that experiencing soreness and stiffness a couple of days following treatment is normal.

Urine therapy

Urine has been used as a therapeutic agent for thousands of years. It's referred to as shivambu kalpa vidhi ("the method of drinking urine in order to rejuvenate") in Ayurvedic texts written over 5,000 years ago. Yogic texts refer to urine therapy as Amaroli ("the practice of ingesting one's own urine.") The Greeks and Romans were acquainted with the use of urine as a medicine, and Hippocrates mentioned its effectiveness. A major German encyclopedia includes various tips concerning the use of urine as medicine. John Armstrong, considered a modern urine therapy pioneer because of his book *The Water of Life,* was exceptionally persistent in his conviction of urine therapy after curing himself of "incurable" tuberculosis through urine therapy. Perhaps the most difficult aspect of urine therapy is the psychological barrier.

Urine contains minute quantities of numerous chemicals including agglutins and preciptins, which have a neutralizing effect on poliovirus and other viruses; antineoplastons, which selectively prevent the growth of cancer cells; and urokinase, a vasodilator that is extracted from urine and sold as medicine. After protein is broken down in the liver, urea is formed. A person normally excretes an average of 25 to 30 grams of urea per day. Some of the urea is converted into glutamine, and intestinal bacteria decompose urea into ammonia. Urea and ammonia have strong antibacterial and antiviral effects.

Therapeutic uses
Urine therapy is reported to be a useful treatment for conditions ranging from aging, allergies, dandruff, diarrhea, morning sickness, depression, fatigue, fever, headache, vertigo, obesity, varicose veins, and warts to bronchitis, arthritis, burns, AIDS, cancer, leukemia, muscular dystrophy, poliomyelitis, syphilis, and tuberculosis.

RESEARCH SUMMARY The concepts behind the use of urine therapy and the claims made regarding its effects haven't yet been validated scientifically. ■

Procedure
Drinking: Several ounces of the mid-stream, first morning excretion are drunk.

Gargling: Urine is gargled and said to help with gum disease or other oral problems.

Drops: Two to three drops are applied to the eye or ear.

Soaking: Urine is used to soak the feet in cases of athlete's foot.

Packing: Cotton gauze saturated with urine is applied topically to minor wounds, snakebites, bee stings, and pest bites.

Massage: Fresh urine is massaged into the skin or hair for topical application.

Capsules: The purified ingredients from 700 ml of urine are packed into a 500 mg capsule, which is taken orally with cold water.

Injection: One bottle containing 5 g in 100 ml of purified ingredients from 7,000 ml urine is mixed with Ringer's solution and administered by I.V. infusion.

Homeopathic preparation: A homeopathic preparation of urine is made by sequentially diluting it in water. The remedy is potentized by succussing (vigorously striking the bottle against a hard surface) the mixture between each dilution. A commonly used potency is a 6×, in which a 1 in 10 dilution is made 6 times (a 1 ÷ 1,000,000 solution). Several drops of the remedy are applied to the tongue a few times each day for a week.

Complications

Urine therapy shouldn't be used when the patient has an active bladder infection or venereal disease. Caution should be used if the patient is taking prescription or recreational drugs because many drugs are metabolized and secreted in urine. Patients with diabetes and kidney diseases can have very low pH readings; checking for acidity is important.

Some people experience a "healing crisis" or "recovery reaction." Common symptoms include diarrhea, itching, pain, fatigue, shoulder soreness, and fever. These symptoms appear more frequently in patients suffering long-term or more serious illnesses, and symptoms may repeat several times. Each episode may last 3 to 7 days, but sometimes it may last for a month, or worsen over 6 months. Urine therapists should make patients aware of such reactions, and stress that they are considered to be normal responses as the body initiates healing.

Nursing perspective

▶ Urine therapy has been used for centuries. Clinicians should be aware of such therapies in case their patients have questions.

▶ There's a significant psychological barrier associated with the use of urine therapy.

Miscellaneous biological cancer therapies

There are numerous unproven alternative therapies aimed specifically at treating cancer. Some of these treatments, such as antineoplastons and shark cartilage, have received a lot of media attention. Others, such as 714X, hydrazine sulfate, hyperoxygenation, immunoaugmentive therapy, and Coley's toxins, are primarily known to alternative practitioners. Many of these therapies are said to work by stimulating the immune system.

Most mainstream health care professionals vehemently reject these treatments and caution patients not to use them before trying conventional medical treatments.

Antineoplastons

Antineoplastons, a cancer treatment developed by Polish-born physician Stanislaw Burzynski, involves the administration of polypeptides that Burzynski claims can convert cancerous cells to normal cells. Burzynski first isolated these substances, which he called "antineoplastons" (meaning anti–new growth), in human urine. He believes patients with cancer are deficient in antineoplastons and for the past 2 decades has offered this treatment (now using synthetic antineoplastons) to thousands of people, first at Baylor College of Medicine and now at his own institute in Houston. Burzynski claims to have produced especially good results in treating prostate cancer and inoperable brain tumors.

> ❝ *In 1997, Burzynski was acquitted of a 75-count indictment charging that his use of an unproven therapy was a violation of FDA and U.S. Postal Service regulations.* ❞

RESEARCH SUMMARY Antineoplaston therapy has been controversial from the start. Some medical researchers have found merit in Burzynski's work, while others attack it. Most of his studies have been presented at conferences outside the United States. Meanwhile, a large devoted following of patients with cancer claims to have been helped by the treatment. In 1997, Burzynski was acquitted of a 75-count indictment charging that his use of an unproven therapy was a violation of FDA and U.S. Postal Service regulations. Several phase II trials, funded in part by the Office of Alternative Medicine, are currently under way.

Phase II clinical trials began in 1993 at Memorial Sloan-Kettering Cancer Center, the Mayo Clinic, and the Warren Magnussen Clinical Center at NIH. Due to inadequate patient enrollment, the studies were closed prior to completion, and no consensus could be drawn regarding the efficacy of antineoplastons. No patient demonstrated tumor regression. Clinical trials are also underway at the Burzynski Research Institute in Houston under FDA Supervision. ■

Shark cartilage

One reason that tumors grow is their ability to develop their own blood supply, a process known as *angiogenesis*. By inhibiting angiogenesis, some cancer researchers reason, tumor growth can be halted. To do this, they have turned to shark cartilage, which contains a protein with antiangiogenic properties.

Shark cartilage comes in powder or capsule form. It's taken orally and sometimes as an enema.

Clinical considerations include:

▶ Shark cartilage shouldn't be used in children or pregnant women because it may adversely affect growth.

▶ It shouldn't be administered to anyone with recent surgery as it may impair healing.

▶ It shouldn't be administered as an enema if a patient has a low white blood cell count. This could result in a life-threatening infection.

▶ Some preparations may contain additives, fillers, or contaminants.

▶ The treatment may cause diarrhea, which may affect the patient's ability to tolerate more conventional cancer treatments.

RESEARCH SUMMARY   Shark cartilage gained much attention after the TV show "60 Minutes" aired a report from a Cuban clinic suggesting that this therapy showed promise against cancer. Although a modest antiangiogenic effect has been observed in laboratory experiments on shark cartilage, reports of similar effects in humans are generally discredited by the medical community. In addition, some researchers say that the oral form of cartilage sold in health food stores is digested by gastric acid before it can be absorbed by the bloodstream; thus it can't provide any benefit. ■

714X

Developed in Quebec by French-born microbiologist Gaston Naessens, 714X is a chemical solution consisting primarily of camphor and nitrogen that is injected directly into the lymphatic system. Naessens' compound is based on his theory that cancer cells require a lot of nitrogen and commonly leech it from healthy cells. By supplying the cancer cells with nitrogen, 714X theoretically "liberates the immune system," enhancing its ability to fight the cancer. In addition, proponents claim 714X "liquefies" the lymph, allowing toxins from the cancer cells to be flushed out.

Using a combination of laser and ultraviolet technology, Naessens developed the somatoscope, which provides significantly greater magnification than the ordinary light microscope. He used this instrument for the diagnosis and monitoring of the disease process by observing basic living particles that he called somatids.

714X is regarded as an alternative therapy in the treatment of autoimmune and degenerative diseases, such as cancer, multiple sclerosis, chronic fatigue syndrome, fibromyalgia, and lupus. It's primarily available in perinodular inguinal injection and sublingual drops, and infrequently is administered by nebulizer.

The treatment appears to cause few adverse effects, although local redness, tenderness, and swelling may occur at the injection site. Because the camphor in the treatment tends to sting, using an ice pack on the area prior to injection is recommended. 714X shouldn't be administered concurrently with vitamins B_{12} or E, chemotherapy, or radiation.

RESEARCH SUMMARY Naessens's studies haven't been published in peer-reviewed literature. In 1989, he was acquitted of health fraud charges in Quebec after many patients (including a former U.S. congressman) testified that they had been helped by 714X. This therapy is offered in Naessens's clinic in Quebec as well as in Mexico and Western Europe. ■

Hydrazine sulfate

In 1968, Joseph Gold, MD, director of the Syracuse (New York) Cancer Research Institute, proposed the theory that hydrazine sulfate, an industrial chemical, could be used to treat cachexia, the progressive weight loss and debilitation that afflicts patients with advanced cancer. He claimed that this chemical, also classified as an MAO inhibitor, could also shrink tumors or even cause them to disappear. Conversely, hydrazine sulfate is thought by some to be potentially carcinogenic.

Possible adverse effects include nausea, vomiting, dizziness, paresthesias of the upper and lower extremities, impaired fine motor function, itching, dry skin, insomnia, and hypoglycemia. Encephalopathy can occur during treatment as well as an altered mental state described as euphoria. The patient must avoid food and beverages high in tyramine to prevent a hypertensive crisis.

RESEARCH SUMMARY Three trials supported by the National Cancer Institute (NCI) demonstrated no benefit attributable to hydrazine sulfate. The largest study found that the quality of life was actually worse in the hydrazine group. Since 1975, several randomized, double-blinded, placebo-controlled clinical trials have found from no improvement to some improved appetite, weight gain, and metabolic measures. In a 1988 interview in the *Washington Post,* former NCI Director Vincent DeVita, Jr., said the NCI was reluctant to study a treatment aimed at preventing weight loss rather than eliminating cancer. ■

Hyperoxygenation therapies

Also known as bio-oxidative therapy and oxidative therapy, hyperoxygenation therapy involves the administration of various forms of oxygen to treat cancer and other diseases. This therapy is based on the theory that cancer is caused by an oxygen deficiency and can be cured by exposing cancer cells to large amounts of oxygen. The most widely used agents include hydrogen peroxide (commonly used to disinfect wounds), ozone, and hyperbaric oxygen.

Hydrogen peroxide may be administered intravenously, injected directly into joints, or absorbed via tub soaks. It's used to kill bacteria, fungi, parasites, viruses, and some types of tumor cells. It has also been used to treat cardiovascular disease and peripheral vascular disease.

Ozone is administered in a variety of ways that include intramuscular injection, rectal insufflation, autohemotherapy and intra-articular injection. It has been used to treat cancer, HIV, hepatitis, and herpes.

Hyperbaric oxygen is administered via a pressurized chamber. It's best known for its effectiveness in treatment of carbon monoxide poisoning, gas gangrene, and tissue decompression.

Adverse effects from oxidative therapies include stomach irritation from hydrogen peroxide and injection site reactions typical of any invasive method. Hyperbaric oxygen may cause seizures, irritation to the inner ear, numbness of fingers, a temporary change to the lens of the eye and inflammation of the optic nerve, which could lead to blindness.

RESEARCH SUMMARY Research in patients with cancer conducted at Baylor University found that hydrogen peroxide injected into a vein could achieve the same effect as hyperbaric oxygen at a much lower cost and with fewer adverse effects. Recent Canadian research showed that ozone kills HIV, hepatitis, and herpes. ■

> ❝ *Stung by the hostile reaction of the medical community, Burton refused to share details of immunoaugmentative therapy with other scientists or publish detailed clinical studies.* ❞

Immunoaugmentative therapy

Developed in the 1970s by Lawrence Burton, PhD, a cancer researcher at St. Vincent's Hospital in New York, immunoaugmentative therapy (IAT) involves the administration of processed blood products containing four protein components obtained from healthy donors. Burton claimed that his therapy, which he patented and later offered at his own clinic in the Bahamas, could stimulate the immune system's ability to detect and destroy cancer cells. However, he maintained that IAT was a way of controlling cancer, not curing it.

RESEARCH SUMMARY Burton, who died in 1993, claimed that IAT achieved tumor reduction or remission in 40% to 60% of his patients. However, stung by the hostile reaction of the medical community, he refused to share details of his treatment with other scientists or publish detailed clinical studies. This lack of documentation has made it difficult for scientists to analyze the treatment or its effectiveness. IAT is still offered at Burton's clinic in Freeport, Grand Bahama. The NCI refused to participate in clinical trials because they wouldn't know what was being tested. ■

Coley's toxins

William Coley, a New York City surgeon in the late 1800s, began searching for alternative treatments for cancer because so few of his patients with cancer were surviving after conventional treatments. Noting that one survivor had suffered two bouts of erysipelas, a severe skin infection caused by *Streptococcus pyogenes,* Coley theorized that this bacterium might have preventive properties and began injecting patients with cancer with a mixture of killed cultures of *S. pyogenes* and *Serratia marcescens.* Although the treatments didn't help everyone, Coley reported dramatic results in patients with various types of cancer. Today, many scientists regard Coley as a pioneer in the study of immunotherapy.

Although other researchers have continued to study Coley's toxins over the years, production of the drug was discontinued in the United States in the 1950s.

During the 1980s, the Coley toxins were tested in mice at Temple University. They compared favorably with other biological response modifiers because of their enhancing effects on the immune response and oncolytic properties at nontoxic levels. Coley toxins have been cited as a promising treatment that may have been prematurely abandoned with the advent of modern radiotherapy and chemotherapy.

Coley's toxins have been used to treat several types of cancer. The treatment is used outside the U.S. in Mexico, Central America, Guatemala, Germany, and China. An adaptation of the treatment is administered at the Waisbren clinic in Milwaukee. The treatment is administered by either subcutaneous or intravenous injections. The most common adverse effects include fever and nausea. Serious infections could result in those patients with compromised immune systems.

As recently as the early 90s, recommendations have been made to reevaluate this treatment in appropriately selected patients. The profile is that of a patient with inoperable soft tissue sarcoma or lymphoma with no prior therapy. The Cancer Research Institute, founded by Helen Coley Nauts, Dr. Coley's daughter, continues to support research in the field of cancer immunology.

Selected references

"Alternative Medicine," *Harvard Health Letter* 25(11):1, September 2000.

Alternative Medicine: Expanding Medical Horizons. A Report to the National Institutes of Health on Alternative Medical Systems and Practices in the United States. Prepared under the auspices of the Workshop on Alternative Medicine, Chantilly, Va., September 14-16, 1992. NIH pub. 94-066. Washington, D.C.: U.S. Government Printing Office, 1994.

Antman, K., et al., "Complementary and Alternative Medicine; The role of the Cancer Center," *Journal of Clinical Oncology* 19 (Suppl. 18):S55-60, September 2001.

Berbari, P., et al. "Antiangiogenic Effects of the Oral Administration of Liquid Cartilage Extract in Humans," *Journal of Surgical Research* 87(1):108-13, November 1999.

Calabresi, P. "Medical Alternatives to Alternative Medicine," *Cancer* 86(10):1887-889, November 1999.

Cerrato, P.L. "A Radical Approach to Heart Disease," *RN* 62(4):65-66, April 1999.

D'Epiro, N.W. "Bee Venom for Multiple Sclerosis," *Patient Care* 33(14):27-28, 31, September 1999.

"FTC Attacks Chelation Therapy," *Nutrition Forum* 16(2):9, March-April 1999.

Green, S. "Autogenous Vaccine: A Defense Against the Bacterial Organism That Causes Cancer," *Scientific Review of Alternative Medicine* 5(2):98-103, Spring 2001.

Leifer, G. "Hyberbaric Oxygen Therapy: Pre- and Posttreatment Nursing Responsibilities Every Nurse Needs to Know About," *American Journal of Nursing* 101(8):26-35, August 2001.

Leviton, R. "Helping AIDS, Cancer, and Multiple Sclerosis with Oxygen," *Alternative Medicine* (23):62-66, May 1998.

Mendelson, G. "A Primer of Complementary and Alternative Medicine Commonly Used by Cancer Patients," *Medical Journal of Australia* 174(11):611-12, June 2001.

Muirhead, G. "CAM Strategies to Promote Wellness," *Patient Care* 33(18):143-45, 149-50, 155-58 passim., November 1999.

Pelletier, K.R. *The Best Alternative Medicine: What Works? What Does Not?* New York: Simon and Schuster, 2000.

Robins, J.L. "The Science and Art of Aromatherapy," *Journal of Holistic Nursing* 17(1):5-17, March 1999.

"The Role of Alternative Treatments for Cancer," *Johns Hopkins Medical Letter Health After 50* 12(6):6-7, August 2000.

Sparber, A., and Wootton, J.C. "Surveys of Complementary and Alternative Medicine: Part II. Use of Alternative and Complementary Cancer Therapies," *The Journal of Alternative and Complementary Medicine* 7(3):281-87, June 2001.

U.S. Congress Office of Technology Assessment. *Unconventional Cancer Treatments.* Washington, D.C.: U.S. Government Printing Office, 1990.

Van Rij, A.M. "Chelation Therapy for Intermittent Claudication: A Double-Blind, Randomized, Controlled Trial," *Circulation* 90(3):1194-199, September 1994.

Wilkinson, S., et al. "An Evaluation of Aromatherapy Massage in Palliative Care," *Palliative Medicine* 13(5):409-17, September 1999.

Internet resources

Alternative Therapies in Health and Medicine: *www.alternative-therapies.com*

HealthWorld on Line: *www.healthy.net*

Journal of Alternative and Complementary Medicine (available online with subscription): *www.catchword.com/titles/1075535.html*

National Center for Complementary and Alternative Medicine: *www.nccam.nih.gov*

Quack Watch: *www.quackwatch.com*

Appendices, glossary, and index

Appendix A
Alternative therapies for specific conditions

The list below gives a sampling of alternative and complementary therapies that practitioners may use for specific conditions, diseases, and signs and symptoms. In many cases, these therapies are used in addition to conventional therapies. Because some of these therapies remain experimental, advise your patients to research any therapy they're considering before beginning it.

Allergies, hay fever
- Environmental medicine
- Homeopathy
- Hypnotherapy
- Juice therapy
- Pancreatic enzyme therapy
- Plant enzyme therapy

Alzheimer's disease
- Art therapy
- Dance therapy
- Music therapy
- Sound therapy

Anemia
- Plant enzyme therapy

Anxiety
- Biofeedback
- Meditation
- Transcranial electrostimulation

Arthritis
- Apitherapy
- Bioelectromagnetic therapy
- Detoxification therapy
- Dietary measures (eliminating nightshade foods, such as potatoes, tomatoes, peppers, eggplant, tobacco) and nutritional supplements (boron, zinc, copper, selenium, manganese, proteolytic enzymes, flavonoids, glucosamine sulfate, evening primrose oil)
- Environmental medicine
- Fasting
- Herbal therapy
- Juice therapy
- Osteopathic manipulation
- Vitamin therapy (vitamins A, B_1, B_6, C, E)
- Yoga

Asthma
- Ayurvedic remedies
- Biofeedback
- Guided imagery
- Herbal therapy (ephedra, mullein tea, passionflower tea)
- Homeopathy
- Hydrotherapy
- Hypnotherapy
- Juice therapy
- Yoga

Atherosclerosis
- Chelation therapy

Autism
- Music therapy
- Sound therapy

Back pain
▶ Bioelectromagnetic therapy
▶ Osteopathic manipulation

Benign prostatic hyperplasia
▶ Herbal therapy (saw palmetto)

Bone fractures
▶ Pulsed electromagnetic fields

Brain injuries
▶ Music therapy

Cancer (all types)
▶ Antineoplaston therapy
▶ Antioxidants (vitamin A, C, and E and trace mineral selenium)
▶ Bioelectromagnetic therapy
▶ Cell-specific cancer therapy-200
▶ Coley's toxins (mixed bacterial vaccine)
▶ Dance therapy
▶ Detoxification therapy
▶ Guided imagery
▶ Homeopathy
▶ Hydrazine sulfate
▶ Juice therapy
▶ Meditation
▶ Pancreatic enzyme therapy
▶ Phytoestrogens (found in soy products, lentils, chickpeas, kidney beans, wheat, corn, rice)
▶ Shark cartilage
▶ 714X therapy

Cancer (breast)
▶ Bioelectromagnetic therapy
▶ Phytoestrogens (found in soy products, lentils, chickpeas, kidney beans, wheat, corn, rice)

Cancer (colon)
▶ High-fiber diet

Cardiovascular disorders
▶ Bioelectromagnetic therapy
▶ Biofeedback
▶ Dance therapy
▶ Detoxification therapy
▶ Humor therapy
▶ Meditation
▶ Osteopathic manipulation
▶ Tai chi chuan
▶ Yoga

Carpal tunnel syndrome
▶ Acupressure
▶ Bioelectromagnetic therapy
▶ Vitamin therapy

Cerebral palsy
▶ Biofeedback

Cerebrovascular disease
▶ Chelation therapy
▶ Music therapy

Childbirth
▶ Hypnosis
▶ Imagery
▶ Massage
▶ Music therapy

Circulation, impaired
▶ Herbal therapy (ginkgo biloba for brain and extremities)
▶ Phytoestrogens (found in soy products, lentils, chickpeas, kidney beans, wheat, corn, rice)

Colds and flu
▶ Guided imagery
▶ Herbal therapy
▶ Homeopathy

Constipation
▶ Colonic irrigation
▶ Herbal therapy
▶ High-fiber diet

Coronary artery disease
- Ayurvedic medicine
- Chelation therapy
- Coenzyme Q10
- Diet therapy (for example, macrobiotic or low-fat diet)
- Meditation, stress-control program
- Polyphenols (found in onions, apples, wine, coffee)
- Trace mineral selenium

Dental disorders
- Bioelectromagnetic therapy
- Hypnosis

Depression
- Saint John's wort

Diabetes
- Bioelectromagnetic therapy
- Detoxification therapy
- Yoga

Diabetic neuropathy
- Bioelectromagnetic therapy

Digestive disorders
- Biofeedback
- Herbal therapy
- Homeopathy
- Juice therapy
- Osteopathic manipulation
- Pancreatic enzyme therapy
- Yoga

Drug and alcohol addiction
- Acupuncture
- Meditation
- Music therapy
- Yoga

Dyslexia
- Auriculotherapy

Emphysema
- Dietary measures (avoiding mucus-producing foods, such as dairy products, salt, junk food)
- Herbal therapy (coltsfoot tea, comfrey or ephedra tea, licorice root)
- Hydrotherapy

Fatigue, chronic
- Bioelectromagnetic therapy
- Biofeedback
- Osteopathic manipulation

Fibrocystic breast disease
- Antineoplaston therapy
- Vitamin E

Fibromyalgia
- Bioelectromagnetic therapy

Genital warts
- Antineoplaston therapy

Glucose, unstable levels
- Spirulina

Gout
- Apitherapy
- Bioelectromagnetic therapy

Hay fever
- Dietary measures (avoiding common allergenic foods, such as dairy products, wheat, eggs, chocolate, peanuts)
- Herbal therapy (nettle, tincture of licorice, comfrey tea)
- Hydrotherapy (hot and cold compresses, steam inhalation)
- Juice therapy

Headaches
- Bioelectromagnetic therapy
- Biofeedback
- Fasting
- Herbal therapy
- Homeopathy
- Imagery
- Meditation

▶ Osteopathic manipulation
▶ Yoga

Head trauma
▶ Music therapy

Hemoglobin, increased
▶ Spirulina
▶ Therapeutic Touch

Hemophilia
▶ Hypnotherapy

Hemorrhoids
▶ High-fiber diet
▶ Hydrotherapy
▶ Qigong
▶ Reflexology
▶ Yoga

Hepatitis
▶ Herbal therapy
▶ Juice therapy
▶ Magnetic field therapy
▶ Oxygen therapy
▶ Vitamin therapy

Herpes zoster
▶ Bioelectromagnetic therapy

Human immunodeficiency virus infection
▶ Dance therapy
▶ Homeopathy
▶ I.V. ozone therapy
▶ Meditation
▶ Yoga

Hyperactivity
▶ Biofeedback

Hypertension
▶ Bioelectromagnetic therapy
▶ Biofeedback
▶ Fasting
▶ Herbal therapy
▶ Meditation
▶ Osteopathic manipulation

▶ Relaxation therapy
▶ Sound therapy
▶ Tai chi chuan
▶ Yoga

Ichthyosis
▶ Hypnotherapy

Immune disorders (general)
▶ Enzyme therapy
▶ Sound therapy

Incontinence (urinary)
▶ Biofeedback
▶ Relaxation therapy

Infection
▶ Herbal therapy (echinacea)

Inflammatory diseases
▶ Fasting
▶ Flavonoids

Insomnia
▶ Aromatherapy
▶ Biofeedback
▶ Herbal therapy (valerian)
▶ Melatonin
▶ Relaxation therapy

Jet lag
▶ Melatonin

Menstrual disorders
▶ Herbal therapy
▶ Osteopathic manipulation
▶ Relaxation therapy

Migraines
▶ Bioelectromagnetic therapy
▶ Biofeedback
▶ Hypnotherapy
▶ Yoga

Motion sickness
▶ Acupressure
▶ Biofeedback
▶ Herbal therapy (ginger)

Reflexology
Relaxation therapies

Multiple sclerosis
Apitherapy
Bioelectromagnetic therapy
Feldenkrais method
Pancreatic enzyme therapy

Muscle and joint pain
Acupressure
Alexander technique
Apitherapy
Bioelectromagnetic therapy
Feldenkrais method
Juice therapy
Reflexology

Obesity
Detoxification therapy
High-fiber diet

Optic nerve atrophy
Bioelectromagnetic therapy

Osteoporosis
Bioelectromagnetic therapy

Pain
Acupuncture
Auriculotherapy
Bioelectromagnetic therapy
Biofeedback
Electroacupuncture
Hypnotherapy
Imagery
Meditation
Music therapy
Osteopathic manipulation
Radiofrequency diathermy
Relaxation therapies
Sound therapy
Stress-control classes
Transcutaneous electrical
nerve stimulation
Yoga

Pancreatitis
Detoxification therapy
Fasting
Juice therapy
Magnetic field therapy
Oxygen therapy
Qigong

Parasitic infection
Light beam generator

Parkinson's disease
Auriculotherapy
Bioelectromagnetic therapy
Music therapy

Phantom limb pain
Bioelectromagnetic therapy

Pneumonia
Acupuncture
Dietary measures (eliminating common food allergens)
Herbal therapy (lobelia, golden seal)
Hydrotherapy

Pressure ulcers
Bioelectromagnetic therapy

Prostate disorders
Juice therapy

Psychological disorders (all types)
Art therapy
Biofeedback
Fasting
Hypnotherapy
Meditation
Music therapy
Psychotherapy

Sciatica
Acupressure
Applied kinesiology
Chiropractic
Hydrotherapy

▶ Osteopathic manipulation
▶ Reflexology

Scoliosis
▶ Osteopathic manipulation

Seizures
▶ Bioelectromagnetic therapy

Sinusitis
▶ Herbal therapy (ephedra, goldenseal, pokeroot, yarrow)
▶ Homeopathic remedies
▶ Hydrotherapy (nasal lavage, hot and cold compresses, steam inhalation)

Sore throat
▶ Aromatherapy
▶ Herbal therapy (such as soothing and astringent gargles)
▶ Hydrotherapy
▶ Light therapy
▶ Pancreatic enzyme therapy
▶ Reflexology
▶ Vitamin therapy

Spinal cord injuries
▶ Art therapy

Sprains and strains
▶ Bioelectromagnetic therapy

Temporomandibular joint syndrome
▶ Bioelectromagnetic therapy
▶ Biofeedback

Trigeminal neuralgia
▶ Bioelectromagnetic therapy

Ulcerative colitis
▶ Relaxation therapies

Ulcers (gastric)
▶ Herbal therapy
▶ Pancreatic enzyme therapy

Urinary problems (chronic)
▶ Acupressure
▶ Aromatherapy
▶ Herbal therapy
▶ Juice therapy
▶ Magnetic field therapy

Viral illness
▶ Detoxification therapy
▶ Fasting
▶ Herbal therapy
▶ Juice therapy
▶ Magnetic field therapy
▶ Oxygen therapy
▶ Pancreatic enzyme therapy

Warts
▶ Herbal therapy (bloodroot paste)
▶ Hypnotherapy
▶ Moxibustion
▶ Vitamin therapy

Whiplash
▶ Bioelectromagnetic therapy
▶ Osteopathic manipulation

Appendix B
Alternative therapy organizations

Acupressure
Acupressure Institute
1533 Shattuck Ave.
Berkeley, CA 94709
1-800-442-2232
www.acupressure.com

Acupuncture
Acupuncture and Oriental
   Medicine Alliance
14637 Starr Rd. S.E.
Olalla, WA 98359
(253) 851-6896
www.acupuncturealliance.org

American Academy of Medical
   Acupuncture
4929 Wilshire Blvd., Suite 428
Los Angeles, CA 90010
1-800-521-2262
www.medicalacupuncture.org

American Association of
   Oriental Medicine
433 Front St.
Catasauqua, PA 18032
1-888-500-7999
www.aaom.org

Bastyr University
14500 Juanita Dr. N.E.
Kenmore, WA 98028
(425) 823-1300
www.bastyr.edu

National Commission for
   Acupuncture Certification
   and Oriental Medicine
11 Canal Center Plaza,
   Suite 300
Alexandria, VA 22314
(703) 548-9004
www.nccaom.org

Alexander technique
American Center for the
   Alexander Technique
39 W. 14th St.
New York, NY 10011
(212) 633-2229

American Society of Teachers
   of the Alexander Technique
P.O. Box 60008
Florence, MA 01062
E-mail: alexandertech@
   earthlink.net
www.alexandertech.org

Alternative medicine
Coalition for Natural Health
1220 L St. N.W., #308
Washington, DC 20005
1-800-586-4264
www.naturalhealth.org

National Center for Complementary and Alternative
   Medicine Clearinghouse
P.O. Box 8218
Silver Spring, MD 20907
1-888-644-6226
www.nccam.nih.gov

Antineoplastons
Burzynski Clinic
9432 Old Katy Rd., Suite 200
Houston, TX 77055
(713) 335-5697
www.cancermed.com

Applied kinesiology
International College of Applied
  Kinesiology
6405 Metcalf Ave., Suite 503
Shawnee Mission, KS 66202-
  3929
(913) 384-5336
E-mail:info@icakusa.com
www.icakusa.com

Aromatherapy
National Association for
  Holistic Aromatherapy
4509 Interlake Ave. N.
Seattle, WA 98103
1-888-275-6242
www.naha.org

Art therapy
American Art Therapy
  Association
1202 Allanson Rd.
Mundelein, IL 60060
1-888-290-0878
www.arttherapy.org

Ayurvedic medicine
Aryurvedic Institute
11311 Menaul N.E.
Albuquerque, NM 87112
(505) 291-9698
www.aryurveda.com

Bastyr University
14500 Juanita Dr. N.E.
Kenmore, WA 98028
(425) 602-3330
www.bastyr.edu

National Institute of Ayurvedic
  Medicine
584 Milltown Rd.
Brewster, NY 10509
(845) 278-8700
www.niam.com

The Raj
1734 Jasmne Ave.
Fairfield, IA 52556
1-800-248-9050
www.theraj.com

Biofeedback
Association for Applied
  Psychophysiology and
  Biofeedback
10200 W. 44th Ave., Suite 304
Wheat Ridge, CO 80033
1-800-477-8892
E-mail: aapb@resourcenter.com
www.aapb.org

Center for Applied
  Psychophysiology–Menninger
  Clinic
P.O. Box 829
Topeka, KS 66601
1-800-351-9058
www.menninger.edu.

Chelation therapy
American Board of Chelation
  Therapy
1407½, North Wells St., 2W
Chicago, IL 60610
1-800-356-2228

Chiropractic
American Chiropractic
  Association
1701 Clarendon Blvd.
Arlington, VA 22209
1-800-986-4636
www.amerchiro.org

World Chiropractic Alliance
2950 N. Dobson Rd., Suite 1
Chandler, AZ 85224
1-800-347-1011
*www.worldchiropracticalliance.
org*

Craniosacral therapy
Upledger Institute
11211 Prosperity Farms Rd.
Palm Beach Gardens, FL 33410
1-800-233-5880
E-mail: upledger@upledger.com
www.upledger.com

Dance therapy
American Dance Therapy
Association
2000 Century Plaza, Suite 108
Columbia, MD 21044
(410) 997-4040
E-mail: info@adta.org
www.adta.org

Detoxification therapies
American College for Advancement in Medicine
23121 Verdugo Dr., Suite 204
Laguna Hills, CA 92653
1-800-532-3688
Fax: (949) 455-9679
www.ACAM.org

Great Smokies Diagnostic
Laboratories
63 Zillicoa St.
Asheville, NC 28801
1-800-522-4762
www.gsdl.com

HealthComm International, Inc.
Clinical Research Center
P.O. Box 1729
Gig Harbor, WA 98335
1-800-692-9400
www.healthcomm.com

International Association for
Colon Hydrotherapy
P.O. Box 461285
San Antonio, TX 78246
(210) 366-2888
www.healthy.net/iact

National Acupuncture
Detoxification Association
P.O. Box 1927
Vancouver, WA 98668
1-888-765-NADA
www.acudetox.com

Electromagnetic therapies
Bio-Electro-Magnetics Institute
2490 W. Moana Ln.
Reno, NV 89509
(795) 827-9099
E-mail: johnz@scs.unr.edu

Environmental medicine
American Academy of
Environmental Medicine
7701 E. Kellogg, Suite 625
Wichita, KS 67207
(316) 684-5500
www.aaem.com

Fasting
International Association of
Hygienic Physicians
4620 Euclid Blvd.
Youngstown, OH 44512
(330) 788-0526
www.iahp.cisnet.com

Feldenkrais method
Feldenkrais Guild of North
America
3611 SW Hood Ave., Suite 100
Portland, OR 97201
1-800-775-2118
www.feldenkrais.com

Gerson diet
Gerson Institute
1572 Seond Ave.
San Diego, CA 92101
(619) 685-5353
www.gerson.org

Guided imagery
Academy for Guided Imagery
P.O. Box 2070
Mill Valley, CA 94942
1-800-726-2070
www.healthy.net/agi

Healing touch
Colorado Center for Healing
    Touch
12477 W. Cedar Dr., Suite 206
Lakewood, CO 80228
(303) 989-0581
www.healingtouch.net

Herbal medicine
American Botanical Council
P.O. Box 144345
Austin, TX 78714
(512) 926-4900
Fax: (512) 926-2345
www.herbalgram.org

Herb Research Foundation
1007 Pearl St., Suite 200
Boulder, CO 80302
(303) 449-2265
www.herbs.org

Holistic nursing
American Holistic Health
    Association
P.O. Box 17400
Anaheim, CA 92817-7400
(714) 779-6152
www.ahha.org

American Holistic Nurses
    Association
P.O. Box 2130
Flagstaff, AZ 86003
1-800-278-2462
www.ahna.org

Homeopathy
National Center for Homeopa-
    thy
801 N. Fairfax St., Suite 306
Alexandria, VA 22314
(703) 548-7790
www.homeopathic.org

Hydrotherapy
Desert Springs Therapy Center
66705 E. Sixth St.
Desert Hot Springs, CA 92240
(760) 329-5066
www.tagnet.org/dstc

Uchee Pines Institute
30 Uchee Pines Rd.
Seale, AL 36875
(334) 855-4764
www.ucheepines.org

Hypnotherapy
Academy of Scientific
    Hypnotherapy
P.O. Box 12041
San Diego, CA 92112
(619) 427-6225

American Board of
    Hypnotherapy
2002 E. McFadden Ave.,
    Suite 100
Santa Ana, CA 92705
1-800-872-9996
www.hypnosis.com

American Guild of
    Hypnotherapists
2200 Veterans Blvd.
Kenner, LA 70062
(504) 468-3223

American Society of Clinical
    Hypnosis
130 E. Elm Ct., Suite 201
Roselle, IL 60172
(630) 980-4740
www.asch.net

Kelley diet
Nicholas Gonzalez, MD
36A E. 36th St., Suite 204
New York, NY 10016
(212) 213-3337
www.Dr-Gonzalez.com

Light therapy
Dinshah Health Society
P.O. Box 707
Malaga, NJ 08328
(856) 692-4686
www.dinshahhealth.org

Society for Light Treatment and
    Biological Rhythms
174 Cook St.
San Francisco, CA 94459
Fax: (415) 751-2758
E-mail: sltbrinfo@aol.com
www.websciences.org/sltbr

Livingston diet
Livingston Foundation Medical
    Center
3232 Duke St.
San Diego, CA 92110
(619) 224-3515
www.lfmc.net

Macrobiotic diet
KUSHI Institute
P.O. Box 7
Becket, MA 01223
1-800-975-8744
www.kushiinstitute.org

Massage
American Massage Therapy
    Association
820 Davis St., Suite 100
Evanston, IL 60201
(847) 864-0123
www.amtamassage.org

National Certification Board for
    Therapeutic Massage and
    Bodywork
8201 Greensboro Dr., Suite 300
McLean, VA 22102
1-800-296-0664
www.ncbtmb.com

Meditation
Insight Meditation Society
1230 Pleasant St.
Barre, MA 01005
(978) 355-4378
www.dharma.org/ims.htm

Institute of Noetic Sciences
101 San Antonio Rd.
Petaluma, CA 94952
(707) 775-3500
www.noetic.org

Maharishi International
    University
Fairfield, IA 52557
1-800-369-6480
www.mun.edu

Music therapy
American Music Therapy
    Association
8455 Colesville Rd., Suite 1000
Silver Spring, MD 20910
(301) 589-3300
E-mail: info@musictherapy.org
www.musictherapy.org

Naturopathic medicine
American Association of
    Naturopathic Physicians
8201 Greensboro Dr., Suite 300
McLean, VA 22102
1-877-969-2267
www.naturopathic.org

Bastyr University
14500 Juanita Dr. N.E.
Kenmore, WA 98028
(425) 823-1300
www.bastyr.edu

National College of
Naturopathic Medicine
049 S.W. Porter St.
Portland, OR 97201
(503) 499-4343
www.ncnm.edu

Osteopathy
American Osteopathic
Association
142 E. Ontario St.
Chicago, IL 60611
1-800-621-1773
www.aoa-net.org

Pritikin plan
Pritikin Longevity Center
19735 Turnberry Way
Aventuro, FL 33180
1-800-327-4914
www.pritikin.com

Qigong
East-West Academy of Healing
Arts
117 Topaz Way
San Francisco, CA 94131
(415) 285-9400
www.eastwestqi.com

Reflexology
International Institute of
Reflexology
5650 1st Ave. N.
St. Petersburg, FL 33710
(727) 343-4811
www.reflexology-usa.net

Reflexology Research
P.O. Box 35820
Albuquerque, NM 87176
(505) 344-9392
www.reflexology-research.com

Rolfing
Rolf Institute of Structural
Integration
205 Canyon Blvd.
Boulder, CO 80302
1-800-530-8875
E-mail: info@rolf.org
www.rolf.org

Sound therapy
Sound Healers Association
P.O. Box 2240
Boulder, CO 80306
1-800-246-9764
www.healingsounds.com

Trager technique
U.S. Trager Association
24800 Chagrin Blvd., Suite 205
Beachwood, OH 44122
(216) 896-9383
E-mail: info@trager-us.org
www.trager-us.org

Vitamin and mineral therapy
American College for Advancement in Medicine
23121 Verdugo Dr., Suite 204
Laguna Hills, CA 92653
1-800-532-3688
Fax: (949) 455-9679
www.ACAM.org

Yoga
American Yoga Association
P.O. Box 19986
Sarasota, FL 34276
(941) 927-4977
*www.americanyogaassociation.
org*

Himalayan International
Institute of Yoga Science and
Philosophy
RR 1, Box 1127
Honesdale, PA 18431
1-800-822-4547
E-mail: info@himalayaninstitute.
org
www.himalyaninstitute.org

Appendix C
Patient teaching aids

Learning about acupuncture and acupressure

Dear Patient:

Acupuncture involves the insertion of very thin metal needles into various areas of the body. Acupressure is deep finger pressure applied to various areas of the body.

Acupuncture and acupressure are both key parts of traditional Chinese medicine. This ancient form of medicine holds that specific body points (called acupoints) are connected or attuned to specific organs. If one of these organs has a problem, such as pain or swelling, stimulating the appropriate acupoints is believed to create balance and restore or improve the flow of *qi (pronounced "chee"),* or energy, thus relieving the problem and restoring health. *Qi* must be in balance to be healthy.

Acupuncture has been used for over 100 conditions, including the following:

- arthritis
- asthma
- back and joint pain
- bronchitis
- conjunctivitis
- constipation
- diarrhea
- gastritis
- headaches
- hiccups
- Ménière's disease
- sinusitis
- trigeminal neuralgia.

Some of the following steps occur during acupuncture:

- The practitioner takes a history of the problem and performs a physical examination.
- You lie on a table and uncover the area to be treated.
- The practitioner inserts thin metal needles — usually no more than 10 or 12 — into various spots of your body and leaves them in from seconds up to one-half of an hour.

▶ The treatment may include electrical stimulation of the needles and, sometimes, the burning of herbs.

▶ You'll feel a small amount of tingling and numbness where the needles are inserted, but the treatment isn't considered painful.

   Some of the following steps occur during acupressure:

▶ The practitioner takes a history of the problem.

▶ Sitting comfortably, you breathe in.

▶ As you slowly exhale, the practitioner applies pressure to the designated acupoint until exhalation ends.

▶ The process is repeated 3 to 5 times, then the entire procedure may be repeated after 10 minutes.

A few tips

▶ If you're considering acupuncture or acupressure, be sure to investigate therapists for proper education and experience with these techniques.

▶ You may obtain a referral for acupuncture from the National Commission for the Certification of Acupuncturists.

▶ Report any signs of infection, such as redness, swelling, heat, or drainage from acupuncture needle sites.

▶ Acupressure shouldn't be applied directly over cuts, sores, scar tissue, or infected areas.

FOR THE PATIENT
Learning about aromatherapy

Dear Patient:
Aromatherapy is the use of essential oils for their effects on the brain. The oils can be inhaled, rubbed on the skin, or placed in bath water. Aromatherapy has been used for the following conditions:

- anxiety
- arthritis
- bacterial and viral infections
- headache; pain
- herpes simplex
- herpes zoster
- indigestion
- muscle disorders
- premenstrual syndrome
- skin disorders.

Basic aromatherapy techniques
Follow these steps:

- Choose the method of aromatherapy that you wish to use — inhalation, massage, soaking, or diffusion. Then, select an essential oil. Shops that specialize in these oils can help you choose.
- For inhalation: Place a few drops of an essential oil in a bowl of steaming water. Place a towel over your head and lean over the bowl, keeping your face far enough away from the steaming water to avoid burning yourself. Inhale the steam for a few minutes.
- For massage: Dilute an essential oil in the appropriate carrier oil. Apply it to the body area in a soothing, rhythmic motion.
- For bathing: Add a few drops of an essential oil to hot bath water. Soak in the tub for 10 to 20 minutes, inhaling the steam as you soak.
- For diffusion: Place a few drops of essential oil on a diffuser and turn on the heat source (such as a candle or light bulb) to diffuse the microparticles of oil into the air. Sit at least 3 feet from the diffuser and inhale the aroma for at least 30 minutes.

A few tips
- Avoid aromatherapy during pregnancy and with infants and children under age 5 because many essential oils may be toxic.
- Keep oils away from your eyes and mucous membranes.
- Don't apply these essential oils before going out in the sun: bergamot, lemon, orange, grapefruit, and other citrus oils.
- These essential oils are unsafe for home use: origanum, sage, savory, thyme, and wintergreen oils.
- Don't use cinnamon and clove essential oils on your skin. Stop using basil, fennel, lemon grass, rosemary, and verbena oils if your skin becomes irritated.

FOR THE PATIENT
Learning about imagery

Dear Patient:
Imagery is a technique used to promote relaxation, relieve symptoms (or help you better cope with them), and heal disease. It can involve visualization (picturing something in your mind), or mentally hearing, feeling, smelling, or tasting something. Imagery is based on the idea that the mind and body are interconnected and can work together to encourage healing. Imagery can benefit almost any medical situation in which problem solving, decision making, relaxation, or symptom relief is useful.

Imagery may help the following conditions:

- asthma
- cancer
- chronic pain
- flu symptoms
- headaches
- high blood pressure
- nausea and vomiting
- recovery from surgery
- smoking cessation.

Basic imagery techniques
Follow these steps:

- Sit comfortably in a quiet, dimly lit room.
- Close your eyes.
- Take a few slow, deep breaths while imagining that you're breathing in calmness and peacefulness and breathing out (decreasing) tension, discomfort, and worry.
- Focus on a mental image of something that would cause relaxation — a calm place, sounds or smells related to feelings of peacefulness, or the like.
- Spend as long as possible on this image. Then, allow the image to fade as you slowly refocus on your external surroundings.

A few tips
- To increase the effect of the image, consider adding a soothing fragrance to the room (such as a scented candle).
- Be aware that if you have a breathing problem, you may have problems controlling your breathing for this therapy.

FOR THE PATIENT
Using herbal therapy

Dear Patient:
Before taking an herbal preparation, you should do the following:

General precautions

▶ Check with your health care provider, especially if you're taking a prescription drug. Review all medicines, vitamins, and herbs you're currently taking, and discuss the herbs you're interested in taking. Review your full medical history. Also, tell your herbalist about prescription medications you're taking. Many herbal remedies contain substances that can interact with other medications.

▶ Be aware that the Food and Drug Administration regulates herbal products only as food supplements, not as drugs; thus, labels on these products don't contain information about risks, adverse effects, or possible harmful interactions with other substances. There's no way to know whether the herb is in a form that the body can absorb or whether the recommended dosage has been tested for safety or efficacy on animals or humans.

▶ Herbal products may contain ingredients other than those indicated on the label; for example, Siberian ginseng capsules were found to contain a weed that's full of male hormone-like chemicals.

▶ The quantity of the active ingredient will vary from brand to brand and possibly from bottle to bottle within a particular brand. Look for the word "standardized" on the label, which means that the dose of herb is the same in each tablet in the package.

▶ When replacing your supply, don't substitute another brand. Different brands may have different amounts of ingredients and, therefore, may produce different effects.

▶ Buying herbs that have been grown organically may be preferable. Herbs that grow naturally in the wild are subject to contamination from pesticides, polluted water, and automobile exhaust fumes.

▶ Most herbal products sold in the United States haven't been scientifically tested. Their alleged benefits are largely based on word-of-mouth.

▶ Be wary of products that promise to cure specific health problems.

▶ Don't use herbal preparations for serious or potentially serious medical conditions, such as heart disease or bleeding disorders.

▶ Avoid herbal preparations if you're pregnant, breast-feeding, or considering pregnancy; herbal effects on the fetus are unknown.

▶ Avoid herbal "cocktails" that contain more than one ingredient; there's little information about the effects of combining herbs.

▶ Research herb suppliers, and go to an established supplier. Avoid products sold through magazines, brochures, the broadcast media, or the Internet.

▶ Remember that the clerk at the health food store is a salesperson, not a trained practitioner.

▶ Follow all instructions for proper herb preparation and dosage. If you don't understand the instructions, ask your health care provider or herbal supplier.

▶ If you experience side effects when taking an herb, stop taking it and contact your health care provider.

▶ As with medications, don't allow other people to use your herbal products, and keep them out of the reach of children.

Warnings about specific products

▶ Bloodroot—promoted as an expectorant, purgative, stimulant, diaphoretic, plaque and cavity preventer, and treatment for rheumatism—is used in such a range of doses that it can be dangerous. It has proved fatal when used as an emetic.

▶ Chan su—a topical aphrodisiac also known as stone, love stone, and rockhard—has caused death when mistakenly ingested.

▶ Chaparral tea, promoted as an antioxidant and pain reliever, has caused liver failure, requiring liver transplantation.

▶ Coltfoot, used for respiratory problems, and comfrey, used for arthritis, have caused liver problems and cancer.

▶ Indian herbal tonics can cause lead poisoning.

▶ Jin bu huan, an ancient Chinese sedative and analgesic, contains morphinelike substances and has caused hepatitis.

▶ Kombucha tea, made from mushroom cultures and used as a cure-all, has caused death from acidosis.

▶ Lobelia, a treatment for respiratory congestion, has resulted in respiratory paralysis and death.

▶ Ephedra, or ma huang, an ingredient in many diet pills, is potentially dangerous because it can raise blood pressure and produce an irregular heartbeat. Also sold under such names as Herbal Ecstasy, Cloud 9, and Ultimate Xphoria to induce a "high" associated with illegal drugs, it may cause heart attacks, seizures, psychotic behavior, and even death.

▶ Mistletoe has been falsely touted as a cure for cancer.

▶ Pau d'Arco tea has been falsely touted to cure cancer and AIDS.

▶ Pennyroyal, used to treat coughs and upset stomach, has shown toxic effects on the liver, inhibiting blood clotting. Its essential oil has been fatal.

▶ Sassafras—used as a tonic for fever reduction, skin disorders, and rheumatism—has been banned in the United States for causing liver damage and is implicated in narcotic poisoning and accidental abortion.

▶ Yohimbe bark, used as an aphrodisiac, has severely lowered blood pressure and caused psychotic behavior.

FOR THE PATIENT
Learning about music therapy

Dear Patient:
Music therapy is the use of rhythmic sound to communicate, relax, encourage healing, and create a general feeling of well-being. Forms of music therapy include creating music, singing, moving to music, and listening to music. Music therapy may work in one of the following ways:

▌ Resonance coming from sound waves restores the body's natural rhythm and encourages healing.

▌ The brain reacts to sound waves by sending out directions to control heart rate, breathing rate, blood pressure, and muscle tension.

▌ Sound impulses cause chemicals to be released which help decrease pain and elevate the mood.

▌ Happy memories occur when certain sounds are created, which reduces stress and increases feelings of well-being.

Music therapy may help with the following conditions:
▌ developmental problems (such as mental retardation)
▌ mental health problems (such as anxiety)
▌ chronic pain
▌ cerebral palsy
▌ stroke and other brain injuries
▌ Parkinson's disease
▌ substance abuse.

Incorporating music therapy
To try music therapy, choose one of the following:
▌ Play a musical instrument or take music lessons.
▌ Dance to music.
▌ Sing, join a choir or music group.
▌ On a radio or CD or tape player or in concert, listen to music that creates a good feeling.

FOR THE PATIENT
Performing relaxation breathing exercises

Dear Patient:
Relaxation breathing can help you cope with stress or pain. You can use it anywhere and at any time. You can also combine it with other techniques to help control pain. Try to practice these simple breathing techniques daily.

1. Sit comfortably with your eyes closed. Inhale slowly and deeply through your nose as you count silently: "In, 2, 3, 4." Notice how your stomach expands first, then your rib cage, and finally your upper chest.

Now, exhale slowly through your mouth as you count silently: "Out, 2, 3, 4, 5, 6." Pretend you're breathing out through a straw to lengthen exhalation. Let your shoulders drop slightly as your upper chest, rib cage, and stomach gently deflate. Repeat this exercise four or five times.

2. Inhale for 4 seconds. This time, *hold* your breath for the count of 4, but don't strain. Then exhale through your mouth for 6 to 8 seconds. Practice this exercise four or five times.

A few tips
▶ Use these breathing exercises for as long as you need to during stressful or painful periods. You may vary the rhythm, but always exhale for 2 to 4 seconds longer than you inhale.
▶ If you feel light-headed or if your fingers tingle, you may be breathing too deeply or too fast. Reduce the depth and speed of your breathing, or breathe into a paper bag until the feeling goes away.

Glossary

acupoints In acupuncture and acupressure, the specific points on the body that are stimulated, either by needles (in acupuncture) or by finger pressure (in acupressure). These points, located along vertical channels known as meridians, are believed to correspond to specific body organs.

acupuncture A form of traditional Chinese medicine that uses thin needles inserted at designated points on the body (acupoints) to restore health. The needles are believed to work by enhancing the flow of energy *(qi)* in the body.

Alexander technique A form of body work aimed at correcting poor habits of posture and movement that are believed to strain the body and result in various ailments. This technique focuses on proper alignment of the head, neck, and trunk.

allopathic medicine A system of health care that treats disease through remedies that produce effects opposite those of the disease. This term is commonly used to refer to mainstream Western medicine in contrast to alternative or complementary medicine.

alternative medicine A broad spectrum of nontraditional medical and nursing practices and healing arts that are neither taught widely in medical or nursing schools nor generally used or endorsed by allopathic practitioners. These clinical interventions lack scientific documentation of safety and effectiveness and aren't usually reimbursable by health care providers.

amino acids Building blocks of proteins.

antioxidants Nutrients, such as vitamin E, that work alone or with a group of other nutrients to destroy disease-causing free radicals.

applied kinesiology A method of assessment and evaluation (also known as "muscle testing") developed within the chiropractic profession in the 1960s that uses the resistance of the patient's muscles to the practitioner's force to assess the relative strength of specific muscles. Particular muscles are associated with specific diseases or organ conditions, so a weak muscle is believed to indicate the cause of the condition.

aromatherapy The therapeutic use of essential plant oils.

art therapy The use of drawing, painting, sculpting, or other artistic expression to provide insight into the patient's feelings. This therapy is primarily used to help treat people with emotional problems and young children, who can't express themselves verbally.

Aston-Patterning An integrated system of movement education, body work, ergonomics, and fitness training. It assists individuals with using their bodies more efficiently to release tension and pain and to improve posture and movement.

Ayurvedic medicine An ancient traditional Indian system of medicine based on Hindu philosophy. This system shares some fundamental concepts with traditional Chinese medicine: the interconnectedness of body, mind, and spirit; the belief that the cosmos is composed of five basic elements (earth, air, fire, water, and space); and the belief in a human energy field that must be kept in balance to maintain health. Ayurvedic medicine also stresses the importance of a person's metabolic body type—*dosha*—in determining his health, personality, and susceptibility to disease. (See also *"doshas."*)

biofeedback A method of promoting relaxation by consciously controlling body functions, such as blood pressure, heart and respiratory rates, temperature, and perspiration. This method involves the use of an electronic device that informs the patient when changes in these functions occur.

biomedicine A system of medicine based on the principles of natural science. This term is used to describe the style of medicine practiced by doctors holding an MD degree.

bipolar therapy A type of magnetic therapy in which both positive and negative magnetic fields are applied to the affected area.

body work Various forms of hands-on body manipulation used to promote relaxation and relieve assorted musculoskeletal complaints, including therapeutic massage, Rolfing, Alexander technique, and Feldenkrais method, among others; also known as manual healing therapies.

carbohydrates Chemical compounds composed of carbon, hydrogen, and oxygen that are an essential part of the daily diet; found mainly in plants.

caring-healing modalities Advanced nursing methods that overlap with alternative therapies, including Therapeutic Touch, Healing Touch, relaxation and stress reduction techniques, nutritional counseling, and imagery and visualization techniques.

centering A technique used before a session of Therapeutic Touch in which the practitioner attempts to become relaxed, calm, and focused on the care that she's going to provide.

chelation therapy A proven treatment for heavy metal poisoning that's also used as an alternative therapy for coronary artery disease and other disorders. It involves the I.V. injection of edetic acid (EDTA) into the bloodstream based on the theory that EDTA will attach itself to coronary plaque or other harmful substances, which will then be excreted in the urine.

chiropractic A manual healing therapy based on the belief that many medical problems are caused by vertebral misalignment and can be corrected by manipulating the spine. Chiropractic is the fourth largest health profession in the United States, with more than 50,000 practitioners.

coenzyme Q10 A lipid-soluble benzoquinone found in every cell in the body. It acts as a free radical scavenger and membrane stabilizer and is a cofactor in electron transport in the mitochondria.

colonic irrigation A form of detoxification therapy and hydrotherapy in which the bowel is cleaned with large amounts of water. This therapy is reported to relieve constipation and detoxify the colon.

craniosacral therapy An offshoot of chiropractic that focuses on keeping cerebrospinal fluid flowing unimpeded from the cranium to the base of the spine.

cupping A component of traditional Chinese medicine that involves placing heated glass cups on the skin to create suction and then removing them. This therapy is believed to dispel dampness, warm the internal energy force *(qi),* and reduce swelling. It's used primarily to relieve bronchial congestion.

detoxification therapies Assorted therapies aimed at ridding the body of "toxic" substances. Proponents believe these treatments, such as colonic irrigation, help to maintain health and prevent disease.

Doctrine of Signatures In herbal medicine, the primitive method of determining which plants should be used for which ailments, based on the plant's resemblance to the ailment—for example, heart-shaped leaves for heart conditions and plants with red flowers for bleeding disorders.

doshas In Ayurvedic medicine, the three basic metabolic body types known as *vata, pitta,* and *kapha.* The *doshas* are believed to determine not only a person's physical characteristics but also his personality traits and susceptibility to disease. Most people are a combination of *doshas.* An imbalance of *doshas* is thought to lead to illness.

electromagnetic therapy A type of energy-based therapy that attempts to diagnose and treat illnesses believed to be caused by disturbances in the body's electromagnetic fields. Many different electric and magnetic devices are used to treat electromagnetic imbalances.

endorphins Endogenous opiates produced in the brain that function as the body's natural painkillers.

energetic healing Any therapeutic technique that focuses on what practitioners call the "human energy field" to promote healing. Practitioners use their hands to transfer energy from themselves or the environment to the patient in an attempt to restore equilibrium to the energy field and thus allow the patient's body to begin the process of self-healing.

enzyme A body substance that initiates or speeds up biochemical reactions.

essential fatty acids Unsaturated fatty acids that aren't synthesized by the human body; essential for optimal health.

essential oils Naturally occurring pure oils that are obtained from the distillation of plants and used in aromatherapy.

fats Along with proteins and carbohydrates, one of the three kinds of food energy; found primarily in animal-based foods, such as meat, fish, poultry, and dairy products.

Feldenkrais method A form of body work intended to help people "unlearn" inefficient patterns of movement and learn new ways of moving freely to optimize health and functioning.

fiber The parts of plants that aren't digestible. In the digestive system, fiber absorbs water and increases fecal bulk, causing feces to move more quickly through the intestine. A high-fiber diet is believed to help lower serum cholesterol levels.

free radicals Molecules containing an odd number of electrons. These substances may play a role in cancer formation by interacting with deoxyribonucleic acid and impairing normal cell function.

gem therapy The use of crystals to bring about a sense of peace and to increase the effects of other healing modalities by detecting and cleansing blockages in the body's energy flow.

Healing Touch A form of energetic healing developed by nurses in the 1980s and based on the concept of the human energy field. By moving her hands over the patient's body, the nurse theoretically realigns the patient's energy flow and reactivates the mind-body-spirit connection that ultimately allows self-healing.

herbal medicine The use of plants for healing purposes, dating back to the ancient cultures of Egypt, China, and India and possibly even to prehistoric times. Today, more than one-quarter of conventional drugs are derived from herbs and about 80% of the world's population use herbal remedies.

holism The belief that an integrated whole has a reality independent of and greater than the sum of the parts. It's the basis for holistic nursing.

homeopathy Based on the theory that "like cures like," a method of healing in which minute quantities of a substance that produces certain symptoms in a healthy person are given to a sick person to cure the same symptoms. Homeopathic remedies are thought to stimulate the body's ability to heal itself.

hydrotherapy Any form of therapy that uses water — hot or cold and liquid, steam, or ice — to treat disease or maintain health. Common forms include whirlpools, Jacuzzis, steam baths, hot and cold packs, and hyperthermia.

hypnotherapy The use of hypnosis to treat medical or psychological problems, such as anxiety, depression, and insomnia; also used to help people stop smoking and overcome substance abuse.

imagery The process of imagining or visualizing an image using any of the senses — sight, hearing, smell, or touch. Imagery is used to change attitudes and behaviors as well as physiologic reactions.

immunoaugmentive therapy Also referred to as IAT, a therapy aimed at augmenting the immune system by balancing four protein components in the blood.

informed consent The process by which a patient is fully informed of the risks and benefits of a proposed medical, surgical, or alternative intervention or treatment and, based on an understanding of these, agrees to proceed with that intervention or treatment.

lipids A group of fats and fatlike substances composed of carbon, hydrogen, and oxygen that are insoluble in water and soluble in fat solvents. Dietary lipids can be converted to essential tissue constituents or transformed into stored energy in adipose tissue.

live cell therapy The administration of live whole cells or extracts derived from living cells to improve or rejuvenate the function of targeted organs.

macrobiotic diet The most widely followed alternative nutritional program in the United States, emphasizing the consumption of whole-grain cereals, organic vegetables, beans, and sea vegetables. This diet, which is used by many cancer patients, is built around the Chinese concept of *yin* and *yang*. When a patient's cancer has been classified as either *yin* or *yang*, depending on its location, the appropriate diet is determined (*yang* foods for *yin* cancers and vice versa).

massage, therapeutic The manipulation of muscles and tissues by rubbing, kneading, tapping, or stroking. This manual healing technique can relieve stress and promote relaxation in nominally healthy individuals. It can also benefit people with health problems by relieving pain and swelling, preventing deformity, and promoting functional independence.

meditation The process of focusing one's mind on a single thought, sound, or image in an attempt to promote relaxation. Regular use of meditation has been shown to produce beneficial changes in physiologic function, such as decreased blood pressure and lower heart and respiratory rates.

mental healing A form of spiritual healing in which the healer attempts to improve a patient's health through mental activity (not necessarily prayer). In one type, the healer (who may be far away from the patient) enters a focused, prayerful state of consciousness in which he tries to "become one" with the patient and the universe. In another type, the healer actually touches the patient, attempting to transfer healing energy from his hands to the patient.

meridians In traditional Chinese medicine, the channels in the body along which the vital energy known as *qi* is believed to flow.

minerals Naturally occurring, organic micronutrients used by the body for bone and tissue formation as well as the activation of enzymes and hormones.

moxibustion A therapy used in traditional Chinese medicine that involves burning a small amount of an herb called *moxa* at specific points on the body or on acupuncture needles that are then inserted into the skin. The heat generated by this process is believed to promote healing by restoring the balance of *qi* in the body. (See also *"qi."*)

myotherapy A noninvasive, therapeutic approach for relief of symptoms associated with muscular pain and dysfunction. It's used to enhance the function of muscles and joints.

naturopathy An alternative system of medical practice combining a mainstream understanding of human physiology and disease with alternative remedies, such as herbal and nutritional therapies, acupuncture, hydrotherapy, and counseling. Naturopathic doctors eschew drugs and surgery in favor of natural treatments aimed at stimulating the body's own healing ability.

neural therapy The injection of local anesthetic agents into nerves, acupuncture points, glands, trigger points, and scars to remove interference fields and promote healing.

oxygen therapy The use of oxygen to promote healing.

prana The ancient Indian concept of a vital energy within the body that must be in balance to maintain good health; similar to the concept of *qi* in traditional Chinese medicine.

proteins Naturally occurring nitrogenous compounds, consisting of different combinations of amino acids, that are found in plants and animals.

qi A form of vital energy, sometimes described as a life force, that's believed to control the functioning of the human body, according to traditional Chinese medicine. *Qi* (pronounced "chee") is believed to flow through the body along invisible channels. Illness occurs when there's an imbalance or obstruction of *qi*.

qigong Pronounced "chee goong," an ancient Chinese health discipline consisting of breathing exercises, deep concentration, and physical exercises and aimed at balancing *qi* to maintain health and prevent disease.

reconstructive therapy Stimulation of the body's own healing ability to regenerate ligaments and tendons. It involves injections into the injured area of a solution that stimulates fibroblast proliferation.

reflexology A form of body work involving the application of pressure to specific points on the feet or hands. These points are believed to be connected to, and have a therapeutic effect on, specific body parts or organs.

relaxation response The decreased metabolism and other physiologic changes seen in people who engage in regular meditation, yoga, or other stress-reduction techniques.

Rolfing A type of deep-tissue massage designed to release kinks in the connective tissues to improve body alignment and functioning; formally known as Structural Integration.

shaman In many ancient cultures, a healer or priest who invokes ancestral spirits and other magical powers to cure the sick.

signature Characteristics of an herb, such as its color or shape.

sound therapy A method of healing in which specific sounds are directed at particular parts of the body for therapeutic purposes. It's based on the theory that everything in the world, including the human body, is in a constant state of vibration and that particular sound frequencies aimed at affected parts of the body can correct vibrational imbalances and thereby restore health.

subluxation A term used by chiropractors to describe vertebral misalignments.

succussion The vigorous shaking of homeopathic remedies that's performed after each dilution to activate the active ingredient in the solution.

tai chi chuan An ancient Chinese exercise program based on the teachings of Taoism and the theory and practice of traditional Chinese medicine. Although originally a martial art, it's usually practiced today as a physical culture regimen to promote health and longevity. Tai chi also includes meditation and breathing exercises.

Therapeutic Touch A method of energetic healing in which the practitioner passes her hands over the patient's body in an attempt to transmit her own energy to the patient; like a number of alternative therapies that originated in the East, Therapeutic Touch is based on the theory that a vital energy flows through all human beings.

Trager approach A body work therapy in which the practitioner gently and rhythmically rocks, stretches, and applies pressure to the patient's body in an attempt to teach the patient how to move freely and without pain. Proponents consider the technique, formally known as Psychophysical Integration, more a movement reeducation process than a therapy.

urine therapy The use of urine as a treatment for various conditions, especially for its antibacterial and antiviral effects.

vegetarianism The practice of avoiding animal flesh and fish in the diet.

vitalism The belief that there's a vital energy permeating the world that's available for healing; the healing power of nature; similar to the concept of *qi* in traditional Chinese medicine.

vitamins Complex organic molecules essential for biochemical functions in the body, including energy production, metabolism, protein metabolism, bone formation, and maintenance. Some vitamins act as antioxidants to protect the body's tissues.

yin and yang In traditional Chinese medicine, the concept used to describe various opposing physical forces in nature and the body, such as hot and cold or active and passive. Each body organ is associated with either *yin* or *yang* characteristics. Good health is believed to require a balance of *yin* and *yang* throughout the body.

yoga An ancient Hindu exercise and health maintenance program that consists of assuming specific positions combined with deep breathing and meditation. It aims to promote relaxation and produce other health benefits.

Index

i refers to an illustration; t refers to a table.

Body-based methods, 9
Body-oriented therapy, 173. *See also*
    Psychotherapy.
Bone fractures, alternative therapy
    for, 431
Boneset, 322t
Boron, 356
Brain injuries, alternative therapy
    for, 431
Brain surgery, acupuncture and,
    241-242
Breast cancer, alternative therapies
    for, 431
Burdock, 322t

C

Calendula, 322t
Cancer. *See also* Breast cancer *and*
    Colon cancer.
  alternative therapies for, 431
  biological therapies for, 421-427
  cell-specific therapy for, 225-227
  diets as treatment for, 361-375
  electromagnetic field exposure and,
    204-205
  hyperthermia treatments and, 269
  static electromagnetic field therapy
    for, 227-229
Capsules as herbal preparations, 311
Cardiovascular disorders
  alternative therapies for, 431
  diets for, 375-381
Care plan, incorporating alternative
    therapies into, 47-48
Carotenoids, 351, 352t, 353-354
Carpal tunnel syndrome, alternative
    therapies for, 431
Cascara sagrada, 322t
Cayenne, 323t
Cell-specific cancer therapy, 225-227
  complications of, 227
  equipment for, 226
  goal of, 225-226
  implementing, 226-227
  mechanics of, 225
  nursing perspective on, 227
  therapeutic uses of, 226
Centering, energy medicine and,
    119, 121
Cerebral palsy, alternative therapy
    for, 431
Cerebrovascular disease, alternative
    therapies for, 431
Chakras
  energy medicine and, 118-119,
    120t
  gemstones and, 145t, 146
  music therapy and, 165
  sound therapy and, 179
Chamomile, 323t
Chamomile oil, 396t
Chelation therapy, 398-401

Chelation therapy *(continued)*
  basis for, 398
  complications of, 401
  equipment for, 400
  implementing, 400-401
  nursing perspective on, 401
  practice standards for, 398
  therapeutic uses of, 399-400
Chicory, 323-324t
Childbirth, alternative therapies
    for, 431
Chinese massage, 236, 238i
Chinese medicine
  diagnostic approach in, 85, 87-89
  Five Phases theory of, 89, 90-91t
  historical perspective of, 84-85
  nursing perspective on, 94
  principles of, 85, 86
  theory of, 85
  therapeutic uses of, 93
  therapies used in, 89-93
  traditional, 3, 84-94
Chiropractic, 253-259
  acceptance of, 254-255
  basis for, 253-254
  benefits of, 254
  complications of, 259
  equipment for, 257
  historical background of, 254
  implementing, 257-258
  nursing perspective on, 259
  spinal manipulation and, 256, 258i
  therapeutic uses of, 255-257
Cinnamon, 324t
Circulation, impaired, alternative
    therapies for, 431
Circulation control, acupuncture
    and, 241
Cleansing. *See* Detoxification.
Cloves, 324t
Coenzyme Q10, 379-381
  complications of, 380
  dosage of, 380
  nursing perspective on, 380-381
  research findings and, 379
  therapeutic uses of, 379-380
Cold laser therapy, 409. *See also*
    Light therapies.
Colds, alternative therapies for, 431
Cold water therapies, 265. *See also*
    Hydrotherapy.
Coley's toxins, 426-427
Colon cancer, alternative therapy
    for, 431
Colonic irrigation, 401-404
  basis for, 401
  complications of, 403
  equipment for, 402
  implementing, 402-403
  nursing perspective on, 403-404
  therapeutic uses of, 402

---

i refers to an illustration; t refers to a table.

---

i refers to an illustration; t refers to a table.

i refers to an illustration; t refers to a table.